Good Thinking:
Test-Taking,
Problem Solving
and Study Skills
for Nursing Students

by

Susan G. Poorman, Ph.D., R.N., C.S.

Cheryl A. Webb, Ph.D., R.N., C.S.

Karen L. Molcan, Ph.D., R.N., C.S.

DEDICATION

To our "good mothers"...

Jeannette L. Poorman
Gwendolyn M. Webb
Blanche B. Molcan

GOOD THINKING:
TEST-TAKING, PROBLEM SOLVING
AND STUDY SKILLS
FOR NURSING STUDENTS

Susan G. Poorman, Ph.D.,R.N.,C.S
Associate Professor
Department of Nursing
Community College of Allegheny County - Boyce Campus
Monroeville, PA
STAT Nursing Consultants

Cheryl A. Webb, Ph.D.,R.N.,C.S.
Associate Professor
Division of Nursing
Mount Aloysius College
STAT Nursing Consultants

Karen L. Molcan, Ph.D.,R.N.,C.S.
Director of Nursing
Western Psychiatric Institute & Clinic
Pittsburgh, PA
STAT Nursing Consultants

STAT NURSING CONSULTANTS
~~6003 DEER RUN DR~~
~~TRAFFORD PA 15085~~

Thank you for spurring my critical thinking
Cheryl

The authors have made every effort to ensure that drug selections and dosage ranges appearing within this text are based on current practice and recommendations at the time of publication. Due to the on-going research in the area of drug therapy and reactions, when questions arise in this area, the reader is urged to check package inserts and current research literature.

All names used in the nursing question review section of this text are fictitious.

All of the questions utilized in this book were tested on samples of associate degree, baccalaureate and diploma nursing students and revised to meet acceptable testing standards.

CONTRIBUTORS

(provided practice questions and rationales used in this textbook)

Theresa A. Brady, MSN, RN, CCRN
Instructor
Mount Aloyius College
Cresson, PA

Julia Greenawalt, BSN, MA
Instructor
Butler County Community College
Butler, PA

Anita Cimino Kerrigan, MSN, RN
Former Instructor
Community College of Allegheny County
Boyce Campus
Monroeville, PA

Anita Andrews Kovalsky, MNEd
Associate Professor
Community College of Allegheny County
Boyce Campus
Monroeville, PA

Melissa L. Mastorovich, MSN, RN, C
Children's Hospital of Pittsburgh
Pittsburgh, PA

Susan G. Poorman, PhD, RN, CS
Associate Professor
Community College of Allegheny County
Boyce Campus
Monroeville, PA

Kim Scheurolucke, BSN, RN, C
Pittsburgh Cancer Institute
Pittsburgh, PA

Kimberly Stephens, BSN, RN
Instructor
Community College of Allegheny County
Boyce Campus
Monroeville, PA

Jeanne M. Thompson, MSN, MBA
Allegheny General Hospital
Pittsburgh, PA

Cheryl A. Webb, PhD, RN, CS
Associate Professor
Mount Aloysius College
Cresson, PA

Rebecca J. Zapatochny, MSN, RN, CCRN
Instructor
Mount Aloysius College
Cresson, PA

TABLE OF CONTENTS

ACKNOWLEDGMENTS

Our appreciation is sincerely expressed to the contributors who wrote the practice questions used in this textbook. We would like to thank Susan Petrie and Jayne C. Guenther for their tremendous efforts in typing and preparing this manuscript for production. Throughout this textbook you will see cartoon drawings of a nursing student whom we have named "Natalie." We used Natalie in our previous textbook to create a user-friendly approach in helping the reader understand some of the major concepts utilized throughout the book. Natalie was created by Silvia Lemus and our heartfelt gratitude is expressed to her for her continued efforts. Finally, we would like to thank all of the clients and staff at STAT Nursing Consultants because without them there would be no book.

ABOUT THE AUTHORS

We wanted to share with you a little bit about our background and how we became interested in helping nursing students become better thinkers. We believe that this will help you in understanding where we are coming from in our approach to study and test-taking skills. All three authors are members of a nurse owned and operated consultation firm located in Pittsburgh, Pennsylvania. The name of our consultation firm is STAT Nursing Consultants. STAT is an acronym for Strategies for Test Anxiety Treatment. STAT Nursing Consultants was founded in 1982, when it was expanded from an individual private practice to a group that now includes five masters and doctorally prepared psychiatric nurses. Although we work with clients with a variety of mental health problems (anxiety, depression, marital discord), we have become specialized in the treatment of performance and test anxiety. Performance anxiety is the pressure to achieve in a situation where a person is being evaluated. Performance anxiety can occur in a variety of situations, e.g. when one has to perform in front of an audience, give a speech, or compete athletically. Test anxiety, the inability to perform to one's capabilities in a testing situation, is one of the major forms of performance anxiety. We developed a treatment program that has been successful in treating this specific form of anxiety. Our treatment program consists of a variety of methods that include cognitive restructuring, problem solving, and behavioral techniques such as visual imagery, progressive relaxation, thought distraction techniques, and test-taking and thinking skills. Over the past 15 years, we have worked with literally hundreds of nursing students, helping them become better students, better test-takers, and enhance their performance on the NCLEX. Over the years, we have become increasingly interested in the way people problem solve and, in general, the way people think. We began by looking at ways to enhance our clients' thinking processes and decrease debilitating thinking patterns. We first saw this problem when we realized that often our clients were not failing exams because of their lack of knowledge or information, but because they were experiencing thinking or reasoning errors. We then began our journey to discover ways to make our clients better thinkers. The impetus for writing this book comes from our belief that learning, practicing and developing problem solving, thinking, and test-taking skills will help nursing students not only enjoy their educational experience, but truly enhance their reasoning ability and become "good thinkers".

Susan G. Poorman
Cheryl A. Webb
Karen L. Molcan

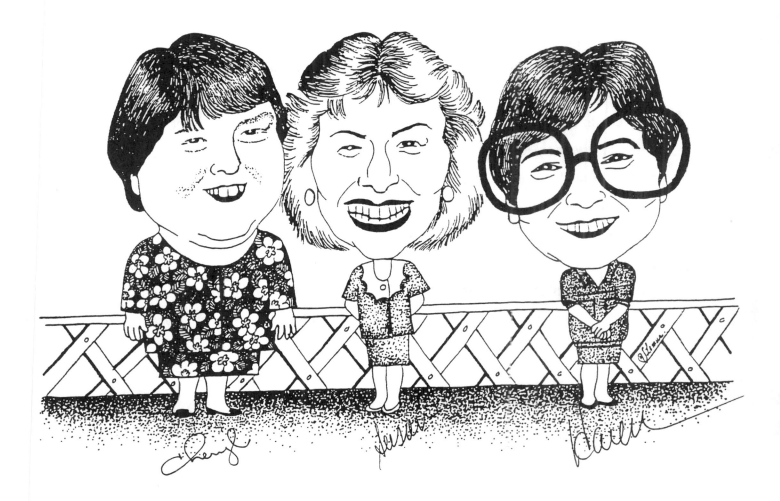

At the risk of sounding like your mothers, this book is good for you. It can help you discover abilities in yourself that you did not know you possessed, help you challenge your negative thinking, and build self-esteem and confidence, all of which have been proven to enhance performance. You can learn to question, problem solve, and utilize the nursing process as a scientific approach to patient care.

1

GOOD THINKING: AN INTRODUCTION

In this textbook we hope to help you develop "good thinking". By good thinking we mean clear, uncontaminated thinking that helps you understand the information you are learning and, most importantly, use it effectively in your nursing practice. It is the ability to think beyond the basics of learning copius amounts of factual knowledge, to having the ability to understand and apply concepts and principles that guide nursing practice.

For some students, academic life is a breeze. For these individuals it comes naturally, almost second nature. They enjoy it. For others, it is a life racked with pain, torture, anxiety, and feels about as natural as a toad without warts. This book is for the latter group. We are not claiming that after reading this book you will learn to love school, but if you practice these skills and techniques you can at least learn to make peace with your academic life.

Entering a nursing education program (associate degree, baccalaureate, or diploma) presents the student with many challenges. Medicine's and nursing's knowledge base is growing and moving faster than a speeding bullet. Even Superman would have trouble just keeping his head above water. Technological advances create a need not only for knowledge, but psychomotor skill. Since

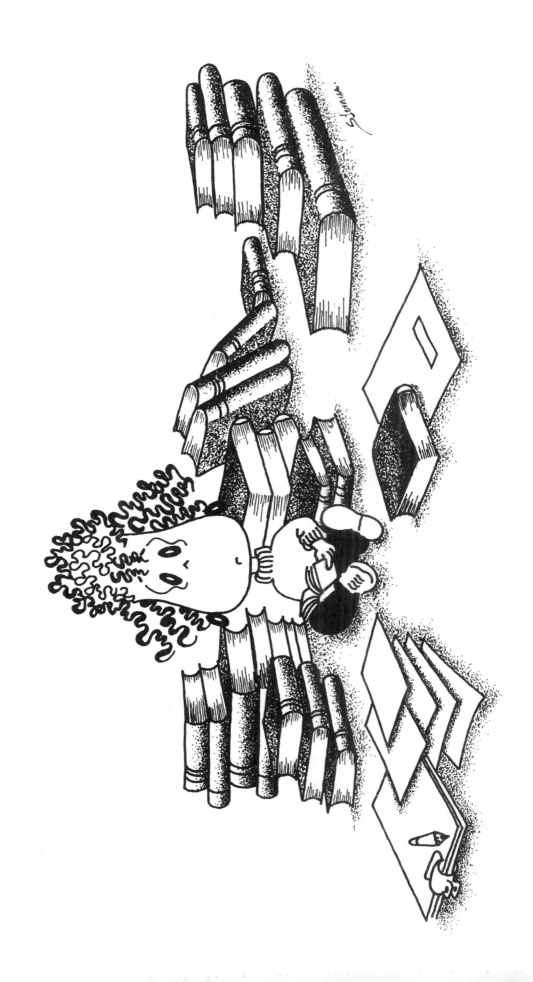

nursing is both an art and a science it demands that nursing students pool resources from every part of their being. Many nursing students are "nontraditional" and have been out of the academic mainstream for over five to ten years. They may have many outside responsibilities beyond their own personal welfare. For these reasons, completing a nursing educational program may appear to be the impossible dream. However, enhancing your problem solving and overall thinking abilities will help you make this dream a reality.

We have tried to write a book that will be helpful to nursing students at all levels of the educational process. The information and techniques that we have included in the first section of this book address the cognitive and emotional aspects of student life. Techniques to restructure your thinking patterns to provide clearer thinking and more effective problem solving as well as chapters on effective study skills and test-taking skills have been included. We have included a chapter on performance and test anxiety to help those students who experience anxiety related to classroom and clinical performance and evaluation. Additionally, we have included several chapters that will help you think like a professional nurse rather than a lay person. You will find chapters that will help you understand the effects of negative thinking on clinical and test-taking performance along with a chapter to help you learn to nurture yourself and seek appropriate nurturance from available support systems.

Basically, this book is divided into two sections. The first nine chapters will help you understand basic principles of thinking, studying, and taking tests more effectively. The second section of the book includes over 500 sample practice test questions divided into practice sessions of 15 to 30 questions each. These questions have been tested on samples of nursing students from all types of nursing programs, at all levels of nursing education. The purpose of this section of the book is to aid you in putting the concepts, principles and skills from the first section of the book into practice. When you are allowed to apply information to simulated clinical experiences such as those in the practice sessions, this helps to cement the information more permanently and make it your own. Extensive rationales for both the correct and incorrect answers have been carefully included to help you understand when you have made an error in reasoning or thinking.

This book has been written in a progressive manner. You can start at the beginning and gradually work your way through the text. The concepts at the beginning are basic and move to a more complex level.

We want to make it perfectly clear that we are not trying to teach you nursing knowledge or content, but rather how to think about the nursing knowledge that you already have and that knowledge that you will continue to gain as you progress through your nursing educational program. It is important

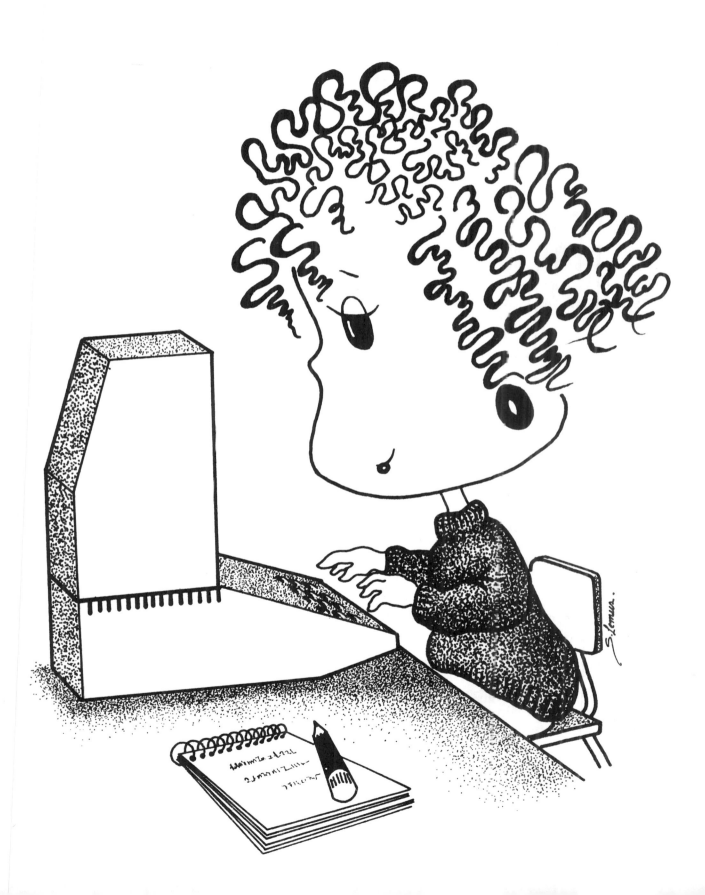

for you to remember that it is not the amount of knowledge that you can gather over the next several years, but how you think about and utilize that knowledge in your nursing practice that will make a difference in your ability to provide quality nursing care.

This book can be an invaluable tool for you as a nursing student if you embrace it with an open mind and dig in; however, it will be a useless collection of tree pulp contributing to environmental waste if you do not actively participate in your reading and then utilize the information contained within it. Every technique and skill within this book may not be appropriate for everyone but, rest assured, there is something of value for everyone. You need to conduct a self-assessment of strengths and weaknesses as a student and thereby pick and choose which parts of this book would be most helpful.

This book does not contain a bag of tricks or secrets of success because, quite frankly, there are none. Nor do we profess to be the fairy godmothers of test-taking, but if you are willing to supply the hard work and effort, there are skills that can be learned and mastered to help you develop "good thinking".

2

STUDY SMART:
THE HORSE BEFORE THE CART

Before we discuss becoming a better test-taker and enhancing test performance, we must examine the process of how you study. Effective study skills are essential for improving test performance. In our experience of working with nursing students, the problem often starts here in study preparation and we would be remiss if we would not take time to discuss and evaluate effective studying habits.

Talking with nursing students about study skills does not usually meet with great enthusiasm. Many nursing students do not want to "waste time" on this topic. Many students comment: "I don't want to spend time talking about study habits. Just tell me how to take the test so I can pass the course." or, "I already know this, I know how to study. I don't need anyone to help me become a better studier. I study all the time." These two responses from students can be equally dangerous. Let's discuss each one separately. First, "I don't want to spend time talking about study habits. Just teach me how to be a better test-taker." For many students, studying and taking tests are two separate entities. This viewpoint allows students to believe that how they study has very little to do with test performance and therefore they do not examine their study skills and habits for potential problems and errors. Regardless of a student's specific test-taking problem, evaluating and enhancing study techniques and habits will usually enhance test grades. For the most part when a nursing student is not taking tests

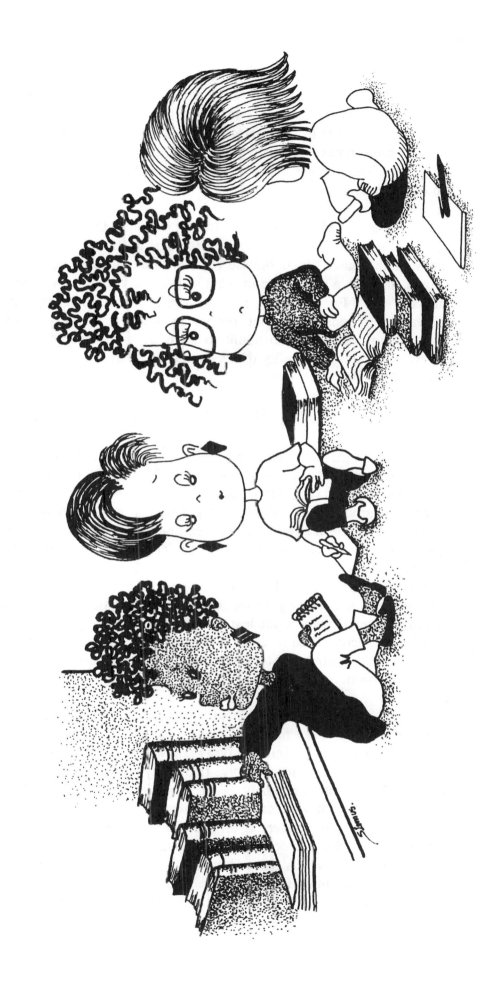

effectively there is usually some connection to their study habits. One common example of this is that students frequently have difficulty understanding the important concepts in their class notes and reading assignments. They read and review their notes repeatedly, however they cannot grasp the main ideas or principles being taught and are often overwhelmed by the volumes of materials to be learned.

The second response, "I already know all this; I know how to study," also has its problems. Often times there is a disparity between what students know and believe about themselves and what students actually do. In other words, there is a difference in what students say they do and what the students actually do. For example, many students report to us that they are easily distracted by noise or other people in the near vicinity when they try to concentrate, yet they also admit to studying with the radio or television on. Many of us are often guilty of not practicing what we know would probably be effective for us.

GOOD STUDY HABITS START BEFORE CLASS

One of the problems that students complain about is the amount of reading that nursing students have to do in school. They aren't use to assignments of 50-75 pages in preparation for a class. There is so much to read that students may become overwhelmed. Most nursing students must learn to be more efficient readers. They need to be able to concentrate, understand, and comprehend what they read. Reading efficiently is an essential skill necessary for effective studying and test-taking. In optimum situations, it is best to read assignments prior to attending class. This will familiarize you with the topic to be discussed. In this way you are not hearing information for the first time. Although some of the reading material may be unclear to you, it often becomes more clear when you hear it the second time in class. If comprehending what you read is a problem for you, the following strategies may help you monitor and improve your comprehension.

As you read the assignment it may help to repeatedly ask yourself, "Am I understanding what I have just read?" so that you are actively involved in the process and become immediately aware when the reading assignment doesn't make sense to you. More simply, frequently stop while reading the assignment and conduct a self-assessment of the material being read. When you are not understanding what was read, several strategies may be implemented. Reading all or part of the assignment again is probably the most common strategy utilized when students don't understand a concept. Sometimes, rereading the material aloud can be helpful. A second strategy is summarizing. When you summarize, you look for the main ideas and details and rewrite them in your own words in a shorter version. A third strategy is looking up the definitions of words you don't understand. Understanding vocabulary is an important part of comprehension. One helpful way to implement this strategy is to always keep a dictionary on your study desk so it is available to you. (Often textbooks have a glossary of items in the back of the book.) Another reason why reading comprehension is sometimes poor, is lack of concentration. Visualization, or visualizing what you are reading is often an effective strategy for this problem. When visualizing, simply create a mental picture in your mind of what you are reading. For example, when reading about the heart, see this fist-sized red pumping muscle in your mind, then fill in the details as you read on. Seeing the concept will help you recall it later. For some individuals, it is easier to add details later as you learn them in class or on clinical. The final strategy is research. This means to use more than one source to get information about a difficult nursing concept. Often students lose concentration while reading an assignment because they lack the background information about that subject. If they continue reading and not comprehending, their frustration grows. Looking up that concept in another text or a basic nursing journal will increase your background knowledge about that subject and increase your concentration and comprehension of that concept (Meltzer & Palau, 1993).

Another complaint that students often report to us is that they do not have time to read all of the assigned readings before coming to class. We caution you here to be honest with yourself. Before this complaint comes from your mouth, take a good long look at how you spend your time. Are you making your nursing education a major priority? Sometimes it's a case of not making the time or taking the time rather than not actually having it. Take a hard look at your daily schedule and ask yourself, "Is it really true that I don't have time to read my assignments before going to class?" Sometimes when we ask that question of our students they reply, "Look, I've got a full-time job and two small children at home. I'm lucky I get to class, let alone read ahead of time!" As nurse educators, we do try to keep our feet firmly planted in reality. We understand that many nursing students are no longer eighteen years old and living in a dormitory, but rather in their mid-thirties with families, children, and work responsibilities. If you fit into this category and, at times, do not have time to read all assignments prior to class, then compromise judiciously. Try to skim or "look over" the major reading assignments prior to class. This includes paying special attention to the introduction and major headings throughout the chapter. Also look for words in special print (italicized or darkened), pictures and diagrams that show a concept in a few words, and reading the summary at the end of the chapter. We realize that this technique is not the best way to prepare for class and should not be used on a regular basis. This can be used in those emergency or rare times when you don't have the amount of time you need to carefully read before going to class. This technique allows you to briefly familiarize yourself with new words or concepts by allowing you to see them prior to attending class.

GETTING THE MOST OUT OF CLASS

One major goal for a student is to become a "cost effective nursing student". By this we mean putting the least amount of energy in and getting the most effective and long lasting rewards. More specifically, if you do not have the luxury of three to four hours every night to study, then make the best use of the time that you do have. Without a doubt the most cost effective improvement in which a nursing student can engage is enhancing actual class time behaviors. If you use your classroom time effectively you can significantly shave hours off your study time. Here are several suggestions:

Always Go to Class! Many nursing students underestimate the importance of classroom lecture and can find numerous reasons and excuses why they should "not go to class today". They rationalize that they can borrow a classmate's notes or have someone tape the lecture, and that they really don't need to be there. The bottom line to all of this is that nothing beats being there. Nurse educators will present the most important and critical information during classroom lecture time. Being there to actually soak in the information first hand is an essential part of your nursing education that cannot be substituted by reading someone else's notes or listening to a taped lecture. Of course, the principle of "always attend class" includes always attending ALL of class. This means getting to class on time and never leaving early, which includes not starting to pack up your books 5 to 10 minutes before the class is over so you can be the first one out of the room. Educators often use the beginning of class to make important announcements and, more importantly, the last five minutes of class to summarize the main points covered in the lecture (Green, 1985).

Listen and Take Notes. In discussing this concept with nursing students it may seem as though the two behaviors cannot be done simultaneously. Students frequently complain this is very difficult so they must do one or the other. They say, "If I sit and listen to a lecture it's hard for me to write it down. On the other hand when I take notes I'm really just writing as fast as I can and it's impossible to pay attention to what the teacher is saying." Contrary to this belief, it is possible to listen and take notes at the same time. We have found that this is a skill similar to learning to ride a bicycle or bake bread, it requires repeated practice. The key to effective listening is that it's almost impossible to write down every word the teacher says. When you attempt to do this you become exhausted, very frustrated, and your hand hurts. The key here is to learn what the main points or principles are. Asking yourself questions such as, "What's really important here?" "What do I need to know to understand this major concept?", will help you in deciding what information is important enough to write down. To be able to do this, however, you must be paying attention and listening to the lecture.

Remember, your notes should not be a re-creation of the lecture itself but rather a summary of the major concepts and principles that were discussed. If the instructor is going too rapidly for you to even pick up the major points of the lecture, leave spaces in your notes with little reminders to yourself. Later review your notes with a classmate and fill in the blanks or ask to speak to the instructor. It is important to make sure your notes are complete because they will be your major vehicle for studying. Your notes will demonstrate to you how well you know and comprehend the information that will be tested. Although some educational experts advise against this, we have found that comparing your notes with other students may sometimes help you enhance the quality of your own note taking skills. For instance, if you are repeatedly missing test questions because of information you do not have in your classroom notes, then you must admit that you're missing major information presented. Check with a classmate who you know takes effective, complete notes, and see if you can see patterns in the types of information that you're missing. One pattern that we have seen in nursing students' class notes is that of limited nursing interventions. Many nursing students will write copious amounts related to assessment data of a specific diagnostic category. However, when they reach important information about interventions they become skimpy in their note taking. This becomes a major problem because it is in this arena where the nurse can apply basic facts into simulated clinical situations. Secondly, many questions on nursing exams deal with the intervention phase of the nursing process. Therefore, it is imperative that the student take complete notes especially during this phase of any classroom lecture.

> **Be Assertive: Sit in the First Row and Ask Questions.**

One attitude that is very important for the student to have during class time is one of consumer rights. Remember, as a student you are a consumer, a consumer of education. Obviously, everyone cannot sit in the first row, but if you know that you are easily distracted when you try to concentrate then you must be careful to get to class early enough to get a first row seat. The further in the front of the room that a student sits, the less chance of being distracted. If you sit near the back of the room, you are not only looking at the teacher and the blackboard, but at the back of everyone else's head; it just makes sense that you can easily be distracted by that, especially in a large class.

Class time is an excellent opportunity to clarify issues that are unclear to you. If the teacher discusses a major point that you clearly do not understand then, by all means, ask. Your education is what you are purchasing and you have every right to know and understand what you are buying. Many students balk at this idea, stating that they are afraid to ask questions and don't want to take up class time, or they're afraid that the question will be dumb and that everyone will laugh at them. Chances are that if you don't understand a concept, someone else

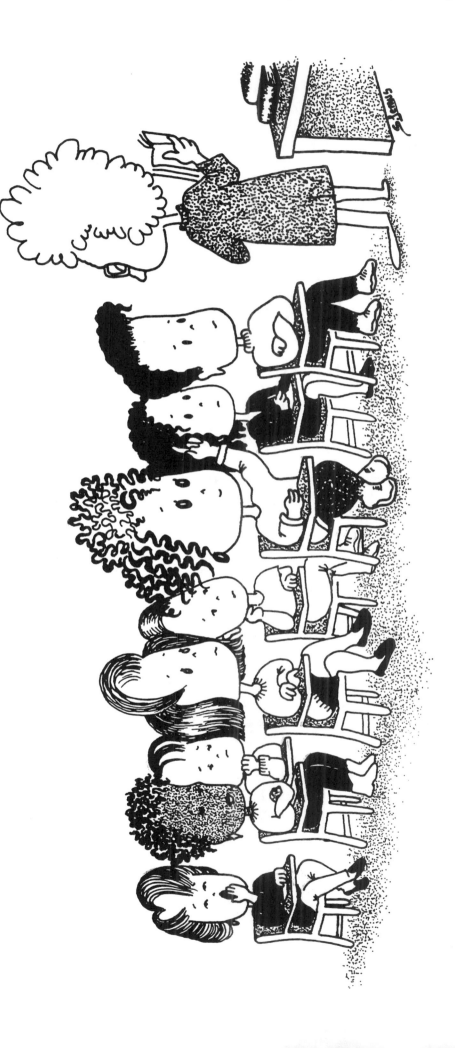

in the room doesn't understand it either and will breathe a sigh of relief because you had the courage to ask the question. It also serves as a gauge for the instructor to know if the class is following the lecture. Of course there will always be individuals who abuse this privilege and will ask a question every five minutes until the entire class is ready to form a lynch mob. But for the most part, occasional questions from students during class time will enhance most lecture presentations. Although asking an occasional question during classroom time is an effective learning tool, resist the temptation to talk to the person beside you. This not only disrupts the class but will provide a break in your concentration as well as that of your classmate and both of you may miss important information. If you are just one of those people who is just too shy to ask questions during a classroom situation, then jot down your question on your note pad and approach the instructor at break time or at the end of class. Remember, the best time to have the question answered is when it is fresh in your mind. If time does not permit you to ask questions after class, make an appointment to see the instructor privately in person or by phone. Most teachers are more than happy to take a few minutes and review questions about lecture material with students.

STUDY PREPARATION FOR A TEST

The following tips are especially helpful for test preparation.

> **Review Classroom Notes as Soon as Possible After Each Class Session.**

One of the most "cost effective" study techniques is to take 15 or 20 minutes and go over your notes from class within the same day that you receive them. For some individuals this may not be until 9:00 o'clock that evening. Regardless of when it happens, reviewing lecture notes on the same day really helps to give you a comprehensive grasp of the material that was presented. You'll be surprised at how helpful this particular technique can be in decreasing the amount of overall study time in the long run. One technique that we have found to be especially helpful is to use a different colored pen or highlighter to underline or star important issues and headings that the instructor has stressed during the actual lecture. Not only will this bring your immediate attention to the important point when reviewing your notes, but it also provides you with the opportunity to test your ability at picking out important principles. This technique has been very useful in helping students who have difficulty knowing what is important from their lecture notes. It will also help you: 1) identify areas of the lecture content that you do not clearly understand or 2) demonstrate noticeable gaps in your note taking. If, when reviewing your notes, you notice that you are missing valuable information from the lecture, it is a perfect opportunity to contact a classmate to go over notes from class together and to check the accuracy of your perceptions. This provides a check and balance system to assure the comprehensiveness of your note taking. This technique also helps if you do find areas in your notes that you do not completely understand. You can go back to the textbook and reread for the second time the information about that particular topic. Often, when combining your class room notes and the textbook, a more complete understanding of the information is available to you.

To Review is to Master.

The best way to obtain mastery over the material is to reread it several times. For example, one week prior to a major exam, start reviewing your notes each night. The more often you review your notes the better the chance of remembering the information long term. Some experts believe that you should take time after each class period and recopy your lecture notes (Green, 1985), while others discourage the general practice of recopying notes as a waste of time (Fry, 1991). Our basic belief about recopying your notes is to know what works for you. If recopying your notes has always been an effective study technique for you then by all means continue to do so. However, recopying classroom notes is not necessarily an essential study technique for everyone. Many students are able to get the same benefit by simply reviewing and highlighting their notes with far less time expenditure.

Create Memory Triggers That Promote Recall of Important Information.

You can create your own jargon or gimmick to help you retrieve important information needed for an examination. (Sides and Cailles, 1989). Several examples include:

1. **Acrostics** - This is a mental tool in which you arrange words into a familiar phrase that triggers the recall of other information to be learned or memorized. For example: "On Old Olympus Towering Top a Fin And German Viewed Some Hops," will help you remember the 12 cranial nerves.

2. **Acronyms** - Using the first letter of several important words to form its own word or symbol, e.g. PEARL - Pupils Equal And Reactive to Light.

Write Your Own Test.

After you have finished studying, developing a hypothetical test may prove to be a rewarding, enjoyable experience. Sit down and try to think of 10 significant questions that your teacher may ask you, then try in a few words to write down what your answer would be. Sometimes when you attempt to develop your own questions and then attempt to answer them, it can really help you identify gaps in your knowledge base. It can also add to increasing self confidence when you are able to answer your own test questions effectively. If you aren't sure of what questions to ask yourself, look at the unit objectives. The objectives show what the teacher thought would be important. Another technique that we suggest to students on a regular basis is to use sample test questions for review and test preparation from the many NCLEX preparation question books. For example, if a student is preparing for a final exam in pediatric nursing, it is often helpful to scan through an NCLEX question book and attempt to answer the pediatric questions. The major concepts of pediatric nursing are the same, so chances are you are going to see some similar questions or at least similar concepts in the review books that will be actually tested on your exam.

STUDY ERRORS

The best way to begin to study for a major examination is to do so in brief, short periods. A short amount of time every day is a much better approach than trying to pull a 24 hour cram session the night before. Basically, in our years of helping individuals become better students and more effective test-takers, we have seen the following study errors occur.

1. Memorization vs. Application.

Probably the most common problem that nursing students encounter when they begin to study for a major exam is that they memorize their notes rather than learning and understanding them. It is not uncommon to hear the following complaint, "I just don't understand it. I studied for hours. I knew my notes inside and out and I still failed the test. I just don't get it. What am I doing wrong?" In a nutshell this problem can best be defined as follows: students study for knowledge level questions and teachers ask application level questions. For example, a student may memorize the peak action of every insulin and expect to see the following question:

The peak action of isophane (NPH) insulin is:
a. 0.5 to 1 hour.
b. 2 to 4 hours.
c. 10 to 16 hours.
d. 18 to 24 hours.

In this question, the correct answer is (c). Onset of action of NPH insulin is 4 to 6 hours, peak is 10 to 16 hours, and duration is 18 to 30 hours. Option (a) is the onset of regular (short acting) insulin. Option (b) is the peak action of regular insulin. Option (d) is the duration of NPH insulin (Karb, Queener & Freeman, 1992; pp. 661-666).

15

Instead, the student may be stunned to see the following application question:

A diabetic client on a mixture of regular and isophane (NPH) insulin is reviewing the diet teaching with the clinic nurse. The nurse ascertains that the client takes his insulin injection at 8 a.m. The nurse evaluates that the client understands the teaching when he chooses which meal plan?

a. Breakfast at 8:30 a.m.; snack at 10 a.m.; lunch at 12 noon; snack at 3 p.m.; dinner at 6 p.m.; snack at 9 p.m.
b. Breakfast at 9 a.m.; lunch at 12 noon; snack at 4 p.m.; dinner at 6:30 p.m.
c. Breakfast at 9:30 a.m.; lunch at 1 p.m.; dinner at 7 p.m.
d. Breakfast at 7:30 a.m.; snack at 9:30 a.m.; lunch at 1 p.m.; snack at 4 p.m.; dinner at 7 p.m.; snack at 10 p.m.

In this situation, the student would not only need to have the knowledge about the peak actions of insulin but would also have to be able to apply that information to a simulated clinical situation. In the above question the correct answer is (a). This meal pattern covers the onset, peak, and duration of both the regular and NPH insulins. The onset of regular insulin is one-half to one hour after the injection. Therefore, a meal such as breakfast should be given 30 minutes after the injection so sufficient glucose is in the system. The peak action of regular insulin is two to four hours. A snack at 10 a.m. (2 hours after the injection) would counteract the regular insulin. At four hours after the injection the regular insulin is still at its peak, plus the NPH insulin is beginning to take effect. Lunch at 12 noon will provide glucose to counter-balance the insulin. The regular insulin has a duration of six to eight hours. A snack at 3 p.m. will provide sufficient glucose. Dinner at 6 p.m. provides glucose during the peak action period of the NPH as does the evening snack at 9 p.m. NPH insulin has a duration of eighteen to thirty hours, so often the morning snack is a little heavier in content to account for this. Options (b) and (c) would only relate to coverage with regular insulin. In option (d), breakfast is eaten before the insulin, lunch is taken after the peak action of regular insulin, but before the peak of the NPH insulin and the 4 p.m. snack is after the regular insulin is active but before the peak of NPH, so the glucose is not covered for breakfast, lunch, or snack (Karb, Queener & Freeman, 1992; pp. 661-666).

Here's where we separate the good thinkers from the not-so-good thinkers. Let's look at some more examples of knowledge versus application level questions.

Knowledge Level:

The most common side effect of prednisone is:
a. nausea.
b. hypotension.
c. hypoglycemia.
d. fat intolerance.

This is a knowledge level question because students can memorize the side effects of prednisone. The correct answer is (a). Prednisone can cause gastrointestinal upset. Adverse reactions include peptic ulcer and intestinal perforation. Hypertension rather than hypotension (option b) would occur since prednisone causes fluid retention by keeping the kidneys from excreting sodium. The extra fluid would increase blood pressure. Hyperglycemia rather than hypoglycemia (option c) would occur because prednisone works against insulin. The drug also alters carbohydrate usage by promoting glucose production resulting in increased glucose in the system. Fat intolerance (option d) would occur with diseases associated with the gall bladder. Fat intolerance is not a problem with prednisone; however, the distribution of fat is changed from the extremities to the trunk (Baer & Williams, 1992; pp. 960-962).

Application Level:

A 66 year old client with chronic obstructive pulmonary disease (COPD) calls the home care nurse. He tells the nurse he has been taking prednisone 40 mg orally every day for the last week. The client states, "Nurse, I get so sick to my stomach 30 minutes after I take my prednisone." The nurse should instruct the client to:
a. continue the medication as ordered and tell the physician about the stomach problem at the next scheduled appointment.
b. discontinue the prednisone immediately because this is an allergic reaction to the medication.
c. take the prednisone after a full meal or with milk.
d. take the prednisone one hour before bedtime to enhance the absorption rate of the medicine.

Remember, for the last question the student probably memorized that prednisone can cause nausea and stomach irritation. How can the same information apply to this situation? If nausea is an expected side effect then it is not an allergic reaction, so option (b) can be eliminated. If nausea and gastric irritation are side effects, then the client shouldn't take it on an empty stomach, so option (d) can be eliminated. If nausea and gastric irritation can lead to the adverse reactions of peptic ulcer and intestinal perforation (probably also information memorized by the student), then ignoring the client's symptoms may lead to the adverse reactions so option (a) can be eliminated since delay can cause further damage to the stomach. Option (c) deals specifically with the known side effects. Taking the prednisone after a full meal or with milk coats the stomach and lessens stomach irritation. If these measures do not assist the client to decrease nausea then the client should call the physician (Vallerand & Deglin, 1991; pp. 359-361). As you can see, the same information is available to the student, but a prudent student would reason through what the information means for the client and how the nurse should care for that client.

Students also tend to miss nutrition questions for the same reasons they miss drug questions. Memorizing certain vitamins and minerals and what role they play in the body is the usual approach. Students believe the question may be something like this:

Knowledge Level:

What nutrients most help wound healing?
a. Vitamins B_6 and K.
b. Vitamin D and calcium.
c. Vitamins A and C.
d. Vitamin B_{12} and zinc.

The correct answer is (c). Although all nutrient requirements are increased during wound healing, vitamins A, C, B, and protein play vital roles in wound healing. Vitamin A is necessary for tissue regeneration. Vitamin C promotes wound healing, collagen formation and helps prevent infection. It may also help to metabolize amino acids which are the foundation of protein. Vitamin B_6 (option a) deals with the integrity of the nervous system and is often ordered with isoniazide (INH) to prevent side effects such as numbness and tingling. Vitamin K (option a) is primarily used for blood coagulation and is used as an antidote for warfarin sodium (Coumadin). Vitamin D and calcium (option b) work together to mineralize bones and teeth and would be needed if fractures occur, but may be limited in clients on prolonged bedrest since excess calcium may form kidney stones. Vitamin B_{12} (option d) is necessary for body cell functioning, particularly red blood cells. However, B_{12} by itself would be passed through the body unless sufficient intrinsic factor is present to promote B_{12} absorption. Intrinsic factor is found in the gastric lining. Zinc (option d) assists in growth and reproduction. Deficiency can cause fetal abnormalities (Whitney & Rolfes, 1993; pp. 308-309, 316, 324-325, 337-338, 350, 358, 418).

Students like these kind of questions because they are so straight forward. However, they do little to prepare you for the real life problems nurses handle on a daily basis, like the following question.

Application Level:

A client is three days post-cholecystectomy and is tolerating a general diet. Which meal would best assist the client's wound healing?
a. Pork, baked potato, green beans, banana.
b. Turkey sandwich with wheat bread, fortified milk.
c. Roast beef, rice, stewed tomatoes, strawberries.
d. Oyster stew, applesauce, tea with milk.

The basic facts that students memorize include that a diet high in protein, carbohydrates, and vitamins A, C, and B is recommended to promote wound healing. But what does this mean to the client? If a nurse tells the client to eat those nutrients, will the client know what to do? Probably not, so the nurse must take the information forward one step to include the foods in which these nutrients are found. Vitamin A is necessary for tissue regeneration and is found in roast beef and tomatoes. Vitamin C promotes wound healing and collagen production and helps to prevent infection. Sources of vitamin C include tomatoes and strawberries. Vitamin C also helps to metabolize amino acids which build protein. Protein is necessary for tissue metabolism. If sufficient protein is not ingested, then negative nitrogen balance occurs in which proteins are broken down by the body so nutrients can be used. Protein sources include meat such as roast beef. Non-protein calories (carbohydrates) are needed so protein can be used for tissue building. Rice would increase carbohydrate calories. With these "facts" at our disposal let's reason through the options. Option (a) contains B_6 (all four foods) and potassium (potato and banana). Vitamin B_6 deals with the integrity of the nervous system. Potassium is an electrolyte that helps with fluid balance. Option (b) contains vitamin D and calcium (fortified milk) plus protein (turkey) and carbohydrate (wheat bread). Remember that vitamin D and calcium are good for fractures. In this meal plan the wheat bread would decrease the absorption of the vitamin D in the milk. Option (d) contains vitamin B_{12} (oysters and milk) and zinc (oysters and applesauce). Remember that vitamin B_{12} is needed for body cell functioning. Zinc assists in growth and reproduction. However, in this meal, zinc absorption would be inhibited by the tea. In option (c), Vitamin A is found in the roast beef and tomatoes, vitamin C is in tomatoes and strawberries, protein is in roast beef and carbohydrates are in the rice. This option contains the most nutrients to promote wound healing (Whitney & Rolfes, 1993; pp. 308-311, 316-317, 324-325, 328-330, 337-338, 346-353, 358-360, 418, 423-424).

Here is another way a nutrition question may be related to client care. The student may memorize how much sodium is in particular foods and expect this question.

Knowledge Level:

What food contains the highest sodium content per serving?
a. One cup of chili con carne with beans.
b. Four ounces of lean ham.
c. One cup of canned tomato sauce.
d. One cup of sauerkraut.

The correct answer is (d). Sauerkraut contains 1560 mg of sodium per cup. Chili con carne with beans (option a) contains 1331 mg of sodium per cup. Three ounces of lean ham (option b) contains 1364 mg of sodium. One cup of tomato sauce (option c) contains 1482 mg of sodium (Whitney & Rolfes, 1993; pp. 1146-1147, 1152-1153, 1176-1179). This type of question is most likely found in a nutrition course examination and provides background for nursing. Information about sodium might be used a little differently in nursing as in the following question.

Application Level:

A client is admitted with right-sided congestive heart failure. The nurse is reviewing information on a low sodium diet. The nurse evaluates that the client understands the diet when he states:
a. "This will keep the water out of my lungs."
b. "I'm glad I'll be able to eat my wieners and sauerkraut."
c. "I know I won't be able to eat oranges and grapefruit."
d. "Maybe my feet will fit into my shoes now."

This question asks the nurse to know the role that sodium plays in the body and what effect the decreased sodium intake will have on the disease process as well as sources of sodium. The correct answer is (d). Right-sided congestive heart failure results in symptoms of fluid volume excess such as edema of hands, legs, ankles, and feet. Excess sodium promotes fluid retention; therefore, lowered sodium allows the fluid to be excreted, thus reducing edema. The end result may be a decrease in the size of feet and allow the client to wear his usual size of shoe. Fluid in the lungs (option a) is related to left-sided congestive heart failure and results in shortness of breath, cough and frothy sputum. Decreased sodium would also promote fluid excretion and improve these symptoms but the question relates to right-sided failure. Wieners and sauerkraut (option b) are high in sodium and would show a need for review of material. Oranges and grapefruit (option c) are high in vitamin C but low in sodium and shouldn't be eliminated from the diet (Lewis & Collier, 1992; pp. 831-834; Whitney & Rolfes, 1993; pp. 322-330, 377-382).

Most students do the same type of memorizing for drug questions. For example, what is the normal dose of a medication? They would expect to see this type of question.

Knowledge Level:

What is the usual daily dosage of meperidine hydrochloride (Demerol)?
a. 1 mg to 4 mg q 3 hours.
b. 5 mg to 15 mg q 4 hours.
c. 15 mg to 60 mg q 4 hours.
d. 50 mg to 150 mg q 3 hours.

The correct answer is (d). Option (a) is the usual dose for butorphanol tartrate (Stadol). Option (b) is the usual dose for morphine sulfate (Morphine). Option (c) is the usual dose for codeine sulfate (Codeine) (Ignatavicius & Bayne, 1991; p. 481). This is straight forward information. Now let's look at a different level of question asking for the same information.

Application Level:

A client is admitted with a compound fracture of the femur and is placed in traction. The physician writes the following orders. The nurse might question:
a. erythromycin (E-mycin) 250 mg PO q 6 hours x 5 days.
b. meperidine hydrochloride (Demerol) 15 mg IM q 4 hours PRN pain.
c. senna (Senokot) 2 tablets PRN constipation.
d. prochlorperazine (Compazine) 10 mg IM q 6 hours PRN nausea.

A student knowing that the normal dose of meperidene hydrochloride (Demerol) is 50 to 150 mg q 3 hours PRN would also know to question option (b). This dose is too low and would not give pain relief to the client. The nurse, as the client advocate, would call the physician to clarify the order. Erythromycin (E-mycin) (option a) is an antibiotic used in prophylaxis and treatment for infections of gram negative and gram positive bacteria. The correct dose is 250 mg PO every 6 hours. Senna (Senokot) (option c) is used for acute constipation or prior to gastrointestinal examinations. It may be used in this client for constipation related to bedrest. Prochlorperazine (Compazine) (option d) is used for nausea and vomiting. The normal adult dose is 5 to 10 mg PO or IM 3 to 4 times per day and 25 mg rectally twice per day (Baer & Williams, 1992; pp. 351, 726, 745, 1036).

In these questions, the same knowledge base was applied to different levels of questioning. Studying must reflect the different situations you might encounter in the classroom (on tests), as a nurse on clinical, and after graduation. Some students have a natural knack, so to speak, for being able to take the knowledge and naturally apply it. However, many students have great difficulty with this and it is in the testing situation where they first understand that they did not study appropriately for the exam. Even more detrimental is when they have no idea how to remedy this very serious studying problem. Unfortunately, the way that they study and answer test questions also shows the way they will think as nurses. Some students may do well on clinical when performing tasks; however, a professional nurse is one who can think and reason, as well as act.

There are several ways to help change your thinking patterns when you study. The first is to try to think like the teacher. For example, "What will the teacher think is important?", or "How might this be put into a test question?" Another very helpful question that the student can ask is, "Why is it important for me to know this?" Secondly, for some individuals, small group study is very effective in moving beyond a knowledge level understanding of material to a much higher level with an application base. In a small group you can ask questions of each other that would stimulate thinking at this higher level. Studying in small groups can provide two other useful purposes. First, it can give you a more realistic understanding of the type of grasp you have on the material. It is easy to fool yourself when you repeatedly memorize page after page of study and lecture notes. However, when you test yourself or test others, by asking them to apply that information into a clinical situation, it forces you to make an accurate assessment of what your true understanding of the material is. Furthermore, group members can "think aloud" in that they can reason through a particular clinical issue or situation and have classmates give them constructive feedback when reasoning errors occur. This can be extremely helpful because then erroneous thinking can be corrected. Memorization is a very costly and energy expending activity. Students need to learn to save their brains for important memorization; to be able to sift through lecture notes and memorize only what is necessary. Remember, nursing is an applied science. It can be the kiss of death to overuse memorization when understanding and application is truly what is necessary to effectively practice nursing today.

---

2. Cramming Cramps Your Style.

Cramming for exams is an interesting phenomena. Although most people will intellectualize that it is not the best study preparation for an exam, many individuals fall prey to its alluring nature. There is something magical in the belief that you can soak up a month's worth of learning into one 24 hour period. Although we consistently tell nursing students to avoid cramming as an effective study method, our advice often falls upon deaf ears. Adding to its allure is the fact that

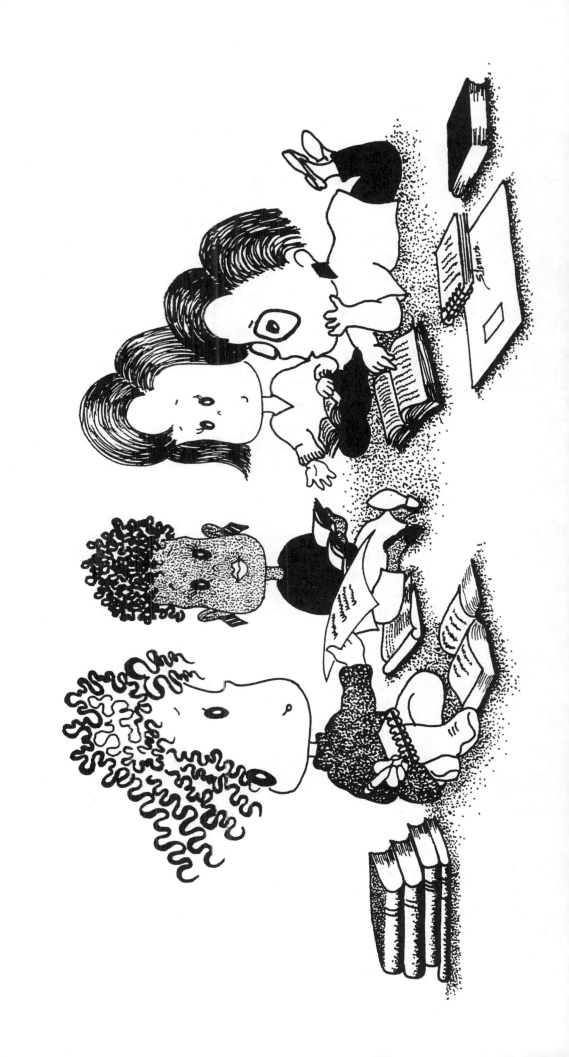

cramming can produce immediate results. Some individuals can do very well by cramming for a test. Once this occurs, it becomes a positive reinforcement to do it again and again. The problem with cramming is that it only works for short term memory. When students cram for every major exam during a semester, they often find themselves in a panic attack before the final exam because cramming is not effective for comprehensive and long term recall (Ellis, 1991). The bottom line here is that, although cramming may appear attractive to many students, it simply does not work in the long haul. This can be especially dangerous for nursing students when they realize that before they become licensed, they must take a licensing exam which tests information that has been learned throughout their entire nursing educational program. Also, complex concepts learned in the senior level nursing courses are built upon the knowledge base of earlier concepts. If you have forgotten the original concepts because you crammed for the test, it will take much more effort to understand and learn the higher level nursing concepts.

---

3. Subjective Meaning of Studying.

Many individuals report that studying on a regular basis is not particularly uncomfortable until they approach the date of the upcoming exam. Almost immediately, the subjective meaning changes; now the meaning of why you are studying, and what is going to happen if it is not effective, changes. Tests have different meanings for everyone. The "meaning" that an individual places on a test is defined in the literature as subjective meaning. Subjective meaning refers to the idiosyncratic interpretation individuals make about their self-referent thoughts based on what they believe about themselves in a particular context (Bruch, Kaflowitz & Kuethe, 1986). In simpler terms, what does the test or test performance mean specifically to you? What do you believe the test is a measure of? Some individuals think that a test measures what you have accomplished in a specific course. Some people believe that tests are a measure of intelligence, while others view tests as a measure of self-esteem and self-worth. Subjective meaning is often expressed by the individual test-taker in the flow of conversation with the cognitions that they repeat over and over to themselves (e.g. "I have to pass this test or I am a complete and total failure."; "If I don't do well on this exam my career is over."). Subjective meaning of your cognitions or thoughts can place an extra burden or excessive baggage on the person to perform well. Research has indicated that the subjective meaning placed on negative thoughts can be detrimental to test performance (Galassi, Frierson & Sharer, 1981). When students study for the purpose of knowing and learning, usually they can remain fairly anxiety free; however, when the act of studying means success or failure on an upcoming test, the ability to remain calm can quickly change. Now studying means success or failure, and sitting down to review your notes and read your textbook can symbolize potential danger. It can often promote cognitions such as, "I'll never learn all of this. I'm going to fail this test. It's impossible.

24

I'll never graduate. I'll never be a nurse. I'll never make anything of myself. This is my last chance." Although the task has remained the same, the student is still studying, the meaning behind the task or behavior has changed. It has gone from an activity to enhance one's understanding to an activity that will predict or determine one's personal success or failure. Thinking more clearly and more constructively during an exam will be discussed in a later chapter. Here it will suffice to say that short, brief periods of study throughout the course will greatly decrease negative, subjective meaning. Cramming, however, can greatly enhance negative subjective meaning.

---

4. Avoid Pre-Study Rituals.

Pre-study rituals are those rituals we engage in to fool ourselves into believing that we are too busy to study. These rituals are almost limitless and quite alluring because almost anything seems like it would be more fun and less anxiety provoking than studying (Jensen, 1989). The pre-study ritual lets us deal with our test performance anxiety through avoidance. Unfortunately, when we begin to start thinking that it's time to study, those thoughts create feelings of anxiety which then create thoughts to avoid studying. We all know what they are. Here are some common examples:

"I'll study after I do the dishes and finish the laundry."
"I'll study after I watch my soap opera."
"I'll study after my aerobics class."

It's not hard to see that pre-study rituals can eat up a lot of our precious study time. Unfortunately, pre-study rituals, although invented to decrease anxiety, only do so temporarily because the entire time we are engaged in the pre-study activity, we are worrying with a common thought such as "I really should be studying, I'll never get everything done." Even though the pre-study ritual was put into action to decrease our anxiety, it ends up increasing our anxiety. Rule of thumb: Keep your pre-study ritual activities to five minutes or less. Make it the same ritual activity each time so it signals the mind that it's time to study. For example, our pre-study ritual in writing parts of this book was to get out our pencils, paper, pencil sharpener, rulers, diet soda, and pretzels. Then we could begin.

AFTER THE TEST: GETTING YOUR GRADE

Most nursing courses include more than one test, each with its own opportunity to perform successfully. Unfortunately, many nursing students have difficulty remembering this. If they receive a poor grade on their first test, they believe that it's all over for them. They begin to have thoughts such as, "I'll never be able to take this teacher's tests, they're too hard." "This is it, it's all over, I'll never be able to get myself out of this hole." "This is a bad sign...if you fail the first test you're not going to do any better on the other ones." The first exam in your nursing course can be a pivotal turning point for how you will do in the remainder of the class. In our experience, we have seen students take one of the two following paths:

| a) **Immobilization and Making Excuses.** |

In this path, the students become immobilized by the test grade. Their drive and motivation for success in the course seem to take a big backslide. They complain that they are now finding it difficult to keep going. They report decreased energy, malaise, and even apathy. Some begin to have thoughts of impending doom such as, "What's the use...I'm just not any good at taking tests." Or, "Why did this happen to me? I worked so hard." In class they report that they are now finding it difficult to concentrate on the lecture material with frequent daydreaming and decreased attention span. When they try to study they make excuses such as, "Why bother? This won't help anyhow." or, "Studying for me is just a waste of time. I do better when I just go in and take the test and don't study."

| b) **Mobilization: Becoming a Detective.** |

Mobilizing yourself after an exam is a much better approach. Right after the test is a perfectly good time to become a detective. In other words, find out where you went wrong. The first step is to ask your instructor if you can see your exam and review it. When you have an opportunity to review an examination with an instructor, you can see where you made your mistakes. Many people will be surprised to see that they made mistakes on their tests that had nothing to do with lack of information. Often students make mistakes such as misreading or misunderstanding the question that was being asked, or simply writing down the wrong answer or filling in the wrong dot on the answer sheet. While going over the exam you have the opportunity to see patterns in your test-taking behavior and will then be able to move forward in correcting those patterns. If you take this approach, these mistakes can often be easily corrected and you can begin immediately to prepare for your next exam, usually with much better results.

REFERENCES

Baer, C. L. & Williams, B. R. (1992). Clinical pharmacology and nursing. Springhouse, PA: Springhouse.

Bruch, M. A., Kaflowitz, N. G. & Kuethe, M. (1986). Beliefs and the subjective meaning of thoughts: Analysis of the role of self-statements in academic test performance. Cognitive therapy and research, 10(1), 51-69.

Ellis, D. B. (1991). <u>Becoming a master student</u> (6th ed.) Rapid City, SD: College Survival, Inc.

Fry, R. (1991). <u>How to study</u>. Hawthorne, NJ: Career Press.

Galassi, J. P., Frierson, H. T. & Sharer, R. (1981). Behavior of high, moderate and low test anxious students during an actual test situation. <u>Journal of Consulting and Clinical Psychology</u>, <u>49</u>(1), 51-62.

Green, G. W. (1985). <u>Getting straight A's</u>. Secaucus, NJ: Lyle Stuart, Inc.

Ignatavicius, D. D. & Bayne, M. V. (1991). <u>Medical-surgical nursing: A nursing process approach</u>. Philadelphia: Saunders.

Jensen, E. (1989). <u>Student success secrets</u>. (3rd ed.) Hauppauge, NY: Barron.

Karb, V. B., Queener, S. F. & Freeman, J. B. (1992). <u>Handbook of drugs</u>. St. Louis: Mosby.

Lewis, S. M. & Collier, I. C. (1992). <u>Medical-surgical nursing: Assessment and management of clinical problems</u> (3rd ed.). St. Louis, Mosby Year Book.

Meltzer, M. & Palau, S. M. (1993). <u>Reading and study strategies for nursing students</u>. Philadelphia: Saunders.

Sides, M. B. & Cailles, N. B. (1989). <u>Nurses guide to successful test-taking</u>. Philadelphia: Lippincott.

Vallerand, A. H. & Deglin, J. H. (1991). <u>Drug guide for critical care and emergency nursing</u>. Philadelphia: Davis.

Whitney, E. N. & Rolfes, S. R. (1993). <u>Understanding nutrition</u>. St. Paul: West.

3

PROBLEM SOLVING:
HOW TO THINK LIKE A NURSE

In our fast paced and quickly changing society, the ability to problem solve in a variety of situations is a necessity for a successful life. Problems ranging from what to wear when you get up in the morning to how to solve major career crises occur on a routine basis. Every individual must learn to solve these problems in order to be able to function effectively in today's society. As both psychiatric nurse clinical specialists and nurse educators, we have seen that the problem solving abilities in both our clients and students vary greatly from one individual to the next. We have also seen that those individuals who have good problem solving abilities seem to function in life at a more proficient level both personally and as nursing students. For years, many researchers and educators have believed that problem solving abilities and thinking skills were innate qualities and could not be taught. However, recent research indicates that teaching general thinking and problem solving skills in specific content areas can substantially increase student's problem solving effectiveness (Nickerson, Perkins, & Smith, 1985).

Research has shown that individuals' appraisals of their problem solving skills will affect their problem solving performance and may be the crucial factor in how and if personal problems get solved (Butler & Meichenbaum, 1981). Self identified effective problem solvers tend to have better self concepts and less self criticism than ineffective problem solvers. The effective problem solvers reported fewer dysfunctional irrational thoughts and coping styles and tended not to blame others for their problems (Heppner, Reeder & Larsen, 1983). They also reported less symptoms of depression and anxiety and showed evidence of a more internal locus of control than those of their counterparts (Nezu, 1985). Effective problem solvers tend to have more confidence about their decision making abilities than that of ineffective problem solvers. Problem solving self appraisal was significantly predictive of study habits regardless of academic ability (Elliot, Godshall, Shrout & Witty, 1990). Research has demonstrated that enhancing one's problem solving abilities will most probably enhance the quality of one's life. Becoming a better problem solver is a skill that is well worth acquiring.

Effective thinking and problem solving skills are also becoming increasingly important to the nursing profession. Problem solving, a dimension of the nursing process, has been acclaimed by many nurse educators as the prevailing model for nursing practice (Holbert & Abraham, 1988). Since problem solving ability is not only important to everyone in general, but is crucial to nurses and their clients, the question becomes, "How can nursing students learn, enhance and enrich their problem solving abilities?" Students need to be able to think like nurses.

HOW TO THINK LIKE A NURSE

Situation: After an exhausting day of clinical practice, Sharon, a first year nursing student, talks over the day with her classmate, Barb.

Sharon:	"What a day I had, my instructor's really on my case!"
Barb:	"What happened?"
Sharon:	"I just couldn't do anything right. I was 25 minutes late for conference because I was so slow at getting finished with my client care. My instructor told me that I'd better get my priorities straight. She told me I have to start thinking like a nurse."
Barb:	"What does she mean by that?"
Sharon:	"You know, I'm not exactly sure. How am I supposed to learn to think like a nurse?"

The above conversation between two beginning nursing students could have been between any two nursing students. When you enter a nursing educational program, you are supposed to start thinking in a different way, a more sophisticated way, a way that is different from a lay person. But what exactly does that mean? More importantly, how do you begin to go about this

29

way of thinking? Hopefully, in this chapter, we will begin to shed some light on this issue and answer some of those questions. In the nursing profession today we struggle with the rapid and continuous emergence of new knowledge and technology. How do you learn and remember all of the information necessary without feeling like a hamster on a treadmill? Although we as a profession make valiant efforts to keep up with new knowledge and technology the fact remains that no nurse can "know it all." The focus for nursing students must shift from what and how much to know to how you think, problem solve and make clinical judgements that create effective nursing care. We may want to cling to our facts and information as we falsely perceive that they will provide a safety net for both the nurse and the client, but the safety net will always have holes in it; holes big enough for us to fall through.

Situation: A nursing instructor overhears a group of graduate nurses discussing the NCLEX which they had just completed.

Bridgette:	"Hey, Did you get that question on Cyclosporine?"
Patrick:	"I don't even remember what that drug is..."
Bridgette:	"They never taught us that drug in nursing school."
Patrick:	"I don't think I learned that drug either. Why didn't they teach us that?"
Bridgette:	"There were several things on this test I never heard of. I'm starting to think I went to a really bad nursing school."

The above conversation demonstrates the frustrations of the new graduates who are coming to terms with the fact that they do not know everything and feel cheated and inadequate because of this. This is not an uncommon phenomena. Many seasoned nurses feel inadequate when they hear of a drug or procedure that they do not know, even if they have intellectually realized that it doesn't matter how much they try, they can't know everything. They have no real problem solving skills to fall back on when the facts don't give them the answers. This issue becomes a real one from the day you enter a nursing educational program when the inundation of information begins. From the first class, first reading assignment, and first time on clinical practice the nursing student is constantly bombarded with feelings of inadequacy at the thought of the tremendous amount of information that is available. The experience of being a nursing student, although rewarding, is often filled with feelings of anxiety, fear, and being overwhelmed. "Will I ever know enough?" "Am I safe?" "Can I really help people?" "Am I smart enough?" "Can I remember enough?" All of these are often questions nursing students live with on a daily basis and, in a way, have to learn to live with forever. The basic reality is that learning never ends. Each day brings new data, new information, and new technology. No matter what nursing school attended, graduates will leave without all of the available knowledge. It simply cannot all be taught or remembered.

So then, what can you expect to be learning in a nursing educational program? This question is a good one. What you really learn in nursing school is far better than a collection of facts. What your nursing education program will teach you is a way to learn, a way to think and reason, and a way to problem solve. You will learn a way of scientifically gathering data, analyzing it, applying that data in clinical practice and evaluating its effectiveness. You will learn the nursing process which is a scientific method that underlies the practice of nursing. You will learn to see and make accurate observations. You will learn to question and where to go to have those questions answered. You will learn to prioritize, evaluate, and reevaluate. you will learn when to listen and when to act. You will learn to base your information on empirical data and also on intuition. You will learn when to judge and when to refrain from judgement. When you have completed your nursing educational program, you may not know everything there is to know, but you will know how to think like a nurse.

What are some of the ways you can enhance your problem solving skills and learn to think like a nurse? That's an interesting question. Socrates, an ancient philosopher, was a master at asking questions. He taught his students to question everything, to look at all the alternatives, to experience what was being taught rather than merely passively hearing the lecturer's voice. If you haven't noticed, nursing instructors tend to ask many questions, particularly in clinical situations and on tests. Listen actively to what they are asking you and learn to anticipate the questions. Enroll the aid of fellow classmates to do the same.

Observe the nurses on your clinical units. Sometimes they'll think out loud, asking and answering questions for themselves. For example, "I wonder why Mrs. Luke spiked a temperature today? She's been normal since the procedure. Well, what could have caused the increase in temperature in a post-operative client? Let's see, she's five days post-operative. What medications is she on? She's not on any medicine that would cause a fever. Does she have any pain? She's not really complaining of any pain anywhere. Okay, what else could cause the problem? Often post-op client's temperatures come from urinary tract infections, wound infections, or pneumonia. Mrs. Luke had a urinary catheter in for 48 hours so urinary tract infection is a possibility. She had surgery so wound infection is also a possibility. She might just be getting a could but maybe I'll check her lungs to assess for pneumonia. I'll go assess for these three possibilities. I wonder if I should call the doctor? I'll ask the unit clerk to page her. She may want to run a few tests or place her on antibiotics. I wonder how Mrs. Luke will feel about this? She won't like it if her discharge is postponed. I must do a careful assessment and explain why this information is necessary so she doesn't dismiss or downplay any of her symptoms." Notice the problem solving here. A lay person may not have even been worried about the elevated temperature, thinking it was a normal occurrence after an operation. Clients often delay reporting problems to the nurse or the physician because the clients may not think they're important, don't want to bother the nurse, or are fearful that something more serious is wrong. Clients don't know or understand the consequences of symptoms or when to call the physician. Nurses have the information to reason this through and should do so as the situation arises.

ANTICIPATORY PROBLEM SOLVING

Often when nursing students have difficulty with problem solving in clinical and classroom situations, they have difficulty with problem solving in their personal lives as well. Unfortunately, difficulty in personal problem solving can have a direct and negative impact on the student's academic life. In these situations it may be very helpful to do some anticipatory problem solving. Anticipatory problem solving is basically looking ahead to possible problems that may occur and then thinking of and preparing for possible solutions that could be employed if these problems actually did occur. Let's look at some examples.

SITUATION 1

Kim has prepared extensively for her upcoming final exam because whether or not she passes the course depends on the grade she gets on this final. On the morning of the exam Kim feels very confident and prepared as she leaves her house. However her feelings quickly turn to dismay when she learns that her car won't start. Kim kicks the car and says, "You old piece of junk. I knew you'd do this to me. Why couldn't you wait just one more day. You've broken down three times in the last month." Kim panics and starts to cry and feels like her life is over. She can't think of any possible solutions because she is so upset. She decides to walk the three miles to school. By the time she gets there, the final exam is over. She tearfully explains to her instructor what happened. The instructor reluctantly agrees to allow her to take a makeup test. Kim is so upset that she finds it difficult to concentrate on the makeup test. She doesn't do well on the test and fails the course.

In the above situation, Kim could have benefitted from using some anticipatory problem solving. Knowing that her car frequently breaks down should have prodded Kim to realize that this was a possible problem. Utilizing

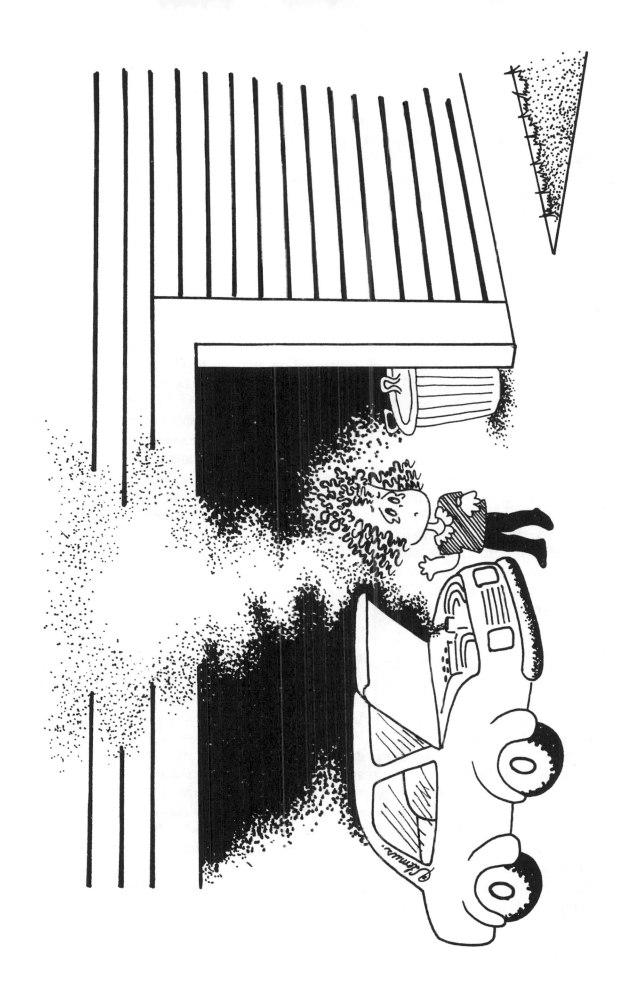

anticipatory problem solving would have allowed Kim not only to look at the possible car breakdown but to prepare for that eventuality. Specifically, she could have gotten bus schedules, the number of the local taxi service or talked with friends and neighbors about emergency rides to school. Once the anticipated problem actually occurred, her mental problem solving could have been put right into play. She then could have acted on one of her possible solutions without having to think of a solution when she was so anxious and upset.

SITUATION 2

John has failed three quizzes in his Introductory Nursing course. He becomes very frustrated because he studies all of the time. "I guess I just have to study harder," he says to himself. John becomes obsessed with studying so that he becomes exhausted. He doesn't discuss the problem with anyone, not even his friends, because he believes he can deal with the problem himself if he just studies hard enough. He decides he doesn't want to waste his time going to test reviews but wants to use the time to study more. He fails two major nursing exams. Totally exasperated the day before the final exam, he decides to ask the teacher for help. The teacher tells John that she has a full schedule of appointments and doesn't have time to meet with him that day. John blows up at the teacher and says, "You don't care about me. I've been trying and studying all term."

John has become a victim of the "study harder, not smarter" phenomenon. Talking over a problem in its beginning stages can keep a small problem from erupting into a massive one. If John had utilized anticipatory problem solving after his first quiz by attempting to find out what specifically went wrong with his testing performance, he may have been able to prevent the recurrence of this problem. Immediately after the first quiz, John should have asked his instructor to go over the exam with him so that together he and the teacher may have been able to identify some testing errors that could have been corrected. Reviewing his tests and study habits could have helped him identify problems and prevented them in the future. By the time John decided to approach his teacher, it was too late to help him even if the teacher had an available appointment time. John could have also talked with his friends and joined them in study sessions to see if he was missing any information or could have learned to study differently. He could also have compared his notes to see if there were problems with his note taking. Most schools have a study skills lab that could have helped him with his study and test-taking skills and possibly paired him with a tutor if needed until John learned better how to deal with the problem.

The above two situations demonstrate how anticipatory problem solving could have avoided problems in both a personal and an academic situation. The skill of learning to use anticipatory problem solving is one of great potential benefit. However, most students don't take full advantage of this skill. The next three situations identify students with problems. Read the situations carefully and see if you can help these students with some suggestions for how they could have used anticipatory problem solving in preventing their problems.

PROBLEM SOLVING EXERCISE 1

Jeanne is trying to prepare for clinical the next day. However, her youngest child becomes ill and she is unable to prepare as much as she likes. She comes to clinical tired because she was up half the night with her sick child. She does not tell her instructor that she is not prepared to pass medications and makes a medication error. The instructor tells Jeanne that a sick child is no excuse for lack of clinical preparation. Jeanne becomes angry and upset and believes that her instructor doesn't understand what it's like to be a mother and try to go to school.

Utilizing anticipatory problem solving, how could Jeanne have handled the above situation differently?

_____

_____

_____

_____

_____

_____

PROBLEM SOLVING EXERCISE 2

Jill is a 19 year old sophomore nursing student who loses her financial aid during her second semester and is forced to get a part time job to help with her expenses. Although Jill worked full time last summer, she did not save any of her money because she knew she was going to have financial aid. Within two months of getting the part time job, Jill's grades start to drop and her instructors notice changes in her behavior. Her written assignments are turned in late and she frequently misses classes and has fallen asleep during two clinical conferences. The instructor approaches Jill about the changes in her academic and clinical performance. She asks Jill to make some decisions about her priorities and then asks her to make a plan to improve her work.

Using anticipatory problem solving how could Jill have prevented this problem? Now that Jill is in academic difficulty how would you help her make a plan for improvement?

_____

_____

_____

_____

_____

PROBLEM SOLVING EXERCISE 3

Donna, a married mother of three children, has returned to school for her nursing degree. In her first semester she experiences much academic difficulty due to several problems. She frequently missed classes because her babysitter was ill. Her husband says he never realized that school would take up all of her time and complains that he and the kids don't ever see her any more. By the end of the semester, Donna is placed on academic probation and decides to drop out of school.

Utilizing anticipatory problem solving, how could Donna have prevented this problem from happening?

_____

_____

_____

_____

Now that you have taken some time to solve these problems, we would like to share with you some of the potential solutions that we came up with. Remember, there is no right or wrong solution here. The goal is to help you search for alternatives to problems that people have encountered and believed were unsolvable. As you can see, there are several ways to approach each problem and, depending upon the individual, the solution may vary.

PROBLEM SOLVING EXERCISE 1

The first possible solution that comes to mind is to have Jeanne try to solicit the instructor's help in solving the problem. She could have approached the instructor before the shift began and asked for some input of what to do. The instructor could then help her identify her level of preparedness and whether a few minutes of reading about the medications would help her be safe. Most students are reluctant to tell an instructor they aren't prepared but the instructor would rather hear that from the student than have to tell students how unsafe they are later. True professionals evaluate themselves and work safely rather than risk another's life. This may mean that the student and instructor together may determine if the student can quickly become prepared and stay on the clinical unit or that it would be unsafe for the student to be on the unit, so the student should return home and make up the clinical day. Most instructors are human enough to realize that children get sick and parents should attend to them. Instructors will also honor a student's professionalism in acknowledging that he/she is not as prepared as they should be.

Other possible solutions could be asking a friend or relative the child trusts to stay with the child while Jeanne prepared for clinical. Then Jeanne could take over when she had finished her preparation. Jeanne would have to watch her level of fatigue, though, because mistakes are often made when a nurse is tired. We realize many parents would be uncomfortable allowing someone else to care for a sick child. Another option would be to call off from clinical that day and make it up later if permitted.

PROBLEM SOLVING EXERCISE 2

In approaching this situation, the old proverb "don't count your chickens before they're hatched" comes to mind. It is never good to make assumptions without firm data to support them. Jill assumed she would get financial aid even though she had no guarantee of this occurring. Anticipatory problem solving involves looking at all possibilities or options. Jill's mistake was letting tunnel vision and wishful thinking guide her behavior instead of planning ahead for alternative sources of financing her education. Jill should have placed her money in the bank for possible unforseen problems such as this.

The first thing Jill should do is cut down on her work hours so she can increase her time on schoolwork to improve her grades. She should then look for alternative funding sources such as loans, financial aid and scholarship opportunities. The immediate short term goal would probably be to try to obtain a loan. Most other financial aid and scholarship opportunities take longer but she could use these to pay off the loan when they come through. Another plan of action could be to drop out of school for a semester, work and save that money, then return to school and finish her education.

PROBLEM SOLVING EXERCISE 3

Anticipating the nursing educational process, Donna could have talked to some upperclass students to see what problems they've had. She could ask questions such as: "What kind of time commitment does nursing school demand? How many hours do you need for clinical, class time, study time, and preparation time?" She could ask what kind of problems they encountered with children, spouse, and time management. What solutions worked for them? Prior to school, Donna could sit down with the family and discuss how Mom entering school would change everyone's life. She could explain that, even though some sacrifices would be made, there would be many benefits. Eliciting support from the family can be planned by talking to them about what Donna is learning. Two ways to do this can be "study time" where everyone studies for an hour then takes a break for a snack or a favorite television show. Donna could also gain interest by making family games from what she has to learn, like naming the bones of the body. She should also schedule "dates" with her husband even for short periods of time when they can be alone. Babysitters become important people and Donna should have several people she can count on in a pinch if the regular babysitter can't be with the children. Having backup babysitters and other support people at hand keeps the spouse from feeling trapped and overwhelmed by having to pick up too much of the slack.

REFERENCES

Butler, L. & Meichenbaum, D. (1981). The assessment of interpersonal problem-solving skills. In P.C. Kendall & S. D. Hollon (Eds.), Assessment strategies for cognitive-behavioral interventions. New York: Academic Press.

Elliott, P. R., Godshall, F., Shrout, J. R. & Witty, P. E. (1990). Problem solving appraisal, self-reported study habits and performance of academically at risk college students. The Journal of Counseling Psychology, 37(2), 203-207.

Heppner, P. P., Reeder, B. L., & Larson, L. M. (1983). Cognitive variables associated with personal problem solving appraisal: Implications for counseling. Journal of Counseling Psychology, 30, 537-545.

Nezu, A. (1985). Differences in psychological distress between effective and ineffective problem solvers. Journal of Counseling Psychology, 32(2), 135-138.

Holbert, C. M. & Abraham, C. (1988). Reflections on teaching generic thinking and problem solving. Nurse Educator, 13(2), 23-26.

Nickerson, R. S., Perkins, D. N. & Smith, E. E. (1985). The teaching of thinking. Hillsdale, NJ: Lawrence Erlbaum.

4

IN SEARCH OF THE "GOOD MOTHER"

Hopefully when growing up most of us had "good mothers" i.e., supportive adults that nurtured, cared for, and helped us build a positive self-image so that we could be productive, successful adults. In part, our "good mothers" were able to nurture and care about us because they were able to nurture and care about themselves. If this nurturing occurred, we should theoretically be able to grow up and nurture others and ourselves in that same manner. The basic belief here is if you are repeatedly told that you are a capable individual while growing up, you will soon come to believe it and act accordingly. You learn to see yourself and your capabilities in a positive optimistic manner. In a perfect world, all of us would have had experienced this and lived happily ever after. However, for any number of reasons, most of us fall somewhere along the "good mother" continuum, in that we received and observed the "good mother" to varying degrees from the important adults in our lives. The less "good mothering" you received, the more difficulty you may have in believing in your abilities to be successful. You may label your abilities and potentials in a negativistic and pessimistic manner. Over the years, in working with individuals to enhance performance, we have noted that these individuals with performance problems often have recurrent negative pessimistic thoughts about their abilities which they have been carrying with them for a long time. Often we find that these people are reacting to the appraisal or pronouncements of another, most often an adult, who evaluated them in a negative way. We struggle with these students to help identify thoughts, their origins, the impact of these thoughts on present behavior, and most importantly ways to change them so that performance can be improved. We have come to use the term "good mother" not because we're trying to blame anyone's biological mother for the behavior of their adult children, but because mothering is a term that most of us believe is synonymous with positive nurturance. This positive nurturance is a method we have found useful to help our students improve their lives. In essence, we are trying to help our students find the "good mother" in the support systems they use in life and, most importantly, to find the "good mother" in themselves.

For those who did not have or take advantage of the "good mother" available to them throughout their lives the question now becomes, "How do those individuals learn to nurture and take care of themselves and learn to view their abilities in a more positive realistic manner?"

The following examples from the authors' files demonstrate how pessimistic negative thoughts related to academic situations cause academic problems for nursing students.

| SITUATION 1 | Meredith reports that she is in danger of flunking out of nursing school. She has to do well on her upcoming comprehensive final or she'll fail the course and be out of school. When we ask her what her thoughts are about the test, she stated, "I've never been a good test-taker as long as I can remember. I keep thinking that this test will make it or break it for my nursing career. I'm just not smart enough." Then we ask Meredith how long she's been thinking like this. She reports that she did not remember when it started but remembers she's always been afraid of quizzes and tests, even in grade school. Her mother told her, "It runs in our family, I've always been scared of tests." Meredith reports that her mother use to help her study for school exams by making her sit down and study for hours for even a small quiz. "My mother use to tell me that she always got real nervous about my tests and believed that if I didn't know everything I might fail the test. My mother was a very strong and assertive woman. I've always admired her. The only time I've ever seen her scared is when she took the real estate exam. She didn't pass the exam until the third time she took it which upset her so much since she spent so much time preparing for it."

| SITUATION 2 | Larry is a first year nursing student who does very well in class and on exams. However, he becomes very ill the night before his clinical experiences, to the point that he's been sent home twice from clinical. When Larry is asked what he thinks about the night before clinical, at first Larry has a hard time identifying his thoughts. After some encouragement, he says he's never felt good in situations where there is pressure to perform. We ask how long he's been thinking like this and he relates the following story. "When I was in junior high I was on the

41

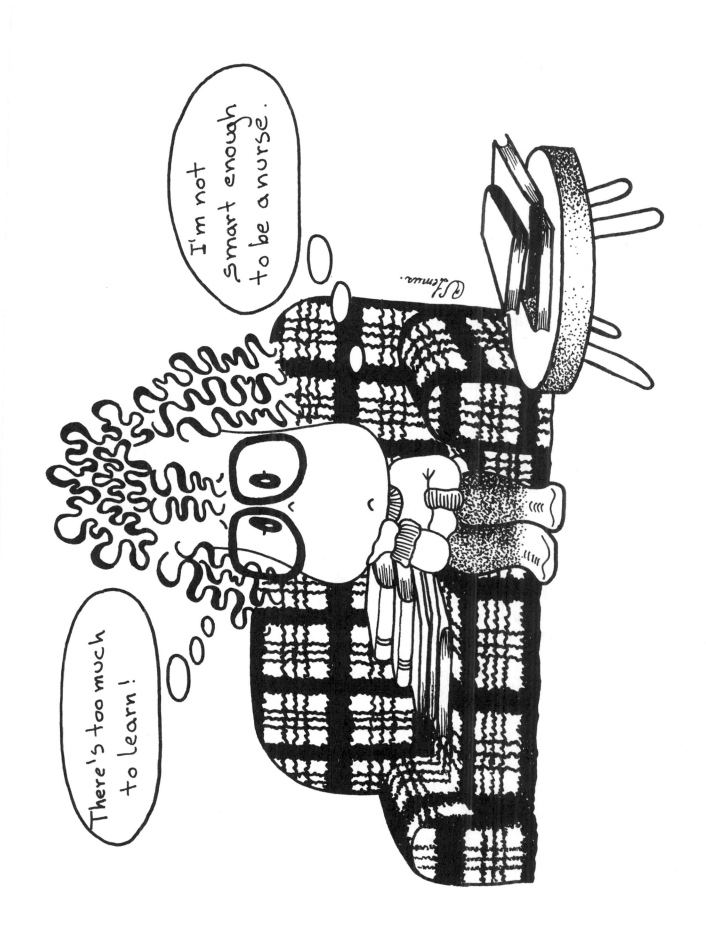

school baseball team. During practice I always did very well. But in the game opener I struck out three times. At the end of the game the coach accused me of folding under pressure. I noticed that throughout the season the coach was reluctant to put me into the games especially when the game scores were close. I kind of lost enthusiasm for baseball. I guess that's where I learned I'm no good under pressure. I feel like when I'm going to clinical it's like I'm stepping up to the plate."

Over the years we have seen hundreds of clients with stories similar to Meredith and Larry's, where situations from their past were interpreted by them to have meaning that encompasses and directs their futures. In working with these clients, we try to help them see their true abilities and be more hopeful and less pessimistic about their performance abilities. In other words, past situations or experiences do not provide global explanations for what occurs in their lives now.

A noted clinician and researcher, Martin Seligman (1990), provides an interesting theory that can be applied in helping individuals to reexamine their performance abilities. Seligman (1990) believes that most individuals view the world in one of two ways and identifies individuals as either optimists or pessimists. The pessimists are characterized as those individuals who tend to believe bad events will last a long time, undermine everything they do and are their own fault. Optimists, on the other hand, think about misfortune in a more positive way. They believe defeat is a temporary setback and is not their fault. Studies have shown that pessimists give up more easily and get depressed more often, whereas optimists do much better at work and academic performance. Seligman (1990) has further theorized that pessimists are more vulnerable to helpless behavior. He also believes that the explanations that individuals give to themselves when bad things happen to them determines their viewpoints in life. This habitual way of explaining bad things to yourself is called your explanatory style and is the hallmark of how you view your place in the world and whether you are an optimist or a pessimist. Your personal explanatory style has three dimensions: permanence, pervasiveness, and personalization. Permanence occurs in those individuals who believe that bad events will persist and will always affect their lives. They think about things in "always" and "never" terms. Pessimistic permanent thoughts include: "You never liked me." "I've always been a loser." "The teacher is trying to get rid of me." "I've always been stupid." The optimist, on the other hand, does not view bad events as permanent, but rather, tends to see them as transient conditions. Examples include: "You can't win them all." "Everyone can't like me." "I'll do the best I can."

The second dimension of explanatory style is pervasiveness. Pervasiveness refers to whether or not individuals are able to come up with specific versus universal explanations as the cause of something bad happening

43

in their lives. For example, if an individual who gets fired believes that the cause is that he is a totally inadequate person, his entire life will suffer. However, if an individual believes he was fired because he did not do a specific job well, he will have the ability to contain the bad event to one situation. Another example would be an individual who, receives a "D" on his first nursing exam, and believes that he is stupid and all of his grades will suffer. In other words, he sees the cause of the bad event as being pervasive in his life. If that same individual saw his "D" grade as part of having a "bad day" and believed he would do better on the next test; his explanatory style is not pervasive.

The third dimension of explanatory style is personalization. Personalization can either be internal or external. If it is internal, when bad things happen, this individual tends to blame himself versus external personalization in which the individual tends to blame other people or circumstances. The optimists style of explaining good events is internal if they believe they cause good things to happen. It is external when explaining bad events if they believe that bad events come from other people or circumstances. The opposite is true for pessimists.

Your explanatory style can have a tremendous effect on the quality of your life. It influences the way you perceive and view the world. It influences your physical health and ability to achieve. This optimism/pessimism style develops in childhood and becomes an habitual way of thinking, becoming crystallized in children as young as age eight. Seligman (1990) has developed these three hypotheses related to the development of explanatory style. The first hypothesis is: mother's explanatory style. The way your mother talked about the world to you when you were a child has a large influence on the way you view the world. The mother's level of optimism and the child's level are usually quite similar. Seligman (1990) found that the child's father's explanatory style did not affect the child. If a child has an optimistic mother, the child will probably be optimistic. Also, if the child has a pessimistic mother, the child will probably be pessimistic. The second hypothesis is: adult criticism. Children listen very carefully to what adults say to them, not only the content but how adults say it. Children believe the criticisms that they get and utilize these criticisms to form their own explanatory style. When a child hears a pessimistic explanatory style that is permanent and pervasive such as, "You're stupid." "You're worthless." or "You're never going to amount to anything." the child finds a way to integrate these comments into his own explanatory style and they become a part of him. The third hypothesis is: children's life crises. A major childhood crisis may give the child a pattern that forms the rest of his life. If the child believes that early losses and traumas will be transient and eventually relent, he will develop a theory that bad events can be conquered. However, if he perceives bad events as permanent and pervasive, the seeds of hopelessness are forever planted.

The importance of Seligman's (1990) work is paramount. Although he believes that individuals are either pessimistic or optimistic in their explanatory style and view of life, he also believes that pessimists can learn to be optimists by learning a new set of cognitive skills. He calls this "learned optimism." There are many different ways in which individuals can learn a more optimistic viewpoint on life. In his book Learned Optimism, Seligman (1990) gives many ways for individuals to change pessimistic beliefs; however, a detailed example of all of these ways is beyond the scope of this textbook. A simple summary of his technique follows. Basically, he states that individuals can learn to speak to themselves from a more encouraging viewpoint. There has been a great deal of research conducted on his techniques and they have been found to be quite effective in changing explanatory style.

One of Seligman's (1990) major cognitive techniques is ABC. "A" stands for ADVERSITY. "B" stands for the BELIEFS we hold about that adversity. "C" stands for the CONSEQUENCES. The beliefs are the direct causes of what we feel and do next. Certain kinds of beliefs set off certain responses. Seligman (1990) teaches his clients to interrupt this vicious cycle by first examining the connections among A, B and C. After identifying each of the categories, Seligman (1990) then teaches clients to dispute their pessimistic beliefs by learning to argue with themselves by asking, "What evidence do I have for this belief? "What are the alternatives to this belief?" "What are the implications of believing this?" "Is this a useful belief?" When individuals are able to successfully dispute these beliefs, they will note that an energy occurs as they successfully deal with their negative beliefs and turn them into more positive ones. Seligman (1990) reports that his techniques for turning pessimistic thoughts into positive ones are based in research. He also differentiates between his techniques and the so-called power of positive thinking. Learned optimism is more than trying to believe upbeat statements in the absence of evidence, but a way of accurately examining beliefs, which helps people cope with their present belief system to create more non-negative ways of viewing their world.

In Chapter 6 we will further examine cognitive techniques which assist you to explore and change negative thinking into realistic thinking, which enhances performance.

REFERENCE

Seligman, M. (1990). Learned optimism. New York: Pocket Books.

5

PERFORMANCE AND TEST ANXIETY

Everyone's life involves performance of some kind, whether we are asked to take part in an athletic competition, get on stage at a dance recital, give a presentation in front of the boss, demonstrate a clinical skill to an instructor, or take a test. Throughout life you will always be evaluated by your performance in one of these arenas. Some people love to perform. They give their best efforts or do their best jobs when they are in front of an audience, under the gun, or feeling the pressure. For others, the pressure to perform means that they are being evaluated and that they cannot cut the mustard. For these people, an upcoming performance can create an overwhelming fear, a crippling pressure and a need to achieve, while at the same time overwhelming feelings of anxiety that they cannot measure up. We are defining this latter group of people as having an evaluation or performance anxiety, which we define as the pressure to achieve in a certain situation where you are being evaluated.

According to Burns (1989), performance anxiety has two causes. The first is obvious: fear of failure. For individuals with performance anxiety, failure is not seen as a natural part of one's life. It is seen in a pervasive and global manner. Failure in performance is translated to failure as a person, in that the individual is not good enough or not smart enough or not worth the love and respect of others. The second cause may be harder to discover. Performance anxiety may occur when an individual has chosen goals that do not fit or are not what that individual really wants out of life. For example, in nursing some individuals may choose the profession because they perceive it to be one that has job security along with a way to pay the bills and receive benefits. When some individuals actually see what nursing is about, especially after starting the clinical portion of the instruction, these individuals may decide that they do not have the constitution for it nor do they like it. Even after this self-revelation they feel trapped into remaining in the profession for a variety of reasons (e.g., too embarrassed they were wrong about a career choice; they believe they have invested too much time and money to change careers now). Sometimes individuals find themselves in a position when they are inadvertently fulfilling a parent's dream. They go into nursing after hearing years of how wonderful it would be to be a nurse and find themselves being lulled into the notion that a nursing career is a great idea. Although both types of individuals may remain in school, their minds may work on other ways of interfering with their progress. Often this is manifested as a performance anxiety. One of the most common types of performance anxiety is test anxiety.

In nursing, tests come in many forms: written exams, clinical performance, or demonstrating psychomotor skills. Nursing students find themselves in a situation where they are being tested or evaluated every day. Students often perceive their lives as being one big test for which there is never adequate time to prepare. For students who have performance and test anxiety, nursing school becomes one relentless nightmare. Because nursing school is an environment that is filled with testing situations which often involve serious or life-threatening consequences, test anxiety can be a widespread problem.

Test anxiety is defined as a "diffuse feeling of dread or unexplained discomfort accompanied by negative cognitive changes in relation to a testing situation resulting in performance below the person's ability" (Spielberger, 1982). Over the years, in our clinical experience, the way people manifest the problem can be varied, but we have noted certain symptoms that are recognizable. Not everybody exhibits all of these symptoms. In fact, some individuals are not aware of any symptoms at all. On the other hand, some individuals can experience mild symptoms which do not interfere with their test performance. The deciding factor is whether or not the anxiety impairs your performance. During a performance you do want to have a certain (mild) level of anxiety. Many great performers get "butterflies" but it tends to enhance performance rather than impair it.

It is important to recognize the signs and symptoms of test anxiety that you may have. Take a few minutes now and think about whether or not these symptoms impair your performance. The following are the signs and symptoms of test anxiety that we have seen:

> **1. Physical symptoms prior to or during an exam or clinical performance.**

This can range from "butterflies" in the stomach to nausea or even vomiting prior to or during the exam. Some testing experts believe that, with all test anxiety, physical symptoms must occur. At our agency, we have not clinically found that to be true. Many test anxious students have no awareness of any physiological responses. In fact, some people will deny any signs of anxiety.

> **2. Decreased ability to concentrate during the performance.**

Some individuals complain that they have difficulty concentrating during the exam. They report that they are bothered by distractions from other students and the testing environment. They notice their classmates tapping their feet and are aware of who gets up to go to the bathroom. These students can frequently be seen popping their heads up and gawking around the room. We call these people "the gawkers." In the literature this is referred to as decreased attention to task (Alting & Markham, 1993; Finger & Galassi, 1977; Wine, 1971). Good test takers are rarely excessively distracted from the task of taking the test, whereas people with test anxiety experience frequent distractions.

You can also see this symptom occur in clinical performance. A student may report she is unable to calculate a medication dosage while being supervised by her instructor. She may make statements such as, "I just can't keep my mind on this, it's too crowded in this med room." This is the very same symptom as decreased attention to task in a clinical performance rather than a testing situation.

> **3. Competitive worries.**

Individuals with test anxiety often spend a lot of time thinking and worrying about whether other people are doing better than they are. They are constantly ranking their own and their classmate's performance in order to establish their self-worth as nurses. They become focused not only on the job they do or how they improved, but on where they ranked in relation to others - or who they beat. Their priorities about their performance or end goal of being a competent nurse become misdirected and their energies are wrapped up in comparing clinical evaluations and test scores, and becoming upset when others do better. Their energies are directed into competitive worries rather than developing an awareness of their own test-taking strengths and weaknesses in order to enhance their own performance.

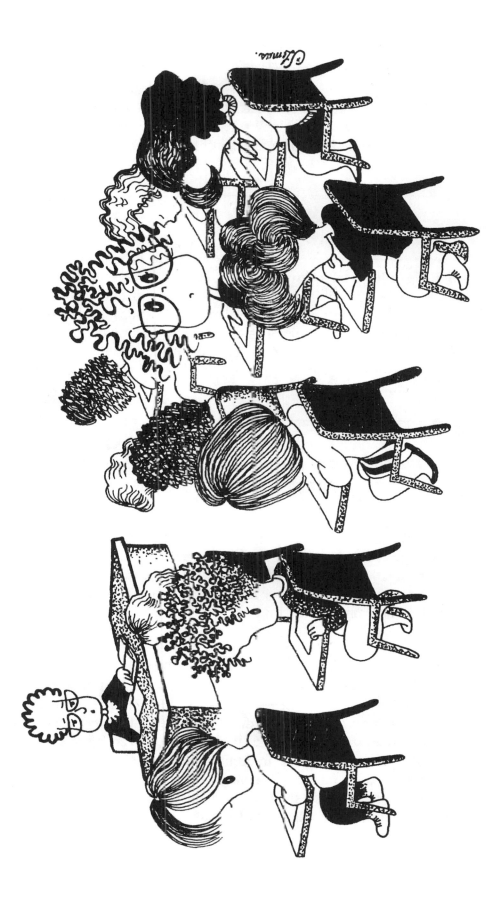

4. Difficulty recalling information during a performance.

Students who have difficulty recalling information they have studied report that they "go blank" during a test or clinical performance. They can go blank if the clinical instructor asks them a question about the pathophysiology of a disease, or they can go blank when they can't "see" the information on a page of their notes when asked to recall information on a test.

5. History of performance and test anxiety.

Many individuals have a history of poor performances on tests and in situations where they fear evaluation. This can be seen in such areas as multiple failures on a driving test, or fear of public speaking, etc. Sometimes it can even be traced to high school or grade school. With some people the performance anxiety may be selective and dependent on the perceived threat of the situation. For example, a student may do well on quizzes and unit exams but do poorly on the final exam, especially if the exam will make the difference between a "good" grade (e.g., "A") or a "poor" grade (e.g., "B").

6. Misreading or misunderstanding verbal directions.

Misreading or misunderstanding written test questions is one of the major problems experienced by test anxious individuals. They misread the situation or the actual stem and therefore answer the question incorrectly. Misreading and misunderstanding test questions happens occasionally for every test taker, however, the test anxious individual often finds that this is a repeated pattern of behavior during examinations. This can also occur in clinical performance. A student may misunderstand the instructor's verbal directions or misread specific directions or instructions in a procedure manual prior to doing a new clinical procedure.

7. Catastrophic fantasy.

Test anxious individuals may worry about what will happen if they fail and have tremendous fantasies of impending doom. Some individuals fantasize that each test they take will be the one that "does them in", or ends their nursing career, or gets them thrown out of school. Often, the more important they perceive the test to be, the more catastrophic their fantasies become. For example, the NCLEX has significant meaning for students, so there is a tendency for students to have excessive catastrophic thinking related to that test.

8. Pressure to be perfect.

Students with a high degree of test and performance anxiety may have a competitive drive that they must be the best, or that they must beat everyone else to win. They believe that "winning is not everything, it is the only thing." They feel pressured to get the very best grades and to always have the best clinical evaluation. Doing well isn't good enough. It has to be the best. For some individuals this may be so ingrained from early in their lives that they are not even aware of their competitive thoughts and behaviors. Interestingly enough, even when the students' competitive nature is pointed out to them by other students or by nursing faculty the students usually have difficulty identifying this behavior in themselves. This behavior has become so habitual that it's almost second nature. Unfortunately, pressure to be perfect can also create a constant feeling of discomfort and tension which the individuals believe is necessary for their survival. For example, a group of students are complaining to their clinical instructor that they feel tremendous pressure in nursing school all of the time. When the instructor asks them to talk more about the pressure specifically, the students say that it started when they tried to enter the nursing program. They state that it was difficult to gain admission and that they needed a high grade point average to enter. The instructor then asked, "If that's where the pressure started and they're already in the program, then why are they still acting so competitively?" The students state that now they have to be competitive because they have to go on to school for their bachelor's degree and that they have to get all "A"s to enter that program. The instructor tells the students that she is not aware of any program that requires prospective students to have a straight-A average to enter. The instructor presents factual data to disprove that belief, including her time on the admissions committee of the local university hoping to alleviate the students' sense of pressure. However, the students state that they have "heard" otherwise so they will try for the grades "just in case" what they heard is true. The instructor offers to contact the admissions office of several programs for the students so they will really know the requirements for entrance into the program. The students decline the offer and decide to trust their own knowledge even though they have no evidence to support it.

Unfortunately it is common not to recognize these characteristics as indicative of a problem. At the point when people do recognize the problem, they won't follow through on suggested proven methods of changing to correct the problem. In fact they'll go back to doing what has not been working thus far such as "studying harder" versus "studying smarter." Most schools have departments which offer assistance or people who can help with academic problems, yet the people who need it the most tend not to go for help even when they are aware this assistance is available.

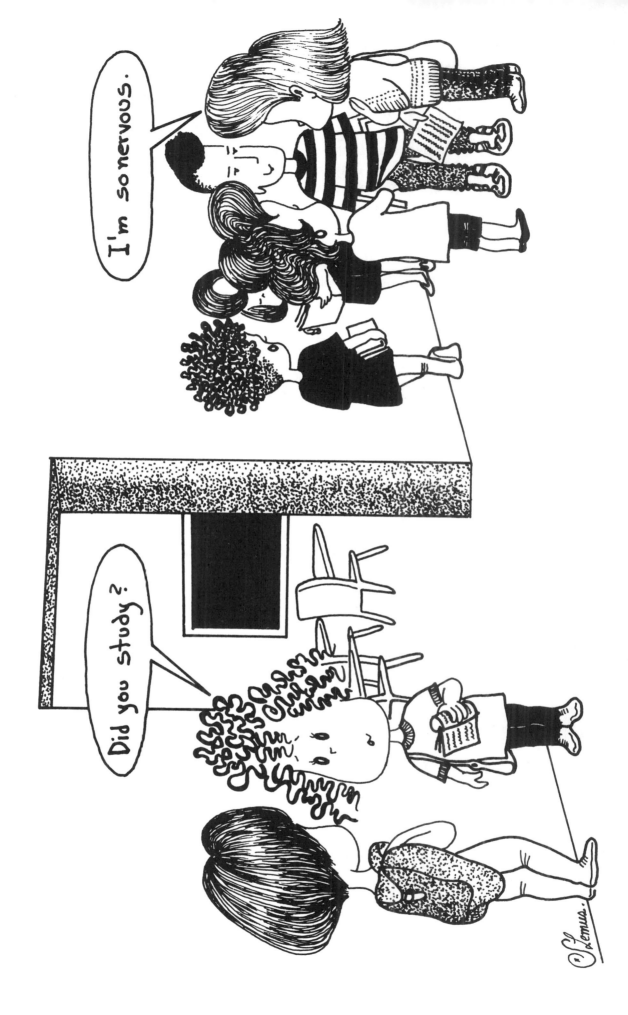

The following techniques have been helpful in alleviating the severity of test and performance anxieties. Two specific techniques that will be discussed here are visualization and progressive relaxation.

Visualization

Visualization is a proven technique that can be powerful in helping people make important changes in their lives. It involves relaxing your body, clearing away distractions, and creating positive mental images (McKay & Fanning, p. 171). Basically, the technique of visualization or visual imagery, as it is sometimes referred, is the ability to create a mental picture in your mind in which you are making a positive change in yourself. The pictures we see in our minds can have real and lasting power. They dictate our reality (Porter & Foster, 1986). According to Simonton, Matthews-Simonton and Creighton (1978), a person forms an image that makes a mental statement about what he/she wants to happen, then when the image is repeated the person soon expects the desired event to occur. The person starts to act in ways that would bring about the desired effect and, in reality, help to make it occur. The authors give the example of a golfer who visualizes the perfect golf swing for a hole-in-one.

Visualization techniques have many uses. They have been utilized in treating many stress related and physical illnesses, anxiety related problems, and in enhancing a variety of performances from athletic competition to test-taking. Due to their effectiveness, these techniques have recently gained increased popularity in the field of athletic competition. In their book, Visual Athletics, Porter and Foster (1990) make the comparison that between athletes of equal and unequal ability, the athlete with the mental edge is most often the winner.

To be effective with visualization techniques, you must create clear vivid specific mental pictures utilizing as many of your senses as possible. For example, visualize a vacation you have taken recently that was particularly peaceful and enjoyable. Try an example of a vacation at the beach and picture it as specifically as you can. Feel the warm sand between your toes and the hot sun touching your back and your arms. Smell the sea air and listen to the sea gulls fly above you. Try to remember what clothes you were wearing and who was with you. Get that mental picture in your mind as clearly and concisely as you can. Put yourself in that situation and feel the good feelings that go with that situation. Sit quietly for a few minutes and feel those peaceful and enjoyable sensations now.......

The above was a brief example of a short visualization that will help you assess your ability to create visual images in your mind. You can use this technique for a variety of situations to practice your ability to imagine and visualize.

Guidelines for Using Visualization

1. Wear loose comfortable clothing and sit back or lie down in a comfortable place. Dim or turn off the lights.

2. Relax your body. Take a deep breath. Hold it for a few seconds then slowly relax and feel the tension leave your body. Starting from head to toe, visualize the muscles from each part of your body relaxing. Imagine your body totally relaxed.

3. Try to visualize the testing scene in vivid detail as it is during the test.

4. Practice makes perfect. Practice your visualization techniques several times daily. The more you practice, the more powerful the visualization becomes. At first, visualizations are usually the easiest at night before going to bed and in the morning when you wake up because this is when your body is most relaxed. After you become proficient at this technique, you will find that you may be able to visualize in many different places; for example, at work, at a restaurant, etc.

A Note on the Use of Affirmations

An affirmation is a strong positive statement that affirms your ability to change your behavior. It uses present tense, avoids negative terms and always starts with the word "I." For example, an affirmation would be, "I am calm" rather than "I am not anxious." Using affirmations during or at the end of a visualization can be extremely helpful in making the image become reality. Some individuals suggest writing the affirmations on index cards and reading them to yourself several times per day. The following are some helpful positive test-taking affirmations:

"I am calm and ready to take the test."   "I am in control."
"I am working toward my goals."   "I am prepared."
"I am confident in what I studied."   "I am a good student."
"I am an effective test taker."

The following is an example of what a visualization exercise might look like for an individual who is trying to enhance test performance. You can use this script by talking it into a tape recorder and listening to it on a daily basis.

Script

Get into a comfortable position and close your eyes. Visualize your body relaxing. Start with the muscles of your head and neck, gradually move down your body relaxing each muscle while feeling the tension leaving your body. (PAUSE) Take a deep breath. Hold it for five seconds (PAUSE) and slowly exhale. (PAUSE) Repeat this again. Take a deep breath hold it for five seconds (PAUSE) and again slowly exhale. Let go of all the tension in your body. As you experience this feeling of relaxation, form a mental picture in your mind. Imagine yourself on the day of your next test. Imagine getting up the morning of the test and getting dressed. Visualize what you will be wearing. Imagine that picture in vivid clear detail. (PAUSE) Picture yourself getting into your car and driving to school. You feel good. You know that you have studied well and are prepared to take the test. See yourself parking the car in the parking lot. Visualize this in your mind. See this clearly in your mind. See yourself getting out of the car and walking into the entrance of the school. You know you are ready to take the test. Feel how good you feel as you know you will be successful. Imagine yourself walking into the classroom and seeing your classmates who are all talking about the test. Visualize yourself walking into the room and taking your seat calmly and quietly. See how you can block out all of the noise. You feel confident. You are able to block the anxiety of the other students because you are prepared and calm. You feel good. You feel successful. You know you will do well. Picture the classroom and the teacher in front of the class. As you visualize this scene you may want to use the following positive statements or affirmations:

"I am prepared and ready to take this test."

"I am in control in this situation."

"I am confident that I will do well."

"I will be able to control my negative thinking during this test."

"I know I have the ability to do well on this test."

As the test is being handed out, you feel calm, you feel good, you can anticipate your success. (PAUSE) You now have the test in your hand and you turn to the first page. If you feel yourself getting anxious, use your techniques to stop the anxiety. You are in control. See yourself taking control and relaxing. See yourself changing the feelings of anxiety into a calm and confident feeling. Imagine yourself taking the test calmly with a feeling of confidence. You feel good. You feel successful. Get that image of yourself firmly and vividly in your mind. (PAUSE) Picture yourself moving through the test, answering the questions one at a time. Moving through the exam at an even pace and in a calm manner. See that exact picture now. Remember if you are feeling anxious as you are taking the test, visualize yourself using your techniques to gain control to decrease your anxiety and feel calm and relaxed. You have gained control of the situation. You feel good. See yourself feeling good as you take the test. See yourself doing well. Get that image in your mind clearly and specifically. You are taking the test. You are doing well. You are able to block out all of your classmates noises. Nothing can bother you. It's as if you are in a clear glass bubble where nothing can bother you. No one can interfere with your successful test performance. Your attention and energy are on the test. No one can distract you from your task. You are focused. You feel good. You are completing the task of taking the test. Experience how good you feel, how successful you feel. Take a moment and feel those good feelings now. (PAUSE) You are finishing the test and getting ready to turn your paper in; visualize the scene of putting your pencil down and picking up your test paper to hand to your teacher. (PAUSE) You feel good because you know you've been successful. You know you passed the test. You were prepared. You were calm. You know that you have done well. Picture yourself walking out of the testing room, handing the test to the teacher. Picture yourself feeling successful as you leave the classroom. Sit quietly for a few moments and enjoy these good feelings. (PAUSE)

Progressive Muscle Relaxation

Progressive muscle relaxation is a technique in which an individual first learns to differentiate the sensation of muscle tension from that of muscle relaxation. It is based on the premise that the body responds to anxiety-provoking thoughts and events with muscle tension. This physiological tension in turn increases the anxiety that the individual experiences. It is incompatible for the body to be relaxed and tense at the same time. Responding to the relaxation can block the habit of responding to the tension (Jacobson, 1974). When you learn to recognize the tension, you can then instruct yourself to release or let go of the muscle tension, thus producing a state of relaxation. The primary purpose of progressive relaxation is to calm the body, promote rest and relieve the individual from daily pressures (Stephens, 1992). Basically, many progressive relaxation exercises start by having the individual tense certain muscle groups starting with the head and working to the toe, then relaxing each muscle group sequentially moving down the body. When a muscle group is tensed, then relaxed, the muscles smooth out and become relaxed (Nugent & Vitale, 1993). Progressive muscle relaxation has been effective in treating anxiety, muscle tension in certain physical conditions such as high blood pressure and back pain (Davis, Eshelman & McKay, 1988). Progressive muscle relaxation techniques can be effective in reducing the anxiety that many students experience related to test-taking situations. Davis, Eshelman and McKay (1988) describe a procedure for progressive relaxation utilizing four major muscle groups which include: 1) hands, forearms, biceps; 2) head, face, throat, shoulders; 3) chest, stomach, lower back; 4) thighs, buttocks, calves, feet. Each muscle group is tensed for approximately 5-7 seconds then relaxed for 20-30 seconds. The procedure of relaxing each individual muscle group can be repeated from one to five times depending upon the tension of that muscle group. Statements such as, "Let go of all of your tension, smooth out the muscles and relax," can be added to the experience to aid in the relaxation process. Progressive relaxation can be practiced with the individual sitting in a comfortable chair with support or lying down in a comfortable position. Individuals may wish to dictate this relaxation exercise or their own variation into a tape recorder to help them create the relaxation response. Another option would be to purchase commercially made "relaxation tapes" which are available in many bookstores. Many relaxation scripts, in a variety of stress reduction books, are available and the individual or someone who has a relaxing voice can read a script into a tape recorder (Davis, Eshelman, & McKay, 1988; Poorman, Molcan & Webb, 1990).

Individuals with any of the following conditions should seek medical clearance before beginning progressive muscle relaxation exercises: organically-based headaches, lower back pain not associated with tension, all medical problems resulting in muscle spasm (Cormier & Cormier, 1985). Other conditions in which a person should seek medical counsel prior to using relaxation include depression, glaucoma, diabetes, heart disease, hypertension, third trimester pregnancy, TIA's, CVA, any recent or serious disorders affecting bones, ligaments or muscles. It is also important to note that progressive relaxation techniques can affect the dosage range of certain medications for some individuals. In general, the need for the medication at the same dosage may be decreased. If you are taking medications on a routine basis, obtain your physician's approval before beginning progressive relaxation (Smith, 1985).

Progressive muscle relaxation techniques and visual imagery techniques are often used in combination, beginning with a brief relaxation exercise then moving to visualization. Some experts believe that the combination of these exercises is more effective than each one separately (Achterberg & Lawlis, 1982). However, a study by Stephens (1992) to compare the effectiveness of visualization alone, visualization with a brief relaxation exercise, and a control group in a sample of first year nursing students found that imagery was as effective alone as it was combined with relaxation. Stephens (1992) believes that these findings are important due to the time constraints of many of today's nursing students. This means that treatments to reduce anxiety, such as imagery, can be used while doing other tasks (e.g. household chores or exercise).

REFERENCES

Achterberg, J. & Lawlis, G. F. (1982). Imagery and health. Topics in Clinical Nursing, 3(4), 55-60.

Alting, T. & Markham, R. (1993). Test anxiety and distractibility. Journal of Research and Personality, 27, 134-137.

Burns, D. D. (1989). The feeling good handbook: Using the new mood therapy in everyday life. New York: William Morrow and Company, Inc.

Cormier, W. H., Cormier, L. S. (1985). Interviewing strategies for helpers (2nd ed). Monterey, CA: Brooks/Cole Publishing.

Davis, M., Eshelman, E. R. & McKay, M. (1988). The relaxation and stress reduction workbook (3rd ed). Oakland, CA: New Harbinger Publications.

Finger, R. & Galassi, J. P. (1977). Effects of modifying cognitive versus emotionality responses in the treatment of test anxiety. Journal of Consulting and Clinical Psychology, 45(2), 280-287.

Jacobson, E. (1974). Progressive relaxation. Chicago: The University of Chicago Press, Midway Reprint.

McKay, M. & Fanning, P. (1987). Self-esteem. Oakland, CA: New Harbinger Publications.

Nugent, P. M. & Vitale, B. A. (1993). Test success: Test taking techniques for beginning nursing students. Philadelphia: F.A. Davis.

Poorman, S. G., Molcan K. L. & Webb, C. A. (1990). A new approach to NCLEX-RN. North Augusta, SC: Arnett.

Porter, K. & Foster, J. (1986). The mental athlete. New York: Ballantine Books.

Porter, K. & Foster, J. (1990). Visual athletics: Visualizations for peak sports performance. Dubuque, IA: William C. Brown Publishers.

Simonton, O. C., Matthews-Simonton, S. & Creighton, J. L. (1978). Getting well again. New York: Bantam Books.

Simonton, O. C., Mathews-Simonton, S., Sparks, T. F. (1980). Psychological intervention in the treatment of cancer. Psychosomatics, 21, 226-235.

Smith, J. C. (1985). <u>Relaxation dynamics: Nine world approaches to self-relaxation</u>. Illinois: Research Press.

Spielberger, C. D. (1982). <u>The state-trait anxiety inventory: A comprehensive Bibliography</u>. Palo Alto, CA: Consulting Psychologists Press.

Stephens, R. L. (1992). Imagery: A treatment for nursing students anxiety. <u>Journal of Nursing Education,</u> <u>7</u>(31), 314-320.

Wine, J. (1971). Test anxiety and direction of attention. <u>Psychological Bulletin,</u> <u>76</u>(2), 92-104.

6

COGNITIVE RESTRUCTURING

In this chapter we will discuss the way your thoughts or cognitions influence your performance in clinical or academic (test-taking) areas. Research has repeatedly demonstrated that continuous negative thoughts during a test or performance can impair that individual's performance, both during the preparation and the actual event (Hunsley, 1987; Poorman & Martin, 1991). Furthermore, since negative thoughts during the performance may impair that performance, changing or restructuring thoughts to more positive ones can facilitate performance (Cooley & Speigler, 1980; Wise & Haynes, 1983). Our overall goal for this chapter will be to help you learn the basic principles of cognitive behavioral therapy and cognitive restructuring techniques to enhance your performance.

BACKGROUND

Aaron Beck (1976) developed the theory of cognitive behavioral therapy for the treatment of depressed patients. The first principle of cognitive therapy is that all of your moods are created by your cognitions or thoughts. A cognition refers to the way you look at things such as your perceptions, your mental attitudes and your beliefs. For example, you feel the way you do right now because of the thoughts you are having at this moment. You may feel anxious if some of your thoughts right now are, "I feel like I'm out of control", "What if I crack up?", or "I'm going to jump out of my skin." The second principle is that when you feel anxious, depressed, or guilty, your thoughts are dominated by a pervasive negativity. You will perceive yourself, events and your performance from a gloomy perspective. Because of that perspective, you'll soon begin to believe that things really are as bad as you've imagined them to be. You'll start thinking the same way about everything that has gone wrong lately. You'll start to think about all the bad things from your past including other failures that you think have happened in your life. This bleak vision can create a sense of hopelessness. You may then believe there is nothing you can do about your situation, you might as well abandon all hope of studying to pass the exam and just go in and fail. The third principle is that research has shown that the negative thoughts which cause the emotional turmoil nearly always contain gross distortions. Although these thoughts appear valid at the time, mostly they're irrational or just plain wrong. Therefore, the anxiety you may feel about the exam is not solely based on accurate perceptions of reality, but on your fears and fantasies concerning the test.

Using cognitive behavioral principles, you can alleviate these distressful feelings by honestly looking at and correcting the distorted thoughts. The first step is to discover and evaluate your thoughts. The second step is to correct distorted thoughts through acquiring new information and recognizing misperceptions. The third step is to restructure the negative thoughts into more positive, facilitative thoughts. If you can change the distorted thoughts from negative to more positive realistic ones, you will experience a change in mood and behavior as well. In simple terms, what we do (behavior) is influenced by what we feel (mood), which is influenced by what we think (cognition).

In summary, cognitive therapy is based on the simple idea that your thoughts or cognitions, not external events, create your moods (Burns, 1989). In the broadest sense, it is based on the concept that cognitions have an enormous impact on feelings and behavior. Specifically, what a person is thinking affects his feelings, which affects his behavior. Although Beck (1976) developed this approach for use with depressed and anxious patients, these basic principles can be used in a self-help format to assist with performance problems frequently experienced by nursing students.

NURSES' COGNITIVE SELF-ASSESSMENT MODEL: A TOOL FOR GOOD THINKING

The nurses' cognitive self-assessment model (NCSAM) based on Beck's theory (1976) is designed to assist nursing students to identify their thoughts, feelings and behaviors related to academic and clinical performance. After identifying thoughts, feelings and behaviors the NCSAM gives the student the opportunity to evaluate any negative or distorted cognition and restructure them to more positive realistic ones. It is a simple tool to help the nursing student restructure cognitions, and improve problem solving and thinking skills. In general terms, the tool helps create "good thinking" on the part of the nursing student. With repeated practice, good thinking will lead to good academic and clinical performance.

The first step in using the NCASM is to write down your behavior, feelings and thoughts in a log type format as seen below so you understand how they are connected.

BEHAVIOR	FEELINGS	THOUGHTS
1. studying for a comprehensive nursing final	overwhelmed, upset, stressed, confused	"I am never going to be able to learn all of this. There's too much information. I'm probably studying the wrong stuff; how can I know what the teacher is going to think is important; I never seem to be able to figure that out. What's the use? Studying never helps."

BEHAVIOR	FEELINGS	THOUGHTS
2. actually taking a comprehensive final	scared, nervous, agitated, hopeless	"I'm gonna fail this test; I don't even know what the first question is asking me. The whole test is hard. Where do they get these questions? It's a waste of time to study for this test. I'll be so embarrassed when everyone finds out I failed. I'm out of the program now. I had no business going back to school.

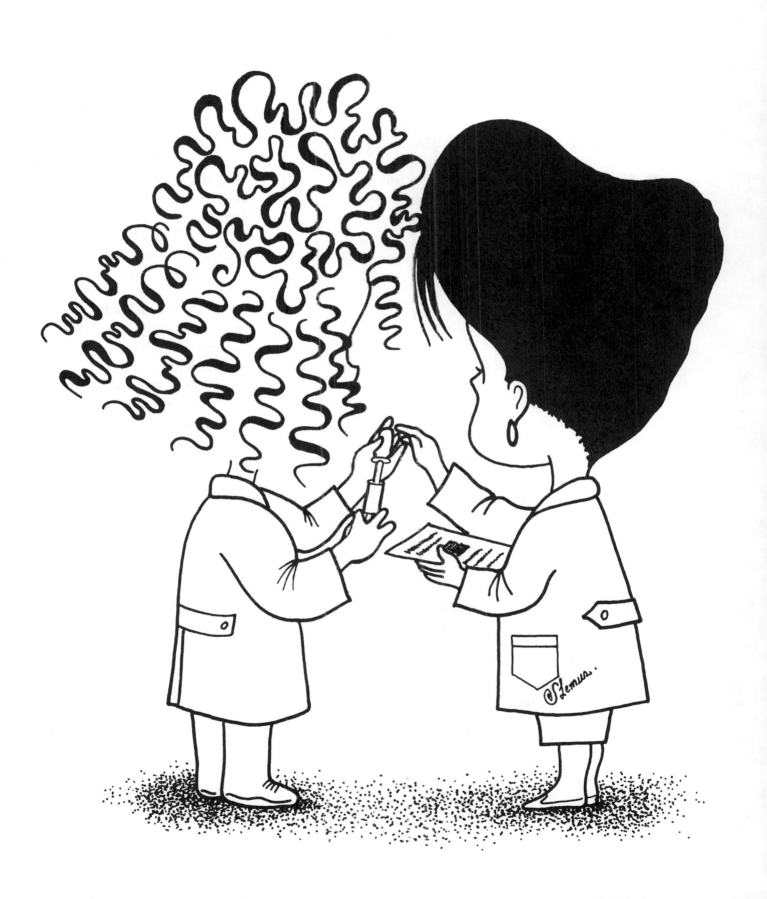

THOUGHTS
(con't)

I'm such an embar-
rassment to my
friends and family;
I'll never be able to
face them."

BEHAVIOR	FEELINGS	THOUGHTS
3. giving medications	unprepared, apprehensive	"The teacher is going to ask me something I don't know. I'm going to give the medication to the wrong patient and the patient is going to die. I'll blank out when she asks the questions and she'll send me home for being unprepared. I'll never be able to handle the clinical and they'll kick me out of school. I can never know enough to be a good nurse."

Step one of the NCSAM may take some practice. Often students have difficulty at first differentiating between feelings and thoughts. Students may focus on the global pervasive feeling of anxiety and are often unaware of the thoughts that accompany these feelings. After you have practiced the three column NCSAM and can clearly identify behavior, feelings and thoughts, you can move to the next step. Step two involves adding a **fourth column** in which you evaluate the cognitions/thoughts by asking the following three questions:

BEHAVIOR	FEELINGS	THOUGHTS	EVALUATION
1. studying for a comprehensive nursing final	overwhelmed, upset, stressed, confused	"I am never going to be able to learn all of this. There's too much information. I'm probably studying the wrong stuff; how can I know what the teacher is going to think is important; I never seem to be able to figure that out. What's the use? Studying never helps."	"I may not be able to learn all of this information, that's true; but I can learn all of the basic concepts and principles. Maybe I need to change the way I study. I need help to know what's important. Maybe I can study with a group of students who seem to do well on the test. Maybe I can go ask the teacher to review my notes and ask what she thinks is important. I know it's **not** true that I shouldn't study because it never helps. Going into a test unprepared is not a

way to help. It won't solve anything. Maybe I need to get help with my study skills at a workshop or at the testing center. Maybe I should learn how to schedule my time differently so that I'm not studying this all at the same time and I won't get so over-whelmed."

Note in the evaluation column that thought evaluation often leads to some action-oriented problem solving. Thought evaluation not only helps you identify when your thoughts are distorted, it helps you to brainstorm and find some answers to the problems. Unfortunately students may admit and know that they should take some kind of action but seem to become immobilized and never follow through on their plans to help themselves. That's why writing it down in the fourth column can help you see that there are alternatives to the way you think and act for better performance. One of the most helpful ways is to keep these thoughts as a log and highlight these plans. If your grade or performance doesn't change you can look back to see if you've followed through on the plans that you've made. The following are several examples that students have reported helped them follow through on their plans. If you feel apprehensive about going to a study skills workshop, then ask someone to go with you. This helps both of you to be accountable for one another. If meeting with a new study group, introduce yourself to some of the people ahead of time so you won't feel so awkward.

BEHAVIOR	FEELINGS	THOUGHTS	EVALUATION
2. actually taking a comprehensive final	scared, nervous, agitated, hopeless	"I'm gonna fail this test; I don't even know what the first question is asking me. The whole	"What evidence do I have that I'm going to fail? Slow down and take a deep breath; read

test is hard. Where do they get these questions? It's a waste of time to study for this test. I'll be so embarrassed when everyone finds out I failed. I'm out of the program now. I had no business going back to school. I'm such an embarrassment to my friends and family; I'll never be able to face them."

the question carefully. I know I can pass. Just because the first question is hard does not mean the rest of the test is going to be impossible. Just take one question at a time. They're trying to get us to understand how the information relates to clinical. I know I can reason this out. Is it really true that they're trying to trick me? What would be their motive? I wouldn't have been admitted if they didn't think I could get through school. When I start to think I'll fail, I know my thoughts aren't clear and I'm being too suspicious. I'm not stupid. I get anxious when I take tests or when questions seem unfamiliar to me, but that doesn't mean I'm stupid. I have no evidence to support not studying. That makes no sense. No one has ever died of embarrassment. It would not be the end of my life if I flunked this test. The worst thing that would happen is that I'll have to work harder the next time. I may not like it but I could deal with it. I'm going to try to have the teacher go over the test with me so I can learn to become a better test taker the next time."

BEHAVIOR	FEELINGS	THOUGHTS	EVALUATION
3. giving medications	unprepared, apprehensive	"The teacher is going to ask me something I don't know. I'm going to give the medication to the wrong patient and the patient is going to die. I'll blank out when she asks the questions and she'll send me home for being unprepared. I'll never be able to	"I know about these medications. I know how to give them. The teacher is going to see that. I learned all of the rules and safety precautions about g i v i n g t h e medication to the right patient. My instructor will be there and won't let m e give this medication to the

THOUGHTS
(con't)

handle the clinical and they'll kick me out of school. I can never know enough to be a good nurse."

EVALUATION
(con't)

wrong patient. If I go blank, I'll explain to the teacher that I'm really nervous and I really did prepare. I'll close my eyes and take a deep breath and try to r e c a l l   t h e information. If I really can't recall the information and the teacher doesn't think I'm prepared and does send me home, I'll make an appointment to talk to the teacher about what happened and what I can do differently about the problem for the next clinical day. I'm going to try to learn some anxiety reduction techniques to keep my anxiety under control next time. No nurse can know everything. I need to learn to solve problems using the knowledge I have and should learn where to go if I don't know something so that I give safe nursing care."

In the above three examples it again becomes apparent that evaluating your negative thoughts and changing them to more positive and realistic ones enhances good thinking and promotes problem solving and action to change behavior. Not only are these students able to challenge their negative thoughts, they are able to determine possible alternatives for their present performance difficulties. When you can learn these techniques, it will not only help you to be a better student but these are also the same problem solving skills that help you to be a better nurse.

Now that you know how to evaluate and change your negative thoughts, we can show you several different methods to stop the negative thinking while it is happening so you can deal with it more effectively.

THOUGHT DISTRACTION TECHNIQUES

THOUGHT STOPPING

Thought stopping is a technique that can be used to help control unproductive, self-defeating thoughts and interrupt thought patterns that become habits. It involves concentrating on the unwanted thoughts and, after a brief period of time, stopping the thought suddenly and distracting yourself from the thought. A loud noise or using a word "STOP" can be used to interrupt these negative thoughts. It is well documented that negative thoughts precede negative emotions. If the unwanted thoughts can be controlled, the individual's stress level can be reduced. This simple but highly effective technique can be utilized with a variety of obsessive and persistent thought processes such as obsessive memories, repeated thoughts of failure, sexual inadequacy and impulses leading to anxiety attacks. This technique is indicated primarily when the problem is cognitive rather than behavioral. These steps have been adapted from the work of Davis, Eshelman & McKay (1988).

The first step is to identify your negative thoughts. (One of the ways we have found to do this is by using the NCSAM.) This allows you to examine whether the thought is realistic, destructive, neutral or self-defeating.

The second step is to imagine the thought. Close your eyes and allow the thought to run through your mind. Bring into your thoughts a stressful situation where the thought is likely to occur. In other words, sit back, shut your eyes and let yourself worry.

Step three is thought interruption. In this step you interrupt the thinking by using a "startle" technique to stop the negative stream of thoughts and empty your mind of all but neutral thoughts. Try to keep your thoughts neutral or your mind blank for at least 30 seconds. If you are unable to do this and the negative thoughts return, use the technique again. Startle techniques include setting an egg timer or an alarm clock or tape recording yourself loudly stating the word "STOP." Other techniques include snapping your fingers or snapping a rubber band that is worn around your wrist.

Step four is unaided thought interruption. After you have practiced extinguishing the thought with the startle technique, you can begin to interrupt the thought by stating the word "stop" in a normal voice. This can progress to interrupting the thought by whispering the word "stop" or imagining the word "stop" in your mind.

Thought substitution is the fifth step. This last step includes substituting the negative thought with a more positive one. One example would be substituting the negative thought: "I will never be smart enough to get through nursing school" to the positive thought, "My nursing education will provide a challenge for me."

Here are some examples of students using the thought stopping technique:

Tracy has decided to apply to a very competitive nursing school. Entrance to this nursing program is largely dependent upon one's QPA accumulated during the pre-requisite courses prior to gaining admission to the nursing program. As Tracy takes her pre-requisite courses, she becomes increasingly anxious with each test. She frequently experiences the following stream of thoughts: "I have to get an A on this test to keep up my QPA. What if I don't get an A? My QPA will drop and I won't get into the nursing program. Every one else in this class has a better QPA than I do. I'll never get accepted into this program. I'll never get to be a nurse." Ironically, the more repetitive these thoughts became for Tracy, the more her grades began to plummet. She was creating her own prophecy. She was making her worst fears come true. Using thought stopping helped Tracy to not only stop the negative thoughts prior to and during the exam, but eventually allowed her to substitute those thoughts with more positive ones, "STOP!........I don't have any evidence to support these thoughts. I'm going to prepare the best way I know how and give it my best shot. I have a good QPA so far and school has been a good experience for me."

Diane is a senior in her last nursing course in leadership before she graduates. She is a solid B-C student who has worked hard and has never been in academic difficulty. For each test in the leadership course, Diane has become increasingly anxious, "This is it. I could really blow it in this course. I think they saved the hardest course for last. What if I don't make it? My life would be ruined." Most of Diane's negative thinking occurs when she is studying for the exam. These negative thoughts have become distracting, decreasing her attention span so that, even though she spends hours studying, she actually is worrying most of the time. Diane begins to use the rubber band technique while she is studying and changes her negative thoughts to, "STOP!........I'm worrying again, I'm not concentrating. This isn't doing me any good. Get back to the information I should be studying. My hard work has paid off up until now and there's no reason to think it will be any different now. If I couldn't do this they wouldn't have waited until now to tell me."

Seligman (1990) suggests combining the technique of attention shifting with thought stopping to get longer lasting results. After snapping the rubber band (or whatever startle technique you decide to use) you now shift your attention in another direction. This will help keep your negative thoughts from coming back after thought interruption. To aid in this attention shifting technique, pick out an object in the room. Describe it in detail. Study it intently. You will find that shifting your attention from your worries to the selected object in the room will keep the negative thoughts from returning so quickly. Thought stopping is a technique that requires practice. Try not to get discouraged if at first when you stop the ruminating negative thoughts and they return quickly. This is a normal occurrence when most people begin to practice this technique. You will find that the more you practice thought stopping, the more effective you will become in stopping your negative thoughts.

WORRY PERIODS

Another technique to control negative thinking is that of the worry period (Borkovec, et. al, 1983). Borkovec recommends the following instructions:

1. First learn to identify your worrisome or negative thoughts that are unpleasant. Distinguish these from pleasant and positive thoughts related to the present moment.

2. Establish a half hour worry period that will occur at the same time in the same place each day. For example, you may determine that your worry period will be from 10:00 p.m. to 10:30 p.m. in the den.

3. Throughout the day when you find yourself worrying, try to postpone your worrisome thoughts until your designated worry period. Then replace the worrisome thoughts by attending to positive or neutral present moment experiences. For example, "I'm not going to worry about the test right now. I'll think about it during my worry period at 10 p.m. Right now I'm going to concentrate on preparing for clinical tomorrow." We have often found it helpful to be very specific when returning to present moment experience. For example, we would follow the above quote with, "The first step is to look up this drug." This helps you to structure your

thinking and become action oriented. At first this may be difficult to do but focusing on specific concrete tasks helps increase the concentration and decrease the worry. Just as in thought stopping, you may need to redirect your thoughts more often, but this redirection becomes easier with practice.

4.   During your worry period, take the half hour and worry about your concerns. Then try to think about ways in which you might problem solve to eliminate these concerns. For example, during a worry period, after you think about all of your worries, you might begin the problem solving process by asking yourself several questions. First, "Which of these worries are interfering with my life? Which of these get in the way of my goal?" Second, "What can I really do about this?" Third, "Who might be able to help me with this and what are my resources to help me resolve it?"

Over the years many individuals have told us that they find the worry period technique as very helpful when combined with thought stopping. For example, after using the rubber band technique or saying "STOP!" they then say, "I'll worry about this at 10 p.m. during my worry period." Often when we teach our students and clients to use the worry technique they look at us with slightly amused and puzzled expressions. They frequently make comments such as, "Are you kidding? I'm not going to sit down every day for 30 minutes and worry. That's silly." or "What if somebody sees me worrying? I'll be so embarrassed." Whether you actually sit down and worry during the worry period isn't the most important issue. The important part of the worry period technique is that the individual not only stops the thoughts but pushes them away during the time when they need to concentrate or perform in something that produces anxiety for them. Remember that negative thoughts create negative feelings that create negative behavior. If you can remove or distance the negative thoughts from the behavior such as test-taking or studying, your test-taking or studying behavior will be enhanced. In summary, whether you actually sit down and worry during your worry period may not matter. What matters is that you take the worry away from the performance.

WORRY BREAKS

Another thought distraction technique is the worry break (Burns, 1989). Worry breaks are especially helpful when you are trying to study. Many individuals often complain that they get distracted and experience many negative thoughts when they are trying to study. Even though they have been sitting at their desks with a book open for three hours, they have really only been studying for 30 minutes. The problem with this is that it feels like you've been studying for three hours and it's easy to fool yourself into believing that you have been.

73

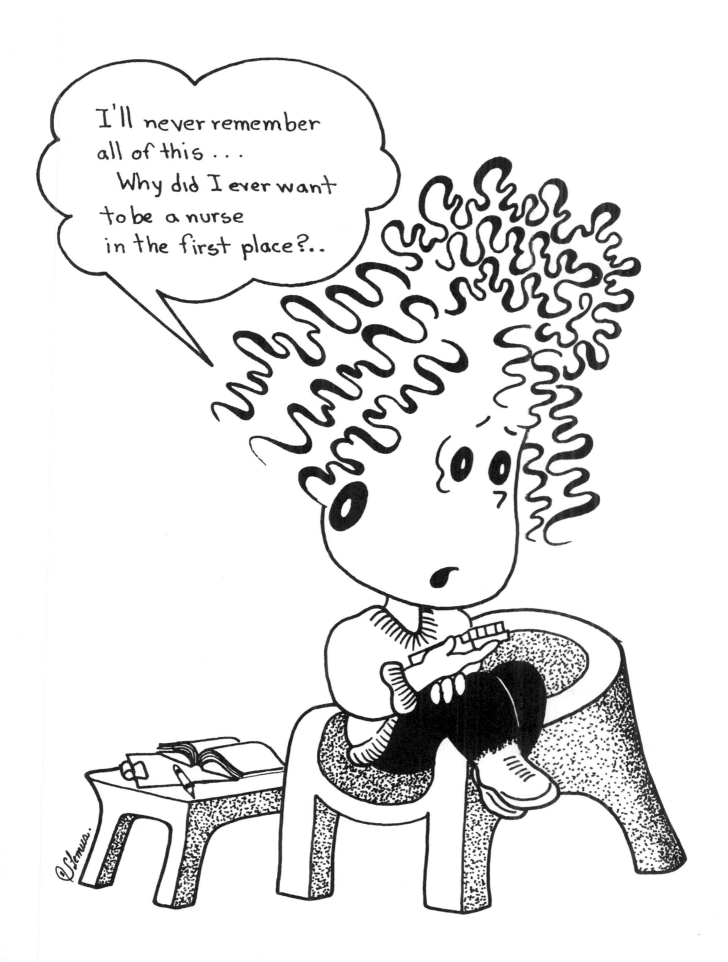

Unfortunately the day of reckoning comes too soon and you can often experience confusion and frustration when your test grades don't reflect the amount of time you thought you studied and prepared. Scheduling worry breaks every so often while studying can help enhance study effectiveness. During your worry break, take a minute to worry or fret about just how awful things are. Let it rip. Don't try to fight it.

Many students find it helpful during the worry break to write these worries down or dictate them into a tape recorder. After you have written your worries or dictated them into the tape recorder, try to go back and study for about 15 minutes and then take another worry break. Repeat the same procedure by either writing down or recording your worries and catastrophic thoughts. At the end of your study period pick up your notebook or tape recorder and read or listen to your negative thoughts and worrisome cognitions. At first, reexamining these thoughts may be painful. After a while most people find that the thoughts lose their sting and even begin to sound funny, silly or even absurd. Often they are the same repetitious thoughts and can become quite boring to listen to or read. When you make the thoughts external rather than internal or stated more simply, from inside of you to outside of you, it's as though they no longer belong to you. Therefore their ability to hurt you has lost its power.

As we stated earlier, when you first hear of these techniques you may doubt they'll be effective. For each individual, some techniques will work better than others. However, whether you use thought stopping, worry periods or worry breaks, or some combination of these techniques, you will probably find them to be extremely helpful. Remember, these techniques will be effective only if you practice them on a regular basis.

REFERENCES

Beck, A. T. (1976). Cognitive therapy and the emotional disorders. New York: International Universities Press.

Borkovec, T. D., Wilkinson, L., Folansbee, R. & Lerman, C. (1983). Stimulus control applications to the treatment of worry. Behavior Research and Therapy, 21(3), 247-251.

Burns, D. D. (1989). The feeling good handbook: Using the new mood therapy in everyday life. New York: William Morrow, Inc.

Cooley, E. J. & Speigler, M. D. (1980). Cognitive versus emotional coping responses as alternatives to test anxiety. Cognitive Therapy and Research, 4, 167-178.

Davis, M., Eshelman, E. R. & McKay, M. (1988). The relaxation and stress reduction workbook (3rd Ed.). Oakland, CA: New Harbinger Publications.

Hunsley, J. (1987). Internal dialogue during academic examinations. Cognitive Therapy and Research, 11, 653-664.

Poorman, S. G. & Martin, E. J. (1991). The role of nonacademic variables in passing the National Council Licensure Examination. Journal of Professional Nursing, 1, 25-32.

Seligman, M. E. P. (1990). Learned optimism: How to change your mind and your life. New York: Pocket Books.

Wise, E. G., & Haynes, S. N. (1983). Cognitive treatment of test anxiety: Rational restructuring versus attentional training. Cognitive Therapy and Research, 1(1), 69-78.

7

TRIUMPH OVER TEST-TAKING: TEST-TAKING STRATEGIES

THE WAY YOU LOOK AT TESTS

Everyone has a preconceived notion when they hear the word "test." They have immediate thoughts and an immediate response to the word, whether they know it or not. You've learned very early in your life a certain perception or framework in which you view a test-taking situation and more importantly your ability in that situation. Some lucky individuals have learned to view tests as a naturally occurring part of life. They believe that you can't escape tests and they have settled into a framework of acceptance. For others, the task is not that simple. Somewhere along the road of life, they learned to view tests as frightening, conquering and devastating. They see tests as an evil monster out to destroy them. The following are some of the cognitions and perceptions that we hear from students about tests and their ability to take tests.

"I know this material. I just don't know what happens to me when I'm taking the test. I just freeze."

"I study very hard but my grades don't show it."

"I do really well clinically but when it comes to paper and pencil tests I just don't show it."

"I've never been a good test-taker."

"My instructor tells me I'm a good nurse, I just don't show it on paper."

"Sometimes I don't know where the instructors are getting the questions."

"I study harder and harder and don't do any better so what's the use?"

"They try to trick us and write hard questions with material from the readings and not from class like they don't really want us to pass."

"I really studied, I knew the material but the instructor asked the question in a funny way so I didn't know what she wanted."

"Every time I take a test, I wonder if this is the one where I'm going to be weeded out."

The first step in becoming a better test-taker is to conduct a self-assessment regarding your views and perceptions at this time. Take a minute and ask yourself what kind of thoughts come to mind when you hear the sentence, "Now you're going to have a test."

List them here:

_____

_____

_____

_____

_____

_____

_____

_____

TESTS: A NEW ATTITUDE

Now that you have identified your thoughts and perceptions about tests, it's time to ask yourself if they are a help or hindrance to your test-taking ability. For many of you, the thoughts and perceptions will be negative and you will need to spend some time as the song says "getting a new attitude." At this point you need to begin to view tests differently. You must learn to view test-taking as a skill in problem solving. Viewing tests as a skill is important because, as any other skill, (riding a bicycle, tying a shoe, giving injections) you can improve with practice. One of the most effective ways to becoming a better test-taker is to simply practice answering test questions. In nursing, this is very easy because there are so many practice NCLEX books. A specific example of this would be a student who is in a pediatric rotation reviewing sample pediatric questions in an NCLEX review book. Many textbooks have questions at the end of the chapters and some books have study guides where you can find questions. Eventually, you can become so good at test-taking, you will think up your own questions and review them with your classmates.

The point we are making here is that before you can become an effective test-taker you must take the sting out of the word "**test**." You must accept the fact that tests are a part of your nursing reality and learn to become skilled at taking them. "**Life is a test. If you woke up alive this morning, it means you got an "A" for yesterday." (Fry, 1992).**

In this chapter we will discuss multiple choice tests and essay exams. At this point most nursing exams are multiple choice because it prepares the student for the NCLEX format. Multiple choice tests will be discussed both in this chapter and in Chapter 8.

When approaching any exam, try to know as much about the test as possible. For you to become test-wise or skilled in the art of test-taking, it is imperative that you learn as much about the testing situation as possible. By this we mean that you should attempt to find out what type of questions (multiple choice, essay, true-false, matching) will be included on the test.

Try to be clear about what content will be tested. What reading assignments and what objectives will be tested. Also, find out if the test will be comprehensive or if certain concepts are tested throughout the curriculum such as communications, safety, oxygenation, etc. You also want to know how much time will be given for the exam. Many tests are timed at approximately one minute per question. Find out approximately how many questions will be on the test. Once you learn the basics of the test, you will be better able to focus and prepare. The following principles suggest ways of approaching multiple choice test items.

STRATEGIES FOR MULTIPLE CHOICE NURSING EXAMS

> **1. Understand how a multiple choice question is written.**

There are three basic components of a multiple choice question. The first part is the **background statement** or the **case situation**. This tells the clinical story. It gives you information about a clinical situation or problem. For example, a case situation would be something like this:

> **Situation: Mr. Henderson is a 20 year old male who was diagnosed with mental retardation at birth. He is admitted to the psychiatric unit because the staff at the group home believes he may be hallucinating and his behavior has become more bizarre. He has also been getting very angry at small disappointments.**

The next part of a multiple choice question is called the **stem**. The stem is the part of the question that actually asks you to solve a specific problem or issue related to the background statement. Stems can be written in a question format or an incomplete sentence format.

> Mr. Henderson is found rocking in his bed and refuses to respond to the nurse's questions. What would be the appropriate nursing diagnosis?
> a. Impaired communication related to inability to ask questions.
> b. Social isolation related to ritualized behavior.
> c. Ineffective individual coping related to low frustration level.
> d. Anxiety related to separation from usual caretakers.

> The nurse is interviewing the caretaker from the group home. The priority assessment data the nurse should ask the caretaker includes the:
> a. events prior to the client's change in behavior.
> b. family's socioeconomic status and support.
> c. family's acceptance of the client's condition.
> d. staff's response to the client's behavior.

Stems can be written in a direct or positive fashion, in that they ask the nurse what the correct assessment, intervention or evaluation would be. Some stems are written in a negative format where they are asking the student what is **not** true, what the nurse would **not** do, what would be wrong or incorrect.

Examples of stems with negative items:

"Which of the following tests would be **contraindicated** in this client?"

"The nurse would assess all of the following **except**:"

"Which nursing action would **not** be included in the plan of care?"

Please note in the above three examples, the word that makes the stem negative is darkened. In some questions it may be capitalized or italicized, however, in some negative stem questions the negative word is not identified in any way and the student must carefully read the stem to identify it.

Some nurse educators try to avoid writing negative stem items. However, occasionally a student may encounter a negative stem item and should know how to approach it because these are easy to misread and answer incorrectly. The third part of a multiple choice question is the **options**. In most multiple choice questions there are three distractors and one correct response. For one of the options to be a correct answer, it must be totally correct, not just partially correct. The correct answer is the response that best completes the stem sentence and solves the problem being asked.

Situation: Donna Alpert, 27 years old, is being admitted for abdominal pain. She looks very tired and pale. She is accompanied by her husband, 3 year old son, and 2 month old infant.

Ms. Alpert says, "I don't know who will care for my children while I'm in here. My husband has to work." The best reply by the nurse would be:
a. "Perhaps you should have made arrangements for the children before you were admitted."
b. "Let me call a social worker. She can call child welfare to take them while you are hospitalized."
c. "Who do you know from your neighbors or church who might be able to help with the children?"
d. "I'm sure your husband can take a few days off from work until you recover."

Please note that you may find that multiple choice questions may be written with the above three parts but some are written just with the stem and four options.

The best way to approach a newly admitted client is to:

a. immediately start on the assessment process.
b. introduce yourself and orient him to the room.
c. introduce him to the other staff and clients.
d. ask him to change into hospital pajamas and robe.

---

2. Identify the stem and the carefully ask yourself: "What are they asking me?"

One of the major mistakes in test-taking is not lack of knowledge of the content being tested but, rather, not understanding what the question is asking you. Try to think of test-taking and trying to answer the questions as solving a mystery. Ask yourself, "What do they want from me?" Then try to paraphrase the stem or put it into your own words so it makes sense to you. This is where the real skill in test-taking comes into play. Here is where we separate the good test-takers from the bad test-takers. Frequently, students become frustrated when they try to put the stem into their own words. This process is difficult at first and students often become angry and project their anger on faculty saying, "This is a stupid question. Why would anyone ask this? I have no idea what she is trying to ask me. Why doesn't she just ask it in plain English?" This can be a crucial period in test-taking because allowing yourself to be distracted from the task and becoming angry will decrease your test-taking effectiveness. Remember, as hard as this is to believe, faculty are the test construction experts, not students. For the most part they know what they are doing. There are no benefits in having an imaginary argument over a test question. Don't fight the process here. Try to learn what they want from you and try to give it to them. Power struggles over who knows best about test-taking only make you the permanent loser.

---

3. Identify key words.

Expert test question writers don't waste words. When they use an adjective or adverb to describe or further define a concept, it is purposeful. You will find that if you can find **key words** in a stem, they will help you answer the question more specifically. Some examples of key words include: initial action, early sign, immediately after surgery.

---

4. Don't "what if" test questions.

Some students have difficulty with inadvertently reading into or adding information to the test situation. They make the assumption from their own thoughts or previous clinical experience that this information is true or applies to this specific test question. They find themselves playing the "what if" game. "What if the client is on bedrest?" "What if the client doesn't have support systems? What if the nurses are too busy to check on him every 15 minutes? After several "what ifs," students find they have created an entirely new test question that doesn't even resemble the one on the page. Remember that your task is taking an objective test and not writing a best selling fiction novel. The rule of thumb here is that, if it isn't written down, you don't have that information about the situation.

5. Reduce your options.

The first time you read your multiple choice options you should eliminate those options you know are wrong. Most students can usually eliminate one or two options. One of the most common problems that students experience during a multiple choice exam is that two of the options look like the correct answer. After you have eliminated the wrong answers, try rereading the stem of the question (not the entire background statement, just the stem). Then try to identify a reason or rationale for each of the remaining answers. Select the option for which you can provide a rationale based on known nursing principles. This technique may take a few minutes at first but, as with all test-taking techniques, you will become more proficient at this skill with increased practice.

6. When all else fail, trust your "glimmer" response.

Sometimes when you are reading a test question over for the first time, for one split second one answer glimmers as the correct response. Most of the time we quickly dismiss this glimmer with statements such as "That couldn't possibly be right, I could never get the answer that fast." We then move on using what we believe is "better" thinking to answer this question when, in reality, the glimmer response is the correct answer. Glimmer responses are not guesses. They are more like unconscious knowing before our mind becomes cluttered with negative cognitions which make us doubt our knowledge and abilities. Try this experiment: complete a series of practice questions, noting both your glimmer response and the answer you would really put down in a testing situation. Next, calculate your percentages with your actual responses and then with your glimmer responses. See which score is higher. If your glimmer score is higher, try this again and pay attention to how often that first glimmer response is correct. Eventually you will learn to trust your glimmer responses and actually select them as the correct answer. Many students find that learning to trust these responses increases test scores.

7. Identify priorities.

In nursing practice, nurses are constantly required to think on their feet; to think quickly and make life and death decisions in a split second. Test questions that ask the nurse to identify priorities are testing this concept. Priority questions are stated as: " What should the nurse do first?," "What is the initial nursing action?" and ask the nurse to simulate how she would think something through in clinical practice. This way the instructors know that the student is a good thinker and can practice nursing safely.

> **8. Answer questions objectively.**

As it is difficult in life not to react and to remain objective, so it is with tests. Certain questions elicit a subjective and highly emotional response from us for a variety of reasons. These are the "button-pushing" questions; when you see a question like this, it pushes your panic button so that you have difficulty thinking or reasoning out the answer objectively. It is important to understand what types of questions elicit this button-pushing response from you because, unless you become aware of when it's happening, you can do nothing to stop and alter the process. Without intervention on your part, these highly emotional reactions often lead to errors in reasoning and incorrect answers. This button-pushing response can be elicited for a variety of reasons. For example, if you see a question on a test about a disease you don't remember studying or a particular problem with which you have had personal experience in friends or family and, in some cases, most of us have questions about certain diseases or concepts that were just difficult to learn. Students consistently tell us that questions about: side effects of medications, chest tubes, communication theory, nutrition, and fluid/electrolyte balance, push their panic buttons. For every student, these button-pushing responses are different. However, it is important for you to know what situations or what type of questions elicit that highly emotional response so that you can learn a more objective, rational way of responding.

> **9. Select answers that encourage expression of feeling without implying judgement by the nurse.**

Some students have difficulty in answering questions where the nurse must respond in a therapeutic manner and have the following two negative cognitions: "Which answer sounds good to me?" and "What would I say if I were at work?" Remember, questions that ask you to respond in a therapeutic manner are based on therapeutic communication theory and should not be based on a "common sense" approach. Those negative cognitions should be changed to: "Which of these responses will encourage the client to express himself?" and "Which option uses therapeutic communication theory?" It is important that you not respond with what you've heard other nurses say to clients or what you would say to a client unless it uses a therapeutic communication response. Judge every situation differently and do not compare them to similar clinical situations you have experienced. Another common mistake that occurs in this type of a question is that, after reading all four options, students indignantly respond to themselves, "I don't like any of these answers." This line of thinking can also lead to troubled waters. Remember, try not to react to the question personally, but rather, respond to the principle being tested. Although you may not phrase the response in the same way as stated in the question, hopefully you would use the same therapeutic principle.

10. Select nonjudgemental responses.

No matter how much we attempt to simulate clinical experience in test writing, tests are never reality. When answering test questions, assume that it is in Hospital USA with Florence Nightingale as the director of nursing and Marcus Welby as the physician. In ideal situations nurses never make negative judgements about their clients even though, in the real world, this is one problem we continue to address.

11. Don't worry about questions you don't know.

Some questions will surprise you or catch you off guard no matter how much time you study or prepare for an exam. This is actually a normal occurrence and not unusual. Do not waste time waiting for divine intervention. Often, the more you stare at a question, the more likely you are to contaminate it and your thinking process with information that clutters your ability to reason effectively. When you have no idea what the correct answer is, take your best guess and move on. Remember, no one knows all of the answers. On any given test it is normal to have to partially guess at several of the answers. When this happens, instead of allowing yourself to become unduly stressed, normalize it; remember that it's normal not to know all of the answers.

12. Remember the scope of nursing practice.

One important concept that is repeatedly tested on nursing exams is whether or not the nursing student can determine what is and what is not within the scope of nursing practice. It is important for the nursing student to differentiate and eliminate options that are not within the nurses' realm. Rule of thumb: do not select options that give away your role as a nurse to another health care professional and do not select options where the nurse would be taking on another health care professional's practice.

13. Do not outsmart the question.

A common nagging consistent theme that runs through the minds of nursing students is that the mean and nasty instructors are writing questions to specifically trick students. As difficult as this may be for you to believe, good test question writers want to test important principles and your ability to use important nursing concepts in simulated clinical experiences. There is no educational purpose in tricking students. If you really believe the answer is option (c), don't change your mind because you think there is some hidden agenda in the test question.

14. Ponder the principle.

As nursing students, you learn a copious amount of factual data. You also learn to treasure these facts and want to believe that the quantity of facts learned is a direct correlation to the quality of nursing care provided. However, quality nursing care is based on basic principles and concepts which embody these facts. You feel secure knowing that you can clutch and hold onto these **facts** but nursing exams really test the **principles** that guide nursing practice. Learning to study and take tests by learning principles helps you organize and understand your information rather than memorizing it for short term test-taking purposes. As you add to your knowledge in nursing school you are adding to those principles. If you learn the basic principles, you will have a sound basis upon which to build nursing theory and practice. Errors are commonly made when you cling to facts by choosing answers according to specific factual policies at one hospital rather than the principles and concepts taught to you in classroom lecture and textbooks. Generalizing from one client to the larger population can be another error. The incident should be related to a principle and learned in the context of that principle rather than as an isolated fact.

15. Maximize strengths and minimize weaknesses.

The best test-taking strategy will always be to maximize your test-taking strengths. Part of maximizing your strengths is identifying and then minimizing weaknesses. For many individuals, these weaknesses become patterns where they commit these errors repeatedly. Every time you participate in a test review or complete practice test questions, look for your test-taking patterns. Common test-taking patterns which cause problems include: **clumping** (missing several questions in a row); **first question freeze** (becoming unnerved when you don't know the answer to the first question and placing undue importance on that question); and **changing answers** indiscriminately or on a whim. A general rule to remember is to change your answer only if you are sure your original answer is incorrect. Ask yourself, "Can I identify a theoretical rationale for changing this answer?"

In chapter 8 we will examine these techniques in actual practice questions.

ESSAY QUESTIONS

Essay questions have become more prominent in nursing education because of the emphasis on thinking and writing skills. Teachers may have several reasons for placing essay questions on a test: 1) Do you know the concept? 2) Can you use the concept? 3) Can you apply the concept by giving examples? 4) How well can you communicate ideas? and 5) How well do you organize your thoughts?

There are two basic types of essay questions: short answer essay and large essay. Short answer essays require a paragraph or less to answer the questions. Large essays require several paragraphs to several pages to answer the questions. Short answer essay questions tend to ask for recall and/or comprehensive knowledge. Larger essay questions generally require knowledge of the concept, analysis, critique and other reasoning skills as well as organization and writing skills. Some basic principles of answering essay questions include:

1. Manage the time wisely.

Read all of the essay questions and how many points each question is worth and assign time accordingly. If the test has three essay questions, each worth 15 points, and you have about an hour of time, you might decide to divide your time by giving 5 minutes for reading through the test, 15 minutes for each essay question, and 10 minutes to read through your answers to make final corrections. Redistribute the time depending on points assigned to the essays. For example, if the test has three essay questions (two worth 10 points and one worth 25 points) and one hour of time, less time should be spent on the essays worth 10 points and more time spent on the question worth 25 points.

2. Understand the question.

Many students answer questions incorrectly because they are unclear about what the question is asking. Often they misunderstand or misread the question. Read the essay carefully. Look for key words such as **compare and contrast** (show how the concepts are alike and different), **differentiate** (show how the concepts are different), **critique** (what is right or wrong according to set criteria) and **debate** (show both sides of an argument). Large essay questions often ask for these more complex answers which require high level reasoning skills. Short answer essays often use such words as **list**, **define** and **identify**. Make sure you understand what is being asked because you don't usually get many points for wrong or unclear answers.

3. Organize your thoughts.

Using an outline as a general guide for answering the question helps to keep you on the subject and keeps you from forgetting ideas. In outline form in a corner or margin of the paper, jot down the major points with key words and examples you might use to illustrate the point. This leaves you free to write and sometimes teachers will give some credit for the outline if the student did not have time to finish the essay. The first sentence of the essay should include rephrasing the question being asked. This shows the teacher that you understood the assignment. Emphasize the major points. If the teacher asks for three concepts, label them as such (e.g., "The first concept is", "The second concept is," etc.). The teacher should not have to look for them. The longer the teacher searches, the fewer points usually given. Illustrate the major points by using examples. This further shows that you understand the concepts. Use the example, then show the connection of the example to the concept. However, make sure the example does illustrate the concept. If you aren't sure of the connection, don't use the example. At the end of the essay summarize the major points in the closing paragraph.

---

4. Use what was taught in class.

The best ideas on what to write come because you attended classes. The teacher generally makes a point of the major ideas, concepts and examples. Therefore, you can probably predict what the essay questions may be and what the teacher will be looking for in an answer. Use the required and recommended readings for backup examples to show that you actually read the assignments.

---

5. Don't give much more or much less than is asked.

For each essay question the teacher will have set criteria on how it will be graded. For example, if a teacher asks a student to define a certain word, a set definition is usually the criteria. If the teacher asks for two arguments against capitalism, the teacher may have five acceptable arguments and the students' answers have to be on the list of acceptable arguments or no points are given. Some students try to give more material than asked. For example, a student unsure of two arguments may give three or four, figuring the teacher will give points for the two correct arguments even if the other two arguments are incorrect. Check with the teacher before the test how this may be perceived by the teacher. Some teachers won't give any points because the directions (for two arguments, not three or four) were not followed correctly. Other teachers will only look at the first two arguments and ignore the others even if they are correct. Also some students try to fool the teacher into thinking that they know the answer to a question by writing a lot of extra words and sentences or will try to change the subject of the test question. Believe it or not, teachers can spot when students are writing "extra thick" or "padding" answers in the hope the teacher gives them credit for trying. Again, teachers know what they want and grade accordingly. On the other hand, make sure you do answer the questions. Don't assume that the teacher knows you understand something. Make sure you answer clearly and give enough information to answer the question completely, as if the teacher never met you and you have to prove you know the material to a stranger. Even if you are unsure of an answer, try to answer the question. If you try to answer a question, you are likely to get some of the points but if you leave the paper blank, you know you won't get any points. It's always worth a try.

6. Use spelling, grammar and writing skills.

Some students believe that attention to spelling, grammar and writing skills should only be true for English composition class. However, these skills were emphasized for a reason. The ability to communicate ideas is essential, no matter what career or field you enter. This means students must pay attention to verb tenses, dangling participles, misspelled words and complete sentences as well as periods, commas and question marks. The essays are easier to read and grade when these rules are followed. Remember, don't make the teacher work too hard for your grade.

Our overall goal in this chapter was to provide you with some basic information to aid you in becoming a better test-taker and therefore moving you toward a more enjoyable educational experience. We have discussed fifteen strategies to utilize when taking multiple choice test questions that, if practiced, will enhance your performance. Essay questions were defined and described as well as ways suggested to meet the teachers' general expectation for answers. Six basic principles for answering essay questions were discussed. Use these ideas to enjoy more success on essay questions.

REFERENCE

Fry, R. (1992). Ace any test. Hawthorne, NJ: Career Press.

8

IMPROVING YOUR THINKING AND REASONING SKILLS ON TESTS

This chapter will address the thinking and reasoning skills most helpful in using concepts and principles to guide nursing judgement. There is so much material that no one is capable of learning every little fact there is to know. A prudent nurse is one who learns to use the concepts and principles at hand to make decisions and to know the limits of your knowledge, or when you need to seek guidance, so the nursing care given is effective and safe.

If you study using concepts and principles by teaching yourself to think ideas through rather than by memorizing facts, these newly found skills will help you more on tests than memorizing facts. The following questions illustrate this point:

> **SITUATION: Mr. Carl Furia, 64 years old, is diagnosed with right-sided congestive heart failure. He is ordered furosemide (Lasix) 20 mg twice a day. (The next three questions refer to this situation.)**

This situation is very short and tells you everything you need to know about this client: 64 years old (not unusual for the condition), right sided congestive heart failure (points you to the process and where questions may be based), and Lasix is ordered twice per day (not unusual for this condition). Now look at the first question.

> The purpose of furosemide (Lasix) in this particular client is:
> a. as a potassium sparing loop diuretic.
> b. to treat edema and hypertension.
> c. to treat acute episodes of pulmonary edema.
> d. as a calcium sparing loop diuretic.

Now you may start out by thinking that this type of question is always hardest to figure out. You have no information to suggest any specific reason for the drug: no vital signs, no lab tests, none of the usual information you go through to find the answer. Well, the answer is one of those four so let's examine the options. Two are about the drug itself and two are about the client. Let's look at the two about Lasix. Lasix is a loop diuretic. You remember it acts on the loop of Henle (in the kidney) to keep the antidiuretic hormone from telling the body to keep the fluid. The major drawback is that it also gets rid of potassium and calcium. That information eliminates option (a), potassium sparing and option (d), calcium sparing. Please remember that if part of the answer is wrong then all of it is wrong even if you like the right part of the answer. However, remember we said Lasix keeps the body from retaining excess fluids. Now look at the last two client centered answers. Options (b) and (c) both deal with too much fluid so the Lasix could be given for either one. That is a problem though, isn't it? The situation says the client has congestive heart failure. It says nothing about edema, hypertension or pulmonary edema. Well, the basic rule is that if the situation or question doesn't offer the information about symptoms, then the symptoms can't be used to answer the question, right? How do you know when to assume information? When usual signs and symptoms are seen in the majority of clients and no information is given to say differently then you can assume the client will show the usual signs and symptoms of the disease process. So the client has right sided congestive heart failure. That means the right side of the heart does not pump effectively so fluid gets backed up. Where does it go? If you've looked at the concept and learned the process of the circulatory system you know that if the fluid backs up, it will flow back into the superior and inferior vena cava which continues back into the body system. If there is extra fluid in the blood vessels, blood pressure increases. If there is extra fluid in the blood vessels, some of it moves into the cells through osmosis. Extra fluid in the tissue is known as edema. Edema and hypertension are parts of option (b) so there is a probability that option (b) is the correct answer. What about option (c)? Pulmonary edema is extra fluid in the pulmonary or lung area. Well, if the fluid backs up into the system because it isn't getting pumped by the right side of the heart, then it never gets to the lungs so it can't be extra fluid in the lungs or pulmonary edema so option (c) is wrong. The correct answer is option (b).

Let's look at the next question.

The furosemide (Lasix) is ordered to be given to Mr. Furia twice a day. The nurse would give the furosemide (Lasix) at:

a. 9 a.m. and 9 p.m..
b. 9 a.m. and 12 noon.
c. 9 a.m. and 5 p.m..
d. 12 noon and 12 midnight.

This is a question to see how the nurse best manages care. It calls for your reasoning skills because there are no absolute time schedules for furosemide (Lasix) so how do we know how to make the decision on this? What factors should we take into consideration? If there are no absolute times then the times are dictated by the nursing care for this client. There are two types of answers for this question. Options (a) and (d) are twelve hours apart. Well, those answers might make sense because the extra fluid would be diuresed throughout the twenty-four hour period to help relieve the symptoms. Let's think this through. If the nurse gives the medication at 9 p.m. or 12 midnight what will be the effect on the client? The client will diurese. What does that mean? He will need to get up or at least wake up to urinate. If the client wakes up during the night several times to urinate, this will interrupt his rest. Good rest periods and sleep are needed because of the extra work the heart is doing to push all of the fluid through the system. If he has to wake up several times during the night to void, he may not be getting the rest he needs for his heart to do its best work. Well, what if the client has a urinary catheter? Some clients do if they have congestive heart failure and are on a diuretic. Then he wouldn't have to wake up to void. STOP! Do ALL clients with congestive heart failure on a diuretic have catheters? No, not all. Does the situation or the question state that Mr. Furia has a urinary catheter? No. If the situation or question does not say he has a urinary catheter then Mr. Furia does not have a urinary catheter. Never add information to the question.

You may then think, "I had a client with congestive heart failure and he got his diuretic intravenously and voided quickly afterward. If that's true then this client wouldn't be up all night either." STOP! Is Mr. Furia's diuretic ordered intravenously? No. The medication is ordered orally so onset of action will not be as rapid as the intravenous dose. Avoid comparing your clinical experience to the client on the theory test. Not all clients are treated exactly the same way. When you think about your clinical client, you may answer questions as if they were being asked about the client in your clinical assignment rather than the client on the test.

Since the client will lose a lot of rest, we can eliminate options (a) and (d). Option (b), 9 a.m. and 12 noon are too close together. The furosemide

(Lasix) may last as long as six hours after oral administration. If the doses are given too close together on a regular daily basis, problems from water and electrolyte depletion may result. That eliminates option (b). Option (c), 9 a.m. and 5 p.m. are eight hours apart. The 9 a.m. dose will be finished working by the time the second dose is given. The 5 p.m. dose will be finished working by 11 p.m. so the client can get a full night's rest. Option (c) is the best answer.

Let's look at the third question.

Mr. Furia is ordered a low sodium diet. The nurse evaluates that Mr. Furia understands his diet when he orders which of the following meals?
a. Fresh fruit salad, broth, saltines.
b. Chicken soup, applesauce, tea.
c. Ham and turkey club sandwich, coffee.
d. Roast beef, garden salad, iced tea.

The key to this question lies in knowing what the question is asking you. The stem reads, "The nurse evaluates that Mr. Furia understands his diet when Mr. Furia orders which of the following meals?" Let's break it down by thinking it through. The nurse wants to know if Mr. Furia understands his low sodium diet. If the client knows the low sodium diet, he'll choose a meal that is low in sodium. It may be helpful to rephrase the question to, "Which meal is low in sodium?" Knowing that this is the question, we will look at each item in the answer to see if it contains sodium. In option (a), fresh fruit salad doesn't have sodium but broth and saltines both have sodium. In option (b), chicken soup has sodium but applesauce and tea do not. In option (c), ham has high sodium but turkey, bread and coffee do not. In option (d), roast beef, garden salad and iced tea do not have large amounts of sodium. Since option (d) has the least amount of sodium, it is the correct answer.

Notice especially in the last two questions that memorizing facts would not give you the correct answer. You definitely had to reason them through. Most nursing questions ask for application of facts which calls for reasoning and nursing judgement. This cannot be memorized.

Let's try another set of questions.

SITUATION: A 65 year old male client is admitted with dyspnea, occasional dry cough and thin build. Test results show a low PaO_2 and increased $PaCO_2$. Admitting diagnosis is pulmonary emphysema. (The next three questions refer to this situation.)

The nurse would expect to find which assessment data?
a. Scattered rales and rhonchi.
b. Diminished breath sounds.
c. Whooshing sound over the lung.
d. Wheezing and congestion.

The correct answer is b. Breath sounds are diminished in pulmonary emphysema. The lungs are hyperinflated because air is trapped in the alveoli. This results in little air exchange to the blood resulting in high CO_2 levels and low O_2 levels. In chronic bronchitis, an inflammatory process takes place which causes rales, rhonchi (option a), and wheezing and congestion (option d). A whooshing sound over the lung (option c) may be present in a sucking chest wound from which an open pneumothorax has resulted where air is rushing into the open wound creating an air pocket between the chest wall and the lung.

The client arrives on the medical unit with the following orders.
Which order might the nurse question?
a. O_2 5 liters by nasal cannula.
b. Bedrest with bathroom privileges.
c. Force fluids to 3000 ml per day.
d. Consult respiratory therapy.

The correct answer is (a). High flow (5 liters) O_2 is not indicated in clients with pulmonary emphysema. These clients retain CO_2 and have persistently low levels of O_2 so the body shifts its drive to breathe and does not trigger breathing with increased CO_2. Low O_2 levels trigger breathing. High levels of O_2 administration slow the breathing and may cause acute respiratory failure. Only low flow O_2 should be used with these clients. Bedrest with bathroom privileges (option b) helps to conserve energy in a client with low O_2. However, range of motion exercises are essential to assist with maintaining good circulation. Fluids are increased (option c) to hydrate the client, increase viscosity of sputum for easier expectoration and to prevent infection. Respiratory therapy consult (option d) is needed to maintain proper ventilation through breathing exercises, postural drainage and chest physiotherapy.

One nursing diagnosis for the client is altered nutrition: less than body requirements. Client teaching should include:
a. exercise before meals to stimulate appetite.
b. avoiding the use of microwave ovens.
c. eating chewy foods to aid in digestion.
d. rest 30 minutes prior to meals.

The correct answer is (d). Eating, especially with foods that require much chewing (option c), is very tiring and has heavy oxygen demands. To conserve oxygen and lessen dyspnea, the client should rest for 30 minutes prior to eating. Exercising before meals (option a) is tiring to the client and usually results in less appetite and less eating because of the effort required. Microwave ovens (option b) may be helpful to clients since food preparation will be less strenuous.

Now that you see how proper reasoning and thinking skills work to help in problem solving, let's try a harder question. Think of it as a challenging puzzle. Honestly try to answer the question before reading the reasoning response in the chapter.

In a client with progressive chronic obstructive pulmonary disease (COPD) the nurse would expect to find which data on assessment?
a. Frothy sputum.
b. Dependent edema.
c. Bronchospasm.
d. Left-sided heart failure.

When a client has COPD, what is restricted? Breathing. When breathing is restricted how much oxygen gets into the lungs? Very little. In COPD, carbon dioxide is high and oxygen is low. This means that there is less oxygen available to any blood vessels, including the blood vessels in the lungs. Less oxygen creates vasoconstriction. The right side of the heart is supposed to push the blood into the lungs. If the blood vessels are constricted, the right side of the heart has to work harder. If there's a problem with the pumping action of the right side of the heart, right-sided congestive heart failure develops, which pushes the fluid back into the system including the extremities. Fluid accumulates in lower extremities showing itself as swollen feet, ankles or legs, often times because the peripheral circulation is more constricted since little oxygen goes to the area. The fluid accumulation in legs and feet is known as dependent edema, option (b). This problem usually carries the medical diagnosis of cor pulmonale which is a complication of COPD. The problem is with right-sided congestive heart failure, which eliminates option (d) (left-sided congestive heart failure). Frothy sputum (option a) is a symptom of left-sided congestive heart failure, not right-sided congestive heart failure. Bronchospasm (option c) is a sign of status asthmaticus, which eliminates it.

Don't be discouraged if you didn't get it right, but, do pay attention to the fact that you can reason it through. Most questions can be answered this way if viewed as a challenge in problem solving and not as an insurmountable mountain. The problem solving principles you learn now will serve you as you continue in school and throughout your career.

We've been dealing mainly with medical/surgical questions. Let's look at a few questions from maternity, pediatrics and psychiatric nursing.

SITUATION: A client has delivered an 11 pound 2 ounce infant boy one and a half hours ago. The physician diagnosed a post-partal hemorrhage and ordered ergonovine maleate (Ergotrate) 0.2 mg intramuscularly to be given immediately. The nurse administers the medication. The client complains of severe cramping 25 minutes after administration.

The correct action of the nurse would be to:
a. suspect that an incorrect dose was administered.
b. inform the client that this sensation is uncomfortable but signifies effectiveness of the medication.
c. notify the labor suite to set up for delivery of an undisclosed twin child the client is carrying.
d. notify the physician of the discomfort and obtain an order for pain medication.

What is important in answering this question? A client has post-partal hemorrhage, is given medication, then complains of cramping. What does the question ask? What should the nurse do in response to this situation? To answer the question, what information do you need? Is cramping normal after this medication? First of all, if you are familiar with this medication you know that it should produce cramping since it causes contractions in the uterus, thus reducing the blood flow. This normally happens automatically after delivery but will cause hemorrhage if the uterus does not contract on it's own. Therefore, if you're not sure of the medication, you can think about what normally happens in the body after delivery. This approach may assist in reasoning through to the answer. Let's examine each of the options. Option (a), incorrect dose, is wrong because this is a normal dose for post-partal hemorrhage. Option (b), medication is effective, is a possibility since cramping of the uterus is the aim of the drug. Option (c), an undisclosed twin, and option (d), order for pain medication, are incorrect because there is not any evidence to suggest a child or that the client has asked for pain medication.

SITUATION: A primipara client is in labor. Her uterine contractions are noted to be inadequate for proper progression. The physician orders oxytocin (Pitocin) to augment labor. The client has been receiving her oxytocin (Pitocin) solution by intravenous piggyback for 30 minutes. The nurse notes the fetal heart rate is 90 beats per minute with a contraction and is not returning to a healthy baseline. The nurse would immediately take which action?

a. Discontinue oxytocin (Pitocin), infuse primary solution, turn client to left side, administer oxygen, and notify the physician.
b. Adjust the monitor as it may be a technical problem.
c. Increase rate of oxytocin (Pitocin) to expedite delivery of the infant.
d. Notify the physician and the operating room staff to prepare for an emergency cesarean section.

What do we know from the situation? A client is on Pitocin. The fetal heart rate is 90 which is below the normal of 120 beats per minute and the fetal heart rate does not return to normal. What does this mean? The fetus is showing signs of fetal distress during contractions which are being initiated by Pitocin. The question asks what the immediate action of the nurse should be. Let's examine the options. Option (d), making the decision about the cesarean section, is not within the scope of practice of the nurse. If the question asked for what order or action the nurse might anticipate by the physician, option (d) might be a possibility. However, the question asks for the nurse's immediate action. Therefore, option (d) is eliminated. Option (c), increasing the Pitocin to expedite delivery would be unsafe. On the present dose of Pitocin, the fetus shows definite distress. Therefore, more Pitocin would create more fetal distress. Also, increasing the dose is not within the scope of practice for the nurse. These reasons eliminate option (c). Option (d), a technical problem, may be true but the safety of the fetus is first priority. Immediate action would be to ensure the safety of the infant through option (a). If Pitocin is producing fetal distress it should be discontinued because it decreases the oxygen supply to the fetus. Turning the client on her left side relieves pressure to the vena cava and optimizes oxygenation of the placenta hence to the fetus. The physician is then notified to determine the next course of action.

An 18 month old toddler is admitted with nephrotic syndrome.
One method of monitoring daily fluid status is by:
a. observing activity level.
b. determining fluid intake.
c. restricting sodium intake.
d. measuring abdominal girth.

This question asks how the nurse can check the client's fluid status which means whether there is too much fluid (edema) or too little fluid (dehydration) in the system. Examine each option using this criteria. Will observing activity level (option b) show if there is too much or too little fluid in the body? No, not directly. The toddler's activity level may change but activity does not directly relate to fluid status. Will determining fluid intake (option b) show edema or dehydration? No, not by itself. Fluid intake should be monitored but fluid output must also be measured to know if too much or too little fluid is being retained.

Will restricting sodium intake (option c) monitor fluid status? No, it is a possible treatment for fluid volume excess. Will measuring abdominal girth (option d) monitor fluid status? Yes, an increased abdominal girth from one day to the next would be indicative of abdominal edema or ascites which would demonstrate fluid volume excess.

The best way to assist children to internalize the discipline necessary for societal adjustment as they become older is to:
a. set consistent limits on activities.
b. allow total exploration of their environment.
c. help them understand the word "no."
d. encourage babies to use the mouth as a sensory organ.

This is an example of a normal growth and development question. Discipline for societal adjustment means to know and follow the rules of society. Will setting consistent limits on activities (option a) help develop discipline? Yes, it may help the child learn that rules must be followed. Inconsistency often leads to adjustment problems and difficulty learning self-control. Allowing total exploration (option b) may teach the child that anything is permitted and does not protect the child from injury or danger. Helping the child understand the word "no" (option c) is important but the child should also understand what can be done or the word "yes." Using mouths as sensory organs (option d) is normal for infants and probably doesn't need to be taught but should be restricted for dangerous objects such as small toys and electrical cords. Notice that even though we believed that option (a) was correct, we did not stop there and just declare it the answer. Always read the four options. Option (a) may be a good answer but better answers could come in later options.

Now that we've completed questions from different areas within nursing, try this practice test. Read each question through and use your reasoning skills to obtain the answer. After you have answered all of the questions look at the rationales following the session. Read each rationale carefully, whether you missed the question or not, since this will help you with your reasoning skills. Don't look at the answers until you have finished all of the questions. Good thinking!

Practice Session

1. A client has just been taught how to use a diaphragm for birth control purposes. The nurse evaluates that the client understands the teaching when the client says:
   a. "I should void after I insert the diaphragm."
   b. "I should remove the diaphragm soon after coitus."
   c. "I will also use a spermicide with the diaphragm."
   d. "I know the diaphragm alters the cervical mucosa."

2. An immunosuppressed client has been admitted to the hospital. The priority area of care would be:
   a. altered nutrition.
   b. impaired skin integrity.
   c. self-esteem disturbance.
   d. potential for infection.

3. During the night shift, the nurse finds a client with congestive heart failure suffering from orthopnea. The client should be placed in what position?
   a. Lithotomy.
   b. Fowler's with legs dangling.
   c. Trendelenberg.
   d. Sims with legs folded.

4. A male client with an indwelling urinary catheter is going to physical therapy for ambulation. The nurse should inform the client that:
   a. bladder distension and pressure may occur.
   b. he will be changed to a condom catheter before going.
   c. he should pull on the catheter to reposition it if discomfort occurs.
   d. the catheter bag should remain below bladder level.

5. The nurse has inserted a nasogastric tube for feeding purposes. The best way of checking proper tube placement is:
   a. instilling air.
   b. tube aspiration.
   c. placing the tube in water.
   d. x-ray film.

6. A client with dehydration complains of severe dizziness upon rising from bed. The nurse should find what changes in vital signs when the client stands?
   a. Decreased pulse, decreased blood pressure.
   b. Decreased pulse, increased blood pressure.
   c. Increased pulse, decreased blood pressure.
   d. Increased pulse, increased blood pressure.

7. A six month old infant is admitted to the pediatric ward. A clean urine specimen is to be collected. The correct action of the nurse would be to:
   a. attach a plastic collection bag to the perineal area.
   b. aspirate the specimen from the infant's diaper.
   c. catheterize the infant.
   d. ask for clarification from the physician.

8. A client with an intestinal obstruction is being assessed by the nurse. Which of the following assessed symptoms is most indicative of intestinal obstruction?
   a. Pain.
   b. Abdominal distension.
   c. Vomiting.
   d. Low grade fever.

9. A client being discharged after cataract extraction demonstrates understanding of instructions with which statement?
   a. "I can get my hair washed at the beauty salon next week."
   b. "I'll increase circulation to my eye when the warm shower water is on my face."
   c. "I'll wear the eye shield during the day but can remove it at night."
   d. "I can't wait to pick up and hold my grandchildren."

10. A client with irritable bowel syndrome (IBS) is given the nursing diagnosis of powerlessness related to unpredictable changes in bowel status. The nurse might suggest that the client:
    a. restrict fiber in the diet.
    b. limit exercise during periods of diarrhea.
    c. keep a diary of bowel changes and life events.
    d. change present coping techniques.

11. A client is admitted to the emergency room with anaphylaxis. The initial goal is to:
    a. help the client stay calm.
    b. check the client's airway.
    c. relieve pruritus.
    d. call the physician.

12. A pregnant woman is found to have gestational diabetes. Education would include which of the following areas?
    a. Insulin pumps are more convenient for a pregnant woman to use.
    b. Clients with gestational diabetes generally use oral hypoglycemics.
    c. Breastfeeding is encouraged and may decrease insulin needs.
    d. Pregnancy will be interrupted close to term for the fetus' welfare.

13. A client with a permanent ileostomy will soon be discharged. The client asks when he can quit wearing a pouch. The best reply by the nurse is:
    a. "Bowel retraining will be started so you will defecate once per day."
    b. "A pouch will always be worn since the drainage will be almost constant."
    c. "Diet will eventually control the ileostomy drainage."
    d. "A representative from the ostomy support group will visit and answer questions."

14. A client is hospitalized for open reduction of a radial fracture. An abnormal finding post-surgery and cast application would be:
    a. palpable pulses.
    b. throbbing pain.
    c. capillary refill in 10 seconds.
    d. warm skin.

15. A client with a decreased cardiac output would probably present with which symptom?
    a. Fatigue.
    b. Palpitations.
    c. Pink face.
    d. Leg pain.

Rationales

1. The correct answer is c. The diaphragm is a dome-shaped cup with a spring which is professionally fitted. A spermicide (option c) should be placed on the surface before inserting the device. To decide about option (a), would it make sense to have a full bladder when inserting a diaphragm? No, it may not fit properly so that would eliminate this option. For option (b), if the diaphragm is a barrier to sperm, should it be removed soon after coitus? Would there be any chance the sperm could still penetrate afterward? It shouldn't be removed for six to eight hours after coitus. For option (d), other birth control methods such as oral contraceptives may alter cervical mucosa but the action of the diaphragm is as a barrier (Lewis & Collier, 1992; p. 1419).

2. The key word here is priority. It means that one or all of the answers may be correct nursing diagnoses but only one is a priority. At this point, look at the possible life threatening or safety issues first, then move into other priority care diagnoses related to the specific problem. Look at the options. Would any of them be life threatening to an immunosuppressed client? Yes, potential for infection since infection in an immunosuppressed client could be fatal. The other three options are possible nursing diagnoses but infection is the major problem (Ignatavicius & Bayne, 1991; pp. 640-643).

3. To answer this question, first define the term "orthopnea". This is difficulty breathing in a reclining position usually related to congestive heart failure. What would aid a client to breathe? When the client lays down, all of the fluid can more easily be pumped towards the heart. The heart cannot handle the extra fluid which may pool to the lungs and against the diaphragm in a reclining position and make it difficult for the client to breathe. Sitting up or standing usually relieves orthopnea since it pulls fluid away from the heart by gravity. Now look at the options. Lithotomy position is reclining with legs up, often in stirrups such as for a gynecology examination. Since the legs are up, gravity will cause even more fluid to go toward the heart so option (a) is eliminated. Fowler's is a sitting position. Legs dangling would keep the fluid from easily returning to the heart so option (b) is a possibility. Should we stop here? No, always read all of the options. A later answer might be even better. Trendelenberg position is with the head down and the client's legs elevated. By gravity, fluid is pulled to the heart. The diaphragm also will have difficulty with getting air into the lungs against gravity. Option (c) should be eliminated. Sims position is a semi-prone position where the client is partially on the abdomen and one leg is flexed. This position does nothing more for the client who is laying down and may obstruct breathing because of the client lying partially on the abdomen. Therefore, option (d) can be eliminated. The correct answer is option (b) (Ignatavicius & Bayne, 1991; p. 2090; Perry & Potter, 1986; pp. 899, 1272).

4. If the client is ambulating, he will be in an upright position. Gravity will help the urine drain better than if the client is laying flat. Therefore, bladder distension and pressure should not occur, thus eliminating option (a). In order to change the client to a condom catheter, the indwelling catheter would need to be removed and there is no order to do so. Condom catheters are not used for the same reasons as indwelling catheters so the two are not necessarily interchangeable, thus eliminating option (b). If the client pulls on the catheter, damage to the urethral meatus may occur. Discomfort should be reported to the nurse for assessment. This eliminates option (c). Placing the catheter bag below the bladder level assists in promoting proper bladder drainage by gravity (option d). This is the correct answer (Perry & Potter, 1986; pp. 786-787, 804).

5. Let's look at the options. Instilling air (option a) and listening for a popping sound as the air comes into the abdomen is not always a correct indication of proper tube placement. Tube aspiration (option b) might show stomach contents but is not failproof. Placing the tube in water (option c) and observing for bubbles may show possible placement in lungs but, again, does not always indicate proper placement. Often options (a), (b), and (c) are performed by the nurse prior to each substance administration through the tube once option (d) is done. The only absolute way to check tube placement is by x-ray to determine that the tube is not in the lung but is in the stomach (Perry & Potter, 1986; p. 743).

6. If a client complains of dizziness only upon rising, this often relates to a change in the heart's ability to pump blood and compensate for the difference in pressure needed to pump blood in an upward direction (toward the head). Therefore the blood pressure is low. The heart tries to start compensating by pumping more often to force the blood into the head and through the body which is in a different position. Therefore the pulse (number of times the heart beats per minute) is increased. This makes option (c) correct (Ignatavicius & Bayne, 1991; p. 255).

7. The order is for a clean specimen rather than a sterile one. Therefore, catheterizing the infant (option c) would be unnecessarily traumatic. Aspiration from the infant's diaper (option b) would not be clean because the urine is contaminated by germs and debris from the diaper. Clarification (option d) is unnecessary since the specimen can be collected. After the diaper is removed, the infant's perineal area should be cleansed and dried. A plastic collection bag (option a) should be attached to include the perineum so the specimen can be easily collected (Perry & Potter, 1986; p. 1154).

8. Clients with an intestinal obstruction may have pain (option a) because the intestine is attempting to move the obstruction. However, abdominal pain may also occur for other reasons. Also, pain may not be present. Cramping is

evident early in the obstruction which then becomes pronounced then actually lessens as the obstruction becomes more severe unless complications such as peritonitis develop. Vomiting (option c) may occur because the body will still try to rid itself of wastes. Since the wastes cannot move past the obstruction, the body forces them upward by reverse peristalsis. Vomiting then occurs which lessens the pain. However, vomiting can also occur with other disorders. Fever of 100° F (37.8° C) generally occurs with obstruction. It may be higher if peritonitis occurs. However, fever may be due to other reasons as well. Abdominal distension is the symptom most significant of intestinal obstruction because it most often is the chief symptom since waste and flatus cause distension of the intestine. Fatigued intestines no longer have the ability to push its contents toward the rectum. All other symptoms (pain, vomiting, fever) result from the fatigued intestines and abdominal distension (Ignatavicius & Bayne, 1991; pp. 1395-1396).

9. The major complications of cataract extraction include increased intraocular pressure, infection, bleeding and retinal detachment. Increased intraocular pressure can cause trauma to the operative site. Ways to increase intraocular pressure include bending and lifting heavy objects such as grandchildren (option d). Retinal detachment and bleeding may also be caused by bending and lifting. Infection may be caused by soap and water from the shower (option b). Trauma and injury to the eye is a problem which can be prevented by wearing protective glasses during the day and the eye shield at night (option c). Hair may not be washed using the conventional method of bending over the sink with the head forward. However the head may be tilted back as in a beauty shop (option a) as long as care is taken to protect the eye (Ignatavicius & Bayne, 1991; pp. 1044-1045).

10. The nursing diagnosis is powerlessness related to unpredictable changes in bowel status. Therefore the nursing goal and actions would relate to that diagnosis. Restricting dietary fiber (option a) is generally unwise since fiber will assist with regular bowel habits. The exception may occur if certain foods cause unpleasant bowel changes so the client should try to keep track of this information. Exercise is an effective way to deal with the stress that may cause diarrhea so limiting exercise (option b) may be counterproductive. Changing coping techniques (option d) may be a way of dealing with the stress related to bowel changes. However, the client will not know what assists and what does not assist with stress reduction until a pattern of coping skills is noted. Predictability and change to promote positive coping cannot occur until a correlation is noted among the life event, coping technique and bowel status. This is probably best accomplished by writing a diary over a period of time to note patterns of what life event (e.g., stress, diet) is related to the bowel changes as well as effective coping skills. Then further changes in coping and lifestyle may be made to

increase predictability and promote feelings of control (Ignatavicius & Bayne, 1991; pp. 1366-1368).

11. Anaphylaxis is a type of shock reaction resulting from a severe reaction to an allergen like an insect bite. The major crisis occurs from airway problems with 70% of death resulting from respiratory failure. The first priority then (notice the key words, "initial goal") is to maintain a patent airway. If the airway is clear on arrival to the emergency room, nasal oxygen should be started at 5 to 10 liters. Very frequent assessment should be continued as the airway problems could worsen rapidly to the point where intubation is necessary. Helping the client stay calm (option a) may be difficult since apprehension is a symptom of anaphylaxis. The anxiety level should be kept as low as possible to assist with airway maintenance and because the client will probably be frightened of the activity in the room and the fear of dying. Pruritus (option c) will be relieved after antihistamine medication is given. Pruritus is not life threatening. The physician will need to be notified (option d) immediately so medication to reverse the anaphylaxis can be ordered but emergency airway procedures should be instituted as a life saving measure until the physician arrives (Ignatavicius & Bayne, 1991; pp. 654-655).

12. In this example, the question is asking which option is true about gestational diabetes. With changing insulin requirements, an insulin pump (option a) may not be as sensitive to the client's needs. Glucose regulation is just as easily managed through traditional glucose monitoring and insulin administration. Oral hypoglycemics (option b) cross placental barriers and can be toxic to the fetus. Pregnancy is continued until term (option d) because of the threat of respiratory distress syndrome. The fetus and mother are closely monitored for problems associated with the pregnancy. Breast-feeding in all clients is encouraged (option c) because of the benefit to mother and baby. Insulin requirements may be lower because glucose is converted to lactose at the breast and increased energy is expended due to production of milk (Olds, London & Ladewig; pp. 457-459).

13. The question here is asking what you know about an ileostomy. Since the contents in the ileum do not have bulk and water has not been reabsorbed (a function of the colon which is below the ileum and no longer functional), the ileostomy drainage will be loose or pasty and will be almost constant. Therefore bowel retraining (option a) will be ineffective. Diet (option c) will not make a difference in the drainage because the function of the ileum will change only slightly. The ileum does some changing over time based on its new role. The small intestine will absorb some water and sodium so the consistency of the stool is less loose and becomes pasty. However, the drainage remains constant and a pouch should be worn at all times (option b). A visit from an ostomy support group (option d) is usually helpful but the nurse can and should answer the question being asked by the client. Option (d) is an example of knowing the

nurse's scope of practice and not giving our practice away. Therefore, option (b) is the correct answer (Ignatavicius & Bayne, 1991; p. 1356).

14. In this question, it is probably helpful to first sequence the events. The client had an arm fracture that required surgery for proper bone realignment (reduction). Following the reduction, an arm cast was applied. The post-operative client is brought back to the unit and the nurse continues to assess the arm every one to two hours. Of the four assessment findings (the four options), one is abnormal and requires intervention by the nurse. Which one is it? Think it through. Would the nurse want to find palpable pulses (option a)? Yes, palpable means the nurse can feel the pulse and circulation is adequate to the area. An abnormal finding would be weak or absent pulses signifying lack of blood flow to the area. What about warm skin (option d)? Yes, because circulation is adequate. An abnormal finding would be skin that is cool or cold to touch since warm blood would be blocked from the area. Would throbbing pain (option b) be normal? Yes. The client has just had surgery with manipulation of bone and tissue. Pain would be expected and is usually described as stabbing or throbbing, usually located at the operative (fracture) site. Capillary refill (option c) should be five seconds so this option would be an abnormal finding. Slow capillary refill might be related to swelling or a tightly applied cast and the physician should be made aware (Ignatavicius & Bayne, 1991; p. 788).

15. A decrease in cardiac output means that the blood is not perfusing well to all parts of the body. Oxygen is carried in the blood so if new oxygenated blood is not perfused and old oxygenated blood stays in the tissues the cells will have difficulty functioning and may need rest periods. The condition is also known as fatigue (option a). Palpitations (option b) occur from a change in heart rhythm or an increased force of contraction. A pink face (option c) would be a normal finding and indicates adequate cerebral circulation. Leg pain (option d) generally occurs from venous insufficiency related to blocked veins or incompetent vein valves (Ignatavicius & Bayne, 1992; p. 2091).

REFERENCES

Ignatavicius, D. D. & Bayne, M. V. (1991). Medical-surgical nursing: A nursing process approach. Philadelphia: Saunders.

Lewis, S. M. & Collier, I. C. (1992). Medical-surgical nursing: Assessment and management of clinical problems (3rd ed.). St. Louis: Mosby Year Book.

Olds, S. B., London, M. L. & Ladewig, P. W. (1992). Maternal-newborn nursing: A family-centered approach (4th ed.). Redwood City, CA: Addison-Wesley.

Perry, A. G. & Potter, P. A. (1986). Clinical nursing skills and techniques: Basic, intermediate, and advanced. St. Louis: Mosby.

9

GETTING READY FOR THE NCLEX

Just when you think that you've conquered test taking and graduation is now the light at the end of the tunnel, you learn there is one more big test: the NCLEX (National Council Licensure Examination). This exam is designed to measure minimum competence, knowledge, skills and abilities that are needed to provide safe, effective nursing care at the entry level (Campbell-Warnock, Jones-Dickson & Fields, 1993). All nursing students must pass this exam before they can become licensed as professional registered nurses.

National Council really stands for the National Council of State Boards of Nursing Inc. (NCSBN). One of the functions of this group is to be responsible for the development and administration of the NCLEX. The NCSBN is a not-for-profit organization composed of 62 boards of nursing. These include the fifty United States, the District of Columbia, and the five U.S. territories. Six states (California, Georgia, Louisiana, Texas, Washington, West Virginia) have two boards of nursing: one for registered nurses and one for licensed practical/vocational nurses.

It is important that you understand both how the NCLEX was developed and the thinking behind the development of the test in order to ensure your success on the test. Students who understand what the exam is supposed to test are more successful in preparing for and actually taking the test. The first step in developing the NCLEX involves collecting data on the nursing activities that are performed by a random sample of newly licensed nurses. This is called a job analysis and is conducted every three years by the National Council. Newly-graduated nurses are asked to rate how often they perform certain nursing duties and how critical these duties are to their jobs. The nursing activities data is then categorized into specific categories of the test plan to provide for a distribution of the questions that will measure competency for job performance (Campbell-Warnock, Jones-Dickson & Fields, 1993).

The Test Plan

The NCLEX-RN test plan currently is composed of two dimensions: 1) the five steps of the nursing process (assessment, analysis, planning, implementation, evaluation), and 2) four categories of client needs. (Each NCLEX question will address one phase of the nursing process and one client need.) These categories of client need include:

1. SAFE, EFFECTIVE CARE ENVIRONMENT: The client needs for this category include coordinated care, quality assurance, goal-oriented care, environmental safety, preparation for treatments and procedures, safe, effective treatments and procedures.

2. PHYSIOLOGICAL INTEGRITY: The client needs for this category include physiological adaptation, reduction of risk potential, mobility, comfort, and provision of basic care.

3. PSYCHOSOCIAL INTEGRITY: The client needs for this category include psychosocial adaptation, coping/adaptation.

4. HEALTH PROMOTION AND MAINTENANCE: The client needs for this category include continued growth and development, self-care, integrity of support systems, prevention and early treatment of disease (National Council State Boards of Nursing, Inc., 1991).

NCLEX TEST PLAN

Category	Percentages of Questions per category
Nursing process	
assessment	15-25%
analysis	15-25%
planning	15-25%
implementation	15-25%
evaluation	15-25%
Client Needs	
safe, effective care environment	25-31%
physiological integrity	42-48%
psychosocial integrity	9-15%
health promotion & maintenance	12-18%

(Campbell-Warnock, Jones-Dickson & Fields, 1993)

The actual questions are written according to this test plan by item writers who are selected based on their expertise in writing questions, their clinical experience and their geographic diversity. Expert clinicians and nurse educators from each of the member boards are selected according to strict criteria and work closely with NCLEX test service staff to write test questions. These questions are then tested, reviewed and revised for accuracy, job relatedness, difficulty level, and possible bias. New questions are often used as experimental items on the NCLEX which do not count when scoring the test.

Computer Adaptive Testing: CAT

Currently, the National Council is moving the NCLEX to the computer. As of this writing, the process will be complete early in 1994 (Megel, 1993). At this time, the way that the test is administered and scored will be changed. Some

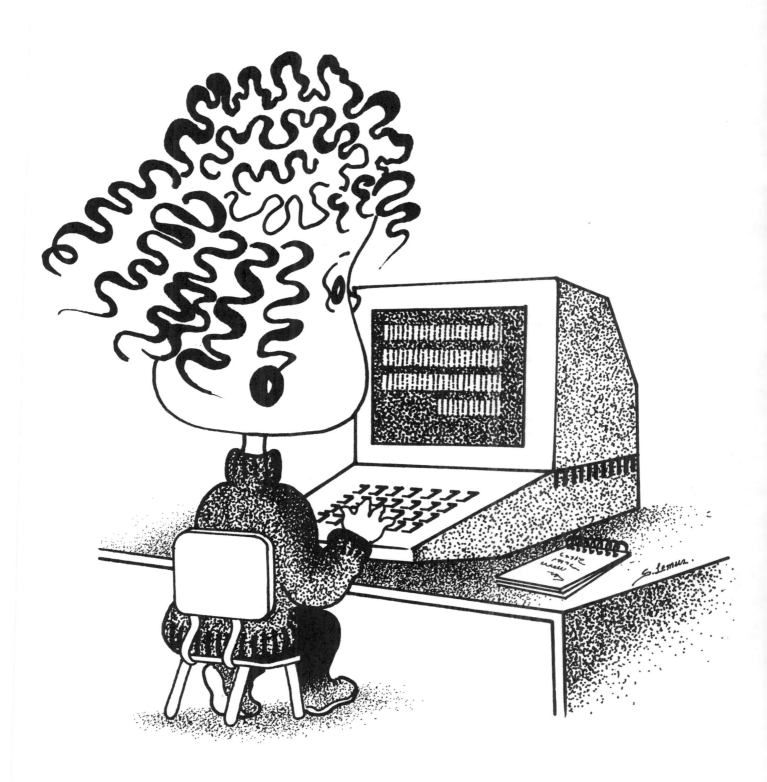

of the basic differences of the computerized test will be the following. The CAT exam is a one day examination which is self-paced and each candidate schedules the test at a specific testing site. Each candidate will sit in an individual carousel with a computer terminal and keyboard. Only two computer keys are needed to take the NCLEX-CAT: the space bar and the enter key. In the beginning, a short tutorial will show you exactly what to expect and what to do. National Council believes that one of the strongest reasons for moving to computer adaptive testing is in the word "adaptive." This adaptive method, in which the test is tailored to each individual candidate, can measure specific information about the true ability level and precise estimate of each candidate's competence. The exam is based on the measurement principle that some questions will be better than others in measuring a candidate's level of competence. Therefore, each candidate's test is unique and is assembled interactively as the person moves through the test. A question is presented on the screen and answered by the candidate. If the question is answered correctly, a higher level question is presented. If the answer is incorrect, a lower level question is given. The level of question given to the candidate is based on the correct and incorrect answers given in the previous questions. In that way, the exam specifically addresses the ability level of each candidate. When the candidate has answered a sufficient number of questions to consistently demonstrate the minimal competence level, the test is completed for that candidate. However, no candidate will answer fewer that 75 questions or more than 265 questions. The maximum time allowed on the computer is five hours. It is important to note that the test plan itself has not changed.

Preparing for the NCLEX

Students often get scared when they prepare for graduation and the NCLEX believing that they must remember everything they learned in their nursing educational program. In actuality, nursing students do begin to prepare for the NCLEX the day they begin nursing school but not in the way they believe. Many students spend many arduous hours and lots of money preparing for the NCLEX. However, preparation does not have to be a horrendous task. Contrary to common belief, the NCLEX is not a test that will measure how much you have memorized in your education. Rather, it is an exam that measures your ability to think and problem solve and put basic principles of nursing into practice in simulated cases. All questions on the NCLEX are multiple choice and most nursing educators attempt to simulate the NCLEX when they create their own tests. Becoming an effective problem solver, thinker and test-taker or learning to think like a nurse, pays the best dividends to help reap the final reward of passing the NCLEX.

In helping students prepare for the NCLEX, we have found that there are certain basic tips that have proven to be most helpful to our students and clients.

1. Practice makes perfect.

As you progress through your nursing educational program, take every opportunity to complete practice NCLEX questions as they pertain to the nursing content you are learning at the time. Remember, you can never do too many NCLEX questions and it is never too soon to start doing them.

2. Know what you need to know.

It is easy to get overwhelmed by the potential amount of material on the NCLEX. Many students make the mistake of trying to go back and relearn every thing they were taught in nursing school. This is an impossible task and will only serve to overwhelm you to the point of being immobilized. Take some time and do a careful and thorough assessment of your strengths and weaknesses and try to develop a plan of action that will specifically help you decrease your weaknesses. First, start with content. What content areas are your strengths? Which areas do you need to review? If at first you are not sure, fall back to Rule 1 and do more NCLEX questions. You will start to see patterns in the questions you miss. For example, while completing comprehensive questions, do you frequently miss pediatric nursing questions? Then just try doing all pediatric nursing questions. Which ones do you miss most frequently? Growth and development? Cardiac? Look for the pattern. Once you have specifically identified those areas you missed, then go back to your textbook and review all of those areas which you have identified. Discriminate in the way you prepare for this test. Use your thinking skills to focus in on the specific areas of weakness to review. If you develop and individualized plan specific to you, you become an active participant in your learning process which will decrease your feelings of being overwhelmed and immobilized.

3. Don't procrastinate.

The earlier you begin to prepare for the NCLEX, the less overwhelming the task will be. We have found that short frequent study periods are much more effective than last minute marathons. It doesn't have to be a separate task. If you reason concepts through as you learn them and do practice questions on those concepts, then you are, in essence, preparing for the NCLEX.

4. Don't study too much.

This may sound like strange advice from nurse educators and, in fact, we are not telling you to forget about your class notes and textbooks. What we are telling you is to review notes and textbooks discriminately. This should only be a part of your study routine. When you spend hours every night reading your class notes and textbooks, you can become what we call "the great pretender;" you are pretending that you really know and understand the information you are reading and can easily apply it to a multitude of clinical situations. In actuality, students are just refreshing this basic factual knowledge at a superficial level and are no closer to being able to apply that knowledge to nursing practice. You are pretending that you really have a good grasp of the information when, in reality, you have become reacquainted with the facts. Often, when we identify students' area of weaknesses, we will ask them to go back and read those areas in their textbooks. Even after they "review" the information, they still have the same difficulties in answering questions or applying the concepts they have just studied. One of the reasons this happens is that it's easier to read the textbook than it is to reason through the concepts and how to apply them. Students feel more comfortable when they are able to spout off many facts they have just memorized or read than when they reason through the facts. It is a more uncomfortable feeling doing the reasoning and yet this is exactly what you have to do on the exam and in real life. One other way students try to pretend is in how they do practice questions. Instead of doing a series of practice questions, sometimes students will do one question and go back to see if the answer is correct. Even if they chose an incorrect answer they may fool themselves by telling themselves they knew that and didn't really miss the question. Do a series of 15 to 30 questions and then check all of the answers (honestly) so you can best decide on a plan of action.

In this chapter we have explained the NCLEX and offered suggestions on how to prepare for it. Remember to plan ahead and stick to your plan of action. Use the techniques from previous chapters in learning how to answer questions and "study smart." Especially remember to use the behavioral and cognitive techniques to decrease your anxiety and control your negative thinking. We wish you well in your career and hope this book is helpful to you now and in the future.

REFERENCES

Campbell-Warnock, J., Jones-Dickson, M. A. & Fields, F. (1993). The NCLEX development process: Some things don't change. Issues, special edition, 5, 9-10.

Megel, M. (1993). NCLEX/CAT coming attractions: The beta test. Issues, special edition, 4, 13.

National Council of State Boards of Nursing, Inc. (1991). The NCLEX Process. Chicago: National Council of State Boards of Nursing, Inc.

PRACTICE SESSIONS

with

ANSWERS and RATIONALES

PRACTICE SESSION: 1

Instructions:

Allow yourself 15 minutes to complete the following 15 practice questions. Use a timer to notify yourself when 15 minutes are over so that you are not constantly looking at your watch while completing the questions.

1. Kurt Feldman, 68 years old, is admitted to the hospital for evaluation of chest pain. After the second day of tests the nurse finds Mr. Feldman crying. Mr. Feldman tells the nurse, "Don't mind me, I'm tired. Just leave me alone for a while and I'll be ok." The best reply of the nurse should be:
   a. "I'm sorry to disturb your privacy. I'll leave now."
   b. "Mr. Feldman, I've seen lots of men cry. I understand."
   c. "It must be difficult to go through these tests, Mr. Feldman."
   d. "Something seems to be troubling you. Let's talk."

2. The nurse is documenting Cheyne-Stokes respirations. Which statement provides the best documentation?
   a. A cyclic pattern of breathing increasing in rate and depth, lasting 30-45 seconds, followed by periods of apnea lasting 20 seconds.
   b. Gasping respirations followed by a 10-15 second duration of apnea.
   c. Consistent shallow respirations 24-26 breaths per minute, during periods of exertion.
   d. Absence of respirations for 10 seconds followed by irregular shallow respirations, rate 12 breaths per minute or less.

3. Mrs. Stacy Jordan brings her four month old daughter Polly to the well-baby clinic for an appointment. The nurse assesses that Polly is demonstrating advanced behavior when she notes that Polly:
   a. sits with adequate support.
   b. turns completely over.
   c. grasps objects with both hands.
   d. holds head erect and steady.

4. Mr. Cyril Benjamin, 84 years old, is being treated on the medical unit for pneumonia. He has refused food since the beginning of the illness and a nasogastric tube has been inserted for feeding and medication administration. After the nurse administers the 9 a.m. medication, the client should be placed in what position?
   a. Semi-Fowlers.
   b. Prone.
   c. Flat.
   d. Position of the client's choice.

Situation: Mrs. Emma Berry, 81 years old, is recovering from a cerebral vascular accident (CVA). She has right-sided weakness with minimal use of her right arm and leg. Upon discharge from rehabilitation she is going to live with her daughter and son-in-law. (The next two questions refer to this situation.)

5. Mrs. Berry's daughter says to the nurse, "My mother will probably be able to function at home just like she did before the stroke. Don't you think so?" The best reply of the nurse would be:
   a. "I'm sure you'll manage very well at home."
   b. "You ought to discuss this with the doctor."
   c. "You believe life will be as it was before the CVA?"
   d. "My mother and I had a difficult time getting along when she came to live with me."

6. Mrs. Berry's daughter tells the nurse she is afraid of what will happen when her mother comes home. She doesn't think she'll be able to handle her feelings of her mother "being helpless." The best referral source to assist Mrs. Berry's daughter with her feelings would be:
   a. American Heart Association.
   b. Easter Seal Society.
   c. Reach to Recovery.
   d. National Multiple Sclerosis Society.

7. A client from a traumatic farm accident is brought to the emergency room. The nurse should prepare to approach the client by wearing:
   a. gloves.
   b. gloves and gown.
   c. gloves and goggles.
   d. gloves, gown, mask and goggles.

8. Miyoko Takahara, 23 years old, is pregnant with her first child. She and her husband are attending a prepared child birth class. The nurse explains that the purpose of this program is to:
   a. provide knowledge of body functioning during pregnancy.
   b. assist in prenatal bonding with the infant.
   c. support the husband-wife relationship during pregnancy and labor experiences.
   d. teach proper parenting techniques to make better parents.

9. The nurse assesses a client scheduled for magnetic resonance imaging (MRI). Which finding should be reported?
   a. History of digitalis (Digoxin) therapy.
   b. Legal blindness.
   c. Permanent pacemaker.
   d. History of a stroke.

10. The physician orders morphine gr ½ p.o. now. Pharmacy supplies morphine sulfate (Morphine) gr ¼ tablet. How many tablets will the nurse prepare to administer?
    a. ½ tablet.
    b. 1 tablet.
    c. 1½ tablets.
    d. 2 tablets.

11. Mr. Miguel Ruiz, 57 years old, is scheduled for a carotid endarterectomy. The night before surgery, the physician had Mr. Ruiz sign the operative consent. The next morning, Mr. Ruiz tells the nurse he's not sure he wants to go through with the surgery. The nurse should:
    a. call the physician to come and speak with Mr. Ruiz.
    b. ask Mr. Ruiz to explain his reluctance to have surgery.
    c. explain to Mr. Ruiz that it's normal to be anxious about surgery.
    d. call the operating room and the surgeon to cancel Mr. Ruiz's surgery.

12. Which of the following clients is most likely to refuse a blood transfusion because of religious convictions?
    a. A Seventh Day Adventist, 42 years old, who has active gastrointestinal bleeding from a duodenal ulcer.
    b. A Jehovah's Witness, 29 years old, who is eight weeks pregnant and hemorrhaging profusely.
    c. A Methodist minister, 34 years old, who is severely anemic related to chronic leukemia.
    d. An Orthodox Jew, 75 years old, severely traumatized and bleeding internally following a motor vehicle accident.

13. Mrs. Darla Stock, 37 years old, has been suffering from headaches with increasing severity. Her physician orders a computerized axial tomography (CAT) scan of the head without contrast. The nurse would do which of the following to prepare Mrs. Stock?
    a. Tell Mrs. Stock to wash and dry her hair thoroughly so there will be no interference with electrode placement.
    b. Ask Mrs. Stock if she is allergic to fish or iodine.
    c. Explain to Mrs. Stock that an x-ray beam will take layered pictures of her head.
    d. Teach Mrs. Stock that images on a screen are formed by bouncing radio waves.

14. The nurse is planning medication discharge instructions for a 62 year old man with congestive heart failure. In order to optimize the client's learning, how should the nurse begin the teaching?

    a. Give the client written information which outline his medication actions and side effects.

    b. Ask the client several questions to assess his baseline knowledge level.

    c. Allow him to visualize each of the four different pills he will take daily.

    d. Explain the action and side effects of each medication.

15. A client who had a cardiac catherization was ordered to have his vital signs, peripheral pulses, and catherization site checked every 30 minutes. The nurse felt the client was stable at 3 p.m. and did not check him again until 4:30 p.m. The client hemorrhaged to death and a tort action subsequently filed against the nurse by his family alleged she committed which of the following?

    a. Invasion of privacy.

    b. Felony.

    c. Negligence.

    d. Assault and battery.

STOP You have now completed Practice Session: 1. Now take a few minutes and correct your answers. Calculate your accuracy rate by dividing the number of questions you completed correctly by the total number of questions you completed (15).

Correct answers ÷ total number of questions completed = accuracy rate.

_____ ÷ _____ = _____

PRACTICE SESSION: 1

ANSWERS AND RATIONALES

1. First look at what is happening with the client. The client is upset, makes an excuse for it and tells the nurse to leave. The question asks what the nurse should say to the client. What theory principles can help with thinking this through? What about communication theory? Principles of communication should help determine what a nurse might say. Let's look at the statements and check whether they help or hinder communication. Option (a) says the nurse will leave the client when he is upset. If the nurse leaves, what will be communicated to the client? Probably abandonment so option (a) can be eliminated. Option (b) focuses on the behavior of crying with the assumption the client is embarrassed about it. First of all, you may or may not make the assumption that the client is embarrassed, but, either way, the crying or the embarrassment is not the point. The point of the conversation is to deal with the client's perception of what is happening to him in the hospital. Focusing on the embarrassment will not foster communication. Focusing on what is wrong will get the client talking. Option (c) makes the same assumption as option (b). Option (c) makes the assumption the tests are the problem. In both cases the nurse is guessing at what is wrong with the client. Again, the client's perception and comments are more important. He may be crying

because of something altogether different than what is happening in the hospital. The only option which allows the client to open up and express the problem without bias is option (d). It makes an observation and suggests collaboration and support in a difficult circumstance (Cook & Fontaine, 1991; pp. 14-15, 60-62).

Nursing Process: Implementation
Client Need: Psychosocial Integrity

2. This question asks for a definition of Cheyne-Stokes respirations so name each definition. The correct answer is (a). Cheyne-Stokes respirations are indicative of bilateral lesions deep in the cerebral hemispheres and basal ganglia that also damage the internal capsules. Conditions causing Cheyne-Stokes respirations include increased intracranial pressure, meningitis, congestive heart failure, drug overdose and renal failure. Gasping respirations (option b) involve damage to medullary centers. Gasping respirations may precede impending respiratory arrest. Tachypnea is shallow breathing exceeding 20 breaths per minute (option c). Tachypnea is associated with fever, anxiety, exercise, respiratory insufficiency and lesions in the pons. Apnea (option d) is absence of respirations. Apnea may be the result of various conditions including sleeping disturbances, thoracic muscle dysfunction, neurologic disorders and cardiac arrest (Craven & Hirnle, 1992;

p. 363; Ignatavicius & Bayne, 1991; pp. 929, 2095; Jarvis, 1992; p. 516; Phipps, Long, Woods & Cassmeyer, 1991; pp. 1756, 1782-1783).

Nursing Process: Analysis
Client Need: Physiological Integrity

3. The question is asking the nurse to identify an advanced behavior for four months. That means three behaviors are true for a four month old or younger and one behavior is true for babies older than four months. So let's look to see what behavior fits each of those categories. Even if you don't remember when each baby normally does each of the behaviors, you can answer this question. Look at the behaviors and try to put them in order of developmental appearance. A baby should hold head erect and steady (option d) before doing any of the other behaviors. Babies can usually sit with adequate support (option a) before turning over. They can usually grasp objects with both hands (option c) before turning over. "Turns completely over" (option b) is the last behavior developed and is the advanced behavior (six months) for a four month old baby (Marlow & Redding, 1988; pp. 552-558).

Nursing Process: Analysis
Client Need: Health Promotion & Maintenance

4. Let's look at what has happened with the client. A client has just had a medication administered through the nasogastric tube. What will happen to the medication if the client is placed in each of these positions? If the client is placed in the semi-Fowler position (option a) the medicine will stay down in the stomach and be absorbed into the system. If the client is prone or flat (options b and c) the medicine may flow back in reflux and the client may aspirate the medication. The client may choose (option d) a position which can be dangerous. After medication administration through a nasogastric tube, a client should be maintained in semi-Fowler's or Fowler's position for a minimum of thirty minutes, thus preventing esophageal reflux of the fluids. All other positions mentioned may not allow proper absorption of the medication as well as cause possible regurgitation and aspiration of stomach contents. If a client is uncomfortable in the semi-Fowler's position, the client may be positioned on the right side with head elevated slightly to prevent aspiration (D'Angelo & Welsh, 1988; pp. 85-88).

Nursing Process: Implementation
Client Need: Safe, Effective Care Environment

5. The question again is focusing on communication principles. Let's look at the options. Stating that the daughter will manage well at home (option a) gives a sense of false reassurance to the situation. The nurse does not know how the new living arrangements will affect the family routine. The daughter may decide she should do well based on the nurse's expectations. When problems arise later the daughter may feel guilty and question her abilities since the nurse basically said nothing should go wrong. Telling the daughter to speak with the physician (option b) gives advice to the daughter and also refers her to the

physician when the nurse should respond to this situation. Telling the client's daughter about the nurse's experience (option d) is inappropriate self-disclosure. The correct answer is (c). The nurse uses slightly different words to rephrase the daughter's comment. This technique assists the nurse to validate what was heard and helps the client reflect on what she just said (Stuart & Sundeen, 1991; pp. 121-123).

Nursing Process: Implementation
Client Need: Psychosocial Integrity

6. This question asks for a referral source for someone who has had a stroke. Well, none of the options say the word "stroke" in it. So let's reason it through. A stroke results from a circulatory problem. Do any of the four groups relate to the circulatory system? Yes. The correct answer is (a). The American Heart Association can assist with the stroke recovery needs of all kinds. They sponsor self-help groups to assist stroke clients and care providers with recovery feelings and activities. The Easter Seal Society (option b) may assist with equipment such as wheel-chairs. Reach to Recovery (option c) assists clients after breast removal. The National Multiple Sclerosis Society (option d) assists clients who suffer from multiple sclerosis (Lewis & Collier, 1992; pp. 1390, 1577, 1599).

Nursing Process: Implementation
Client Need: Health Promotion & Maintenance

7. This question asks the nurse how best to approach this client's care. This means the action will be something dealing with the preparation of the nurse. The client has had a traumatic injury resulting in probable contact with blood through invasive procedures and splashing. What guidelines are available to assist with deciding how the nurse should approach the client? The Centers for Disease Control (CDC) suggest gloves, masks and goggles or face shields and gowns (option d). Options (a), (b) and (c) would be insufficient protection against possible transmission of human immuno-deficiency virus (HIV) (Smith & Duell, 1993; p. 15).

Nursing Process: Planning
Client Need: Safe, Effective Care Environment

8. This question asks why a couple should attend a childbirth class. This is a prepared childbirth class so it deals only with pregnancy and birth. Since parenting techniques occur after birth, option (d) can be eliminated. The parents' relationship during pregnancy and labor would involve more than just childbirth such as the changing roles of the family, feelings about the pregnancy, financial considerations, etc., so option (c) can be eliminated. Prenatal bonding is also outside of the scope of childbirth classes so option (b) can be eliminated. The correct answer is (a). The purpose of prepared childbirth classes includes teaching about body changes during pregnancy, labor and birth which has

been proven to provide a more positive attitude towards the whole experience. According to research, improved parent-infant bonding (option b), more stable husband-wife relationship (option c) and teaching parenting techniques (option d) are not supported as resulting from the childbirth classes (May & Mahlmeister, 1994, p. 422).

Nursing Process: Implementation
Client Need: Health Promotion & Maintenance

9. The question states that a client is getting ready for a diagnostic test. If a finding should be reported, then there is probably an answer that is contra-indicated in relation to the diagnostic test. Examine each option to determine if it would interfere with magnetic resonance imaging (MRI) or if an MRI would interfere with the option. Digitalis (Digoxin) therapy (option a) would not interfere with the MRI nor would the MRI do anything to jeopardize a client who is on digitalis (Digoxin) so this option could be eliminated. Legal blindness (option b) or history of stroke (option d) would not constitute a problem so these options could be eliminated. The correct answer is (c). Clients with permanent pacemakers should avoid magnetic fields including nuclear magnetic resonance imaging. The magnetic forces can interrupt functioning of the pacemaker. Medications including digitalis do not affect MRI testing. Clients who are able to communicate and comprehend verbal instructions are candidates for MRI regardless if they are legally blind or have had a stroke. MRI is used frequently to diagnose a stroke

(Ignatavicius & Bayne, 1991; pp. 731, 860).

Nursing Process: Analysis
Client Need: Safe, Effective Care Environment

10. This question is asking for a drug calculation. First look at the two amounts. Try to visualize a circle in your mind and divide it in half and then in quarters. One quarter grain is less than one half grain so you will need more than one tablet. This eliminates options (a) (one half tablet) and (b) (one tablet). It takes two quarters to equal one half so you need twice as many tablets as are supplied by the pharmacy. This means the nurse should administer two tablets (option d) thus eliminating option (c) (one and one half tablets). The actual calculation would be:

desired dose x volume = correct dose
on hand dose

gr ½ x 1 tablet =
gr ¼

gr 0.5 x 1 = 2
gr 0.25

(Weaver & Koehler, 1992; p. 65).

Nursing Process: Implementation
Client Need: Safe, Effective Care Environment

11. The question concerns a client who has previously consented to surgery and now may not want to have the surgery. What is the nurse's responsibility here? Let's look at the options. The nurse may have to call the physician to come speak with

the client (option a) so we'll keep that as a possibility and see if one of the other options is better. Option (b) says the nurse will ask the client more about his decision. Is it within the nurse's scope of practice to explore the client's decision with him? Yes, communication theory states nurses can do this and it will not alter any circumstances. Should the nurse do this before or after notifying the physician? Well, if the nurse talks to the client, the nurse may assess some information which will be helpful to the physician and client in making any decisions about surgery so calling the physician could wait until after talking to the client so option (a) can be eliminated. Option (c) is a correct statement, it is normal to be anxious about surgery and the nurse could explain that to the client but should also still deal with that anxiety so option (c) can be eliminated. Canceling the surgery (option c) is up to the physician, not within the scope of practice of the nurse so option (d) can be eliminated. The correct answer is (b). The nurse's role is to explore this client's seemingly sudden decision not to have surgery. The nurse may be able to handle this situation by assisting the client to express his concerns, correcting any misinformation and dealing with questions and anxiety of the client and his family. The physician would only need to be called if the client continues to refuse the surgery although the incident should be noted on the chart (Phipps, Long, Woods & Cassmeyer, 1991; pp. 446, 451).

Nursing Process: Implementation
Client Need: Physiological Integrity

12. This question asks who would not consent to a blood transfusion. A key element here is also that the question states the refusal is related to religious convictions. Each of the options states a religion and the client's condition. First eliminate the client conditions and choose an answer based on the religion. If more than one client would refuse based on religion then look at the medical conditions for clarification. The correct answer is (b). Jehovah's Witnesses oppose the use of blood or blood product transfusions as forbidden by God. Each of the other religious denominations (options a, c and d) allow for blood transfusions (Taylor, Lillis & LeMone, 1989; p. 1102).

Nursing Process: Analysis
Client Need: Safe, Effective Care Environment

13. This client is going to have a computerized axial tomography (CAT) scan of the head done and there is preparation involved. Let's reason this through. What will happen in the test? Is any special preparation involved? A CAT scan involves x-ray so she shouldn't have any metal on her head or the film may show it as an abnormality in the head. Nothing else should interfere. Let's look at the options. Option (a) can be eliminated because there are no electrodes with a CAT scan. These instructions may be given to a client undergoing an electro-encephalogram (EEG) which picks up the electrical activity of the brain. The nurse would ask a client if there is an allergy to fish or iodine if a contrast dye will be used with the test. The order is

for a CAT scan without contrast so no dye will be given thus eliminating option (b). Taking layered pictures of the head is what will happen with a CAT scan and client teaching is important so we will consider option (c) until we read the next answer. Images formed by bouncing radio waves is true for a magnetic resonance imaging (MRI) scan thus eliminating option (d). The correct answer is (c). A computerized axial tomography (CAT) scan of the brain is a noninvasive procedure which x-rays the head in successive layers. The test may be accomplished with or without a contrast dye. If the client suffers from claustrophobia, medication may be necessary since the machine surrounds the client's head (Bullock & Rosendahl, 1988; pp. 828-829).

Nursing Process: Implementation
Client Need: Safe, Effective Care Environment

14. The situation is about a 62 year old man receiving discharge teaching. What theory principles are available to help guide our thinking and reasoning in this situation? Teaching-learning principles can be used here. The question also stipulates that this is the beginning of the teaching. That means one answer should happen before all of the others. Giving written information (option a) might be a correct answer but may not be first so we'll go on to the next option. Assessing what the client knows (option b) is definitely a principle and would happen very early in client teaching. Assessing present knowledge would occur before giving written information so we can eliminate option (a). Visualizing the medications (option c) is a good principle but would also come after assessing baseline knowledge so we can eliminate option (c). Explaining action and side effects (option d) would also be a part of teaching but would occur after assessing baseline knowledge so option (d) is eliminated. The correct answer is (b). Before beginning formal teaching, the nurse must first assess many factors including: developmental aspects of functioning, level of education, past experiences with learning, physical condition, and emotional well-being (Taylor, Lillis & LeMone, 1989; pp. 362-364).

Nursing Process: Assessment
Client Need: Health Promotion & Maintenance

15. This question describes a situation where a nurse was supposed to check a client every 30 minutes. A one hour and 30 minute gap occurred between 3 p.m. and 4:30 p.m. when the nurse did not check the client. This nurse did not properly supervise her client's care and the client died as a result. Which of the options is defined by this lack of supervision? Invasion of privacy (option a) is an intentional tort wherein confidential information is imparted to an inappropriate third party. There was no breach of confidentiality described as part of the situation so this option is eliminated. A felony (option b) is a charge brought by the state against a defendant. In this case the lawsuit was filed by the deceased client's family as a civil tort so option (b) is eliminated. Assault and battery (option d) is an intentional tort wherein a person threatens and carries out unlawful

touching. This was not described in the situation so option (d) is eliminated. The correct answer is (c). Negligence, an intentional tort, is an act of omission, not acting in a reasonably prudent manner. In this case, a reasonably prudent nurse would have assessed the client as ordered (every 30 minutes) following the procedure (Craven & Hirnle, 1992; pp. 49-51).

Nursing Process: Evaluation
Client Need: Safe, Effective Care Environment

PRACTICE SESSION: 2

Instructions:

Allow yourself 15 minutes to complete the following 15 practice questions. Use a timer to notify yourself when 15 minutes are over so that you are not constantly looking at your watch while completing the questions.

---

1. A client is diagnosed with malnutrition. Which nursing diagnosis should be included on the nursing care plan?
   a. Fluid volume excess related to overhydration.
   b. Potential for infection related to decreased immune response.
   c. Alteration in nutrition: more than body requirements related to dysfunctional eating patterns.
   d. Alteration in body image related to weight gain.

2. An adult female client is admitted to a rehabilitation unit with the diagnosis of polymyositis. A serum creatinine phosphokinase (CPK) was ordered along with other serum enzymes. When the laboratory calls the results to the unit, the nurse will expect the serum CPK level to be:
   a. elevated.
   b. within the normal range.
   c. decreased.
   d. dependent upon other enzyme levels.

3. A 36 year old female comes into the outpatient clinic for a baseline mammogram. A breast exam and teaching of self breast exam were performed by the nurse. Which of the following responses demonstrates an understanding of regular self breast exams?
   a. "I seldom check myself in the shower."
   b. "I will check my left breast with my left hand using small circles."
   c. "I'll start again one week after I have my baby."
   d. "I should check my breasts a few days after my period."

4. The nurse is charting a narrative note on a woman admitted with vascular insufficiency. As she completes the note, the nurse realizes that she forgot to assess the client's right groin pressure dressing from the arteriogram of the previous day. The appropriate action of the nurse would be to:
   a. leave the nurse's note unsigned, assess the dressing, then complete the note with assessment findings and signature.
   b. draw a single line through each line of the nurse's note, write "error" and her signature, then assess the dressing.
   c. sign the note she has written, then assess the dressing and add an additional timed entry with a new signature.
   d. destroy the entire note by tearing it up, then write a new note after properly assessing the client.

5. A 72 year old male states he wants to stay mentally and physically active especially since his spouse has "passed on." The nurse would plan to discuss which activity with the client?
   a. Bowling with a group from church.
   b. Walking while listening to music.
   c. A subscription for large print books.
   d. Stretching exercises to a videotape.

6. The nurse is speaking to a senior citizen's group. A 56 year old woman asks how to prevent becoming a "hump back" like her mother. The nurse's best response would be:
   a. "After menopause there is no way to prevent osteoporosis."
   b. "Estrogen supplements tend to decrease calcium reserves."
   c. "Daily exercise helps to increase bone strength."
   d. "This disease is almost the same as rickets."

7. Many personality development theorists believe that individuals with antisocial personality disorders have difficulty with the separation-individuation stage of development (18-36 months) and therefore do not obtain object constancy. The nurse knows that object constancy is the ability to understand:
   a. that the self and mother are two separate entities.
   b. that mother still exists even when the child cannot see her.
   c. that withdrawal of emotions is a means of manipulation.
   d. that they are physically able to walk away from mother.

8. The nurse administers isophane (NPH) insulin 15 units subcutaneously to a client at 7 a.m. What is the approximate time of onset for isophane (NPH) insulin?
   a. 1-1½ hours.
   b. 2-5 hours.
   c. 4-6 hours.
   d. 7-15 hours.

9. Mrs. Susan Blake, 42 years old, is admitted for tests for abdominal pain and fever of unknown origin. She is ordered a cholecystogram. The nurse administers the radiopaque drug. The client asks why she has to take these pills. The best reply of the nurse would be that the pills:
   a. help decompress the liver to improve its function.
   b. prevent bile leakage during the test.
   c. are given to people who are allergic to iodine.
   d. help to determine functioning of the gall bladder.

Situation:
Jerry Maddux, 7 years old, has come to the pediatric clinic with complaints of a sore throat, cough, malaise and low grade fever. He is accompanied by his mother and 4 year old sister. (The next three questions refer to this situation.)

10. The physician orders a throat culture. The nurse would take the throat culture from the:
    a. papillae.
    b. uvula.
    c. pharynx.
    d. sinus.

11. Jerry's mother should be given which of the following instructions for Jerry's care?
    a. Encourage activity to distract Jerry from throat pain.
    b. Jerry can play freely with his younger sister.
    c. Jerry should not be given cough syrups or analgesics.
    d. Jerry should drink fluids of at least 2500 ml per day.

12. Jerry's mother calls for the throat culture report. The nurse notes that the causative agent is group A streptococcus and that Jerry is on penicillin. The priority action of the nurse would be to:
    a. tell Jerry's mother to continue giving the penicillin to Jerry.
    b. instruct Jerry's mother to bring all family members to the office for throat cultures.
    c. suggest to the mother that Jerry's sister should begin taking penicillin until she can be checked.
    d. inform Jerry's mother that testing for kidney and heart problems will be necessary after Jerry recovers.

13. The nurse performs a urine specific gravity every four hours on a post-operative client. The nurse is assessing for possible:
    a. infection.
    b. blood volume loss.
    c. dehydration.
    d. urine output.

14. An elderly woman is being returned to home after hospitalization for debridement of a decubitus ulcer. The nurse should teach the family that the best way to prevent a decubitus ulcer is to:
    a. maintain proper body alignment.
    b. do passive range of motion exercises.
    c. keep the skin clean and dry.
    d. place tincture of benzoin on reddened pressure areas.

15. A client hospitalized for two weeks in the rehabilitation unit says to the nurse, "I don't know what I'll do without you when I go home." The best response by the nurse would be:
    a. "You've been doing very well here in the hospital and will do well at home, too."
    b. "I expect you'll function as well at home as you do here in the hospital."
    c. "You can call here as much as you want after you go home."
    d. "What specific kinds of problems do you think you'll have at home?"

STOP You have now completed Practice Session: 2. Now take a few minutes and correct your answers. Calculate your accuracy rate by dividing the number of questions you completed correctly by the total number of questions you completed (15).

Correct answers ÷ total number of questions completed = accuracy rate.

_____ ÷ _____ = _____

ANSWERS AND RATIONALES

1. When addressing this question, keep in mind the signs and symptoms of malnutrition. Remember that both parts of the nursing diagnosis will have to be right for the answer to be correct. If part of the answer is wrong, even if you like the other part, the whole answer is wrong. Let's look at the options. Would fluid volume excess (option a) be related to malnutrition? Probably not. Malnutrition usually results in a fluid volume deficit due to dehydration so option (a) can be eliminated. Potential for infection (option b) is a possibility since there would be a lowered immune capacity so we can save that until we look at the other answers. There would be an alteration in nutrition (option c) and there would probably be dysfunctional eating patterns for malnutrition but it would be less than body requirements (not more than) related to an inadequate caloric intake. Option (c) is eliminated because part of the answer is wrong. An alteration in body image (option d) would be true but it would be related to weight loss and muscle wasting. The client does not gain weight in a malnourished state so this option is eliminated. The correct answer is (b). A major complication of malnutrition is a decreased immune response. The client is at high risk for infection due to decreased lymphocyte production, primarily T-cells. Lymphocytes are proteins. When protein is deficient, this leads to decreased cellular immune function. Medical and surgical asepsis are extremely important in the malnourished client (Carpenito, 1992; pp. 390-396, 503-513, 610-613, 719-723; Jarvis, 1992; p. 148; Phipps, Long, Woods & Cassmeyer, 1991; pp. 1256-1257).

Nursing Process: Analysis
Client Need: Safe, Effective Care Environment

2. This question deals with a client who has polymyositis and is ordered a laboratory test. The two must be related so let's figure out how. Well, poly means many. Myositis means an inflammation of some type. The client is on a rehabilitation floor so maybe the skeletal or neuromuscular system is involved. Myo may mean muscles. That means the client has an inflammation of the muscles. Now let's look at the laboratory test ordered. Serum means blood so that's a blood test. Creatinine phosphokinase (CPK) is probably in the muscles since that is what is wrong with the client. If there is an inflammation of the muscles where the CPK is, then there should be some change which means it won't be normal and that eliminates option (b). CPK is not dependent on other enzymes to function so it would be reasonable to assume that its measurement would not be dependent on those enzymes either. That eliminates option (d). The last two options to be considered are elevation of CPK (option a) and decrease of CPK

(option c). In inflammation there is increased activity in the muscle so elevated would be the better choice. The correct answer is (a). Polymyositis is a muscle disorder therefore the CPK level would be increased. The CPK is an enzyme found in high concentrations in the heart and skeletal muscles and in much smaller concentrations in the brain tissue. Since CPK exists in relatively few organs, this test is used as a specific index of injury to the muscle. CPK is a reliable measure of skeletal muscle disease and serum levels are most useful in indicating muscular cellular destruction (Fischbach, 1992; pp. 342-345).

Nursing Process: Analysis
Client Need: Physiological Integrity

3. The question asks which statement shows an understanding of regular self breast exam. This means to choose the one statement that is true about regular self breast exam. The other three will be false. Let's look at the options. The first option, seldom checking self in the shower, is false. Breasts can be checked in the shower. The woman should use circular motion over the breast while it is wet and soapy. Breasts should then be checked in front of the mirror, palpated in upright and supine positions. That eliminates option (a). Checking the left breast with the left hand would be awkward (picture doing this in your mind) and would not allow for a thorough examination of the breast. Using the right hand to check the left breast would be more thorough and easier so option (b) is eliminated. Starting one week after having the baby (option c) implies that the person hasn't

checked her breasts while she was pregnant. Pregnancy does not make a person immune to breast cancer so the woman should continue to perform self breast exams while pregnant, thus eliminating option (d). Checking breasts a few days after the menstrual period would be correct. The correct answer is (d). Regular self breast exam should be performed monthly between the fifth and eighth day of the menstrual cycle with the first day of menses counted as day one (Lewis & Collier, 1992; pp. 1380-1381).

Nursing Process: Evaluation
Client Need: Health Promotion & Maintenance

4. The situation is that the nurse charted the day's note on the client but forgot to assess the dressing. The nurse needs to assess the dressing then chart on it. How should the nurse accomplish this? What would be legally correct in charting this new information? Let's look at the options. The first option (option a) says to leave the note unsigned in the chart while the nurse leaves the chart and goes back to the client's room to check the dressing. There would be no reason to leave the chart unsigned. Besides, documentation should occur chronologically and not be a summation of events so there would be no reason not to sign the note then attend to the client. Option (b) says to draw a line and write "error." Well, the situation doesn't say the note was wrong, just that something more needs to be charted. If there was no error then it shouldn't be documented as an error thus eliminating option (b). Option (c) says to sign the note presently being

written, attend to the client, then chart the new assessment findings. There wouldn't be anything wrong with that so this option is a possibility. Option (d) says to tear up the note and that's illegal to destroy a hospital document so this option is eliminated. The correct answer is (c). Each individual entry into the nurse's note of a client's record should document the time of entry as well as the nurse's signature (Craven & Hirnle, 1992; pp. 153-154; Taylor, Lillis, & LeMone, 1989; p. 310).

Nursing Process: Implementation
Client Need: Safe, Effective Care Environment

5. This question relates to an older adult who wants to stay alert when he no longer has his spouse to be with him. Which activity will meet this client's developmental needs? Criteria here should be based on a physical activity that involves interaction with other people. Let's look at the options. Bowling would be a physical activity and a group from church would be social interaction. Option (a) is a possibility then and we'll keep it in mind as we look at the other options. Walking is a physical activity, listening to music is a mental activity but he's doing it by himself. There is no social interaction so option (b) is eliminated. Large print books will keep him mentally active (option c) but we have no information to suggest he needs large print books. There is also no social interaction nor physical activity so that eliminates option (c). Stretching exercises to a videotape (option d) would be physical activity but there is no social interaction so this option can be eliminated. The correct answer is (a). Bowling is a recreational activity which can provide physical exercise and a source of accomplishment. The church group can provide companionship and social stimulation. Both bowling and group interaction may help fill voids and assist the client toward meeting his goals of mental and physical activity (Bomar, 1989; pp. 226-227).

Nursing Process: Planning
Client Need: Health Promotion & Maintenance

6. In this question the woman doesn't want to become a "hump back" like her mother. Before we can respond to the woman we have to first figure out what this means. A "hump back" would probably relate to a loss of bone mass from osteoporosis. Let's see how we could respond to this person. Option (a) says that after menopause there is no way to prevent osteoporosis. Osteoporosis can be prevented through an intake in dietary calcium before or after menopause so this option is eliminated. Estrogen supplements assist in keeping calcium reserves rather than decreasing them so option (b) is eliminated. Daily exercise tends to strengthen the bone so option (c) is a possibility. Rickets (option d) is not quite the same as osteoporosis. Vitamin D deficiency in adults is known as osteomalacia and is similar to rickets in children. Both diseases result in decreased bone calcification which creates bone softening and deformities. The difference between the two diseases is that epiphyseal growth plates are still open in children but not in adults. The correct answer is (c). "Hump back" or

kyphosis in older adults is usually related to osteoporosis which is a loss of bone substance. The loss results in fractures and wedging vertebrae which may eventually manifest as kyphosis. Osteoporosis may be prevented through increased calcium intake, daily exercise and estrogen replacement (Lewis & Collier, 1992; pp. 1714-1715).

Nursing Process: Implementation
Client Need: Health Promotion & Maintenance

7. This question is asking for the definition of object constancy. In looking at the words we might determine that the person would know an object would remain real whether the person could continue seeing it or not. Let's look at the options. Self and mother being two separate entities (option a) would not define object constancy. The child can begin to differentiate that the mother and the child are two separate entities at approximately six months of age. Option (b) says the child knows the mother is still around even if the child cannot physically see her. This option is close to what we defined as our principle so we'll save it as we go through the other options. Option (c), withdrawal of emotions as a means of manipulation, explains the behavior of the mother that thwarts the child from moving towards healthy individuation. This is opposite to what we are looking for and eliminates this option. Option (d), the child can physically walk away from the mother, occurs prior to the development of object constancy (three to eighteen months) and is a sign of independence so this option is eliminated. The correct answer is (b). Object constancy is the

ability for the child to have a consistent mental image of the mother even when she is not present (Haber, Leach-McMahon, Price-Hoskins & Sideleau, 1992; p. 482).

Nursing Process: Analysis
Client Need: Psychosocial Integrity

8. This question asks in a straightforward way what the onset of action is for isophane (NPH) insulin. This is a knowledge question. You would either know the information or not. If you know the information, choose the answer and move on. If you don't know the answer then make your best guess and move on. Don't waste a lot of time in trying to guess but try to eliminate answers and make an educated guess. Never leave an answer blank. Use your glimmer response or make a guess but always answer it. That way you have at least a 25% chance of getting the answer right instead of a 0% chance of getting it right if you leave it blank. Something is better than nothing. In this case you may know that isophane (NPH) is a long acting insulin so that may help. Notice also that it asks for onset of action, not peak time and not duration time. The correct answer is (a). Onset of time refers to the time frame that it takes for the medication to enter the bloodstream and start to take effect. The onset of subcutaneous isophane (NPH) insulin is one to one and a half hours. Option (b) (2-5 hours) is the peak time for subcutaneous regular insulin. Peak time refers to the time frame that the drug concentration in the plasma increases from zero level and continues to rise until the elimination rate of the drug is equivalent to its rate of absorption.

Option (c) (4-6 hours) is the onset time for ultralente insulin given subcutaneously. Option (d) (7-15 hours) is the peak time of lente insulin given subcutaneously (Reiss & Evans, 1990; pp. 20, 610).

Nursing Process: Analysis
Client Need: Physiological Integrity

9. This client has been given tablets of radiopaque dye and wants to know why she must take them. The question is asking you what the radiopaque dye does. Let's look at the options. The dye is being given for a test: cholecystogram. Chole means gall bladder so this would have nothing to do with the liver which eliminates option (a). Bile leakage shouldn't occur as part of a cholecystogram since this is a noninvasive test, thus eliminating option (b). There is no evidence to suggest this client is allergic to the iodine so option (c) is eliminated. Radiopaque dye might be given to visualize the gall bladder so the correct answer is (d). The pills are a radiopaque dye which is placed for storage in the gall bladder by the liver. If the gall bladder stores the dye in sufficient quantity, then it will be easily visualized on the x-ray. If stones are present, they will be seen as non-visualized areas in the gall bladder. If the gall bladder is not visualized, it is possible that the gall bladder is dysfunctional or more dye needs to be given. Percutaneous trans-hepatic cholangiography is a procedure where the dye is injected straight into the bile duct within the liver and is used to pick up other types of pathology such as an obstructive jaundice. Decompression of the liver may happen as a result of this test which would serve to improve function (option a). Bile leakage, peritonitis and hemorrhage may occur as complications to percutaneous trans-hepatic cholangiography (option b). If allergies to iodine or fish are present, radiopaque dyes are usually contra-indicated (option c) (Phipps, Long, Woods & Cassmeyer, 1991; pp. 1359-1360).

Nursing Process: Implementation
Client Need: Physiological Integrity

10. The question asks specifically from which part of the throat the nurse would take the culture. Let's look at the options. The sinus (option d) is a cavity in the face and is not directly accessed from the mouth so this option can easily be eliminated. Papillae (option a) are the taste receptors (taste buds) located on the tongue, not the throat, so this option can be eliminated. The uvula (option b) is a soft tissue protrusion from the upper portion of the mouth rather than the posterior and is less likely to be infected so this option can be eliminated. The pharynx is often another name for the throat so the correct answer is (c). To take a throat culture, cotton swabs are rubbed over each of the tonsils as well as the posterior of the pharynx. In acute pharyngitis areas of infection generally include the pharyngeal membranes and the tonsils so these areas are necessary to culture (Smeltzer & Bare, 1992; pp. 335-387).

Nursing Process: Implementation
Client Need: Physiological Integrity

11. The mother wants to know how to care for someone with a sore throat. What should the nurse tell her? Let's look at the options. Encouraging activity (option a) might be contraindicated since Jerry is sick so this eliminates option (a). Usually rest periods are encouraged. Jerry could probably play somewhat with his sister (option b) but children of these ages should be supervised. They should not eat or drink from the same cup or utensils. Jerry should be cautioned not to put his fingers in his mouth. He should use tissues when sneezing or coughing to prevent spread of infection. Since there is no evidence of virus, aspirin could be given for throat pain relief. Cough syrups are often used to control cough which further irritates the throat. This eliminates option (c). If Jerry has a fever (remember the situation stated he has a low-grade fever and a sore throat) and an infection he probably should be encouraged to increase his fluids so the correct answer is (d). Jerry's mother should force fluids as much as Jerry can tolerate with a minimum of 2500 ml per day (Smeltzer & Bare, 1992; p. 387).

Nursing Process: Implementation
Client Need: Physiological Integrity

12. There are two key words in this situation. Jerry has streptococcus which is dangerous and contagious; and the stem asks for the priority action. This means several actions may be correct but there is one action that should be performed before the others. Let's look at the options. Option (a) would be true. The nurse would tell Jerry's mother to continue giving the penicillin to Jerry so this is a correct answer.

Let's look to see if there is a higher priority. The nurse probably would instruct that all family members should be tested. Since streptococcus can lead to other problems if not properly treated, option (b) would be the priority over option (a). Let's continue. Telling the mother to give Jerry's penicillin to his sister (option c) would be incorrect. Sharing prescription medications should not be encouraged unless the physician gives specific instructions to do so. Also, other family members are not usually treated with penicillin unless they have positive cultures so option (c) can be eliminated. Family members should be given information about signs and symptoms of complications of streptococcal infections which may include rheumatic fever and nephritis. However, testing would be unnecessary unless these symptoms occur thus eliminating option (d). The correct answer is (b). When one family member is diagnosed with a streptococcal infection all family members should be examined due to the severe complications that can accompany this infection if it is left untreated. Jerry should remain on the penicillin as ordered by the physician (option a) but the priority is to also get other infected family members onto medication since Jerry is already being treated (Smeltzer & Bare, 1992; pp. 386-387).

Nursing Process: Implementation
Client Need: Health Promotion & Maintenance

13. This question asks why urine specific gravity is done on a post-operative client. Urine specific gravity would show if a person has a fluid volume

deficit or a fluid volume excess so let's examine the options. Direct signs of infection would not be evident in a urine specific gravity so option (a) is eliminated. A white blood cell count might show that an infection would be present although this does not usually occur this soon in a post-operative client. Blood volume loss (option b) would be measured by a hematocrit and hemoglobin thus eliminating option (b). Dehydration (option c) might show as a high urine specific gravity since there would be more solute to less water so option (c) is a possibility. Urine output itself would not be measured in a urine specific gravity so option (d) is eliminated. The correct answer is (c). When liquids have been withheld from a diet for a number of hours because of surgery, specific gravity will measure the kidney's ability to concentrate the urine. A high specific gravity can indicate dehydration (fluid volume deficit) (Fischbach, 1992; p. 149-153).

Nursing Process: Assessment
Client Need: Physiological Integrity

14. The question asks what the best way is to prevent a decubitus ulcer. Again, this means that more than one answer may be correct but the best is what we look for. Let's look at the options. Maintaining proper body alignment, option (a), might help but this wouldn't be the first defense against decubiti. Passive range of motion exercises (option b) would help a little with circulation. Actually the primary reason body alignment and range of motion exercises are done is to prevent contractures, thus eliminating options (a) and (b). Keeping the skin clean and dry

(option c) would keep it from being irritated so this is a possibility. Tincture of benzoin (option d) is a medication and it is not within the nurse's scope of practice to suggest medications to a client so option (d) is eliminated. The correct answer is (c). The best way to prevent decubitus ulcers is to make sure the skin is clean and dry so breakdown doesn't occur from noxious substances (Smith & Duell, 1993; pp. 932-935).

Nursing Process: Implementation
Client Need: Health Promotion & Maintenance

15. This question deals with the nurse-client relationship. The client comments about reluctance to leave the nurse. The last phase of the relationship is the termination phase so principles guiding communication in that phase should help us answer this question. Option (a) seems to dismiss the client's concerns. It blocks communication by telling the client everything will turn out alright which is false reassurance. Option (b) does not allow the client to voice what problems she thinks might occur at home that might be different than those encountered in the hospital. This blocks communication thus eliminating option (b). Telling clients to call as much as they want (option c) promotes dependence on the nurse and the hospital. A client should be told how to obtain help if needed but should be encouraged to be independent so option (c) is eliminated. Option (d) asks an open-ended question that keeps the client talking and fosters communication. The correct answer is (d). This answer places the focus back on the client by asking the client to identify specific areas of concern so the

nurse and client can work out the problems (Smith & Duell, 1993; pp. 75-77).

Nursing Process: Implementation
Client Need: Health Promotion & Maintenance

PRACTICE SESSION: 3

Instructions:

Allow yourself 15 minutes to complete the following 15 practice questions. Use a timer to notify yourself when 15 minutes are over so that you are not constantly looking at your watch while completing the questions.

1. Mr. Harry Williamson, 72 years old, is a resident in a nursing home. He is suffering from incontinence. The nurse is planning care. An appropriate nursing order for the plan of care would be:
   a. offer the urinal every two hours.
   b. restrict fluids outside of mealtimes.
   c. change adult diapers at least three times per shift.
   d. keep urinal in place.

2. The nurse is using a hoyer lift to assist a client into a bedside chair. The initial position of the bed should be:
   a. flat in the high position.
   b. flat in the low position.
   c. raised to a sitting position with knee gatch flat.
   d. flat with the client rolled on the side away from the lift.

3. Ms. Marsha Roy, 22 years old, calls the clinic to make an appointment for a gynecological examination and a pap smear. The nurse should instruct her:
   a. to make the appointment during her menstrual period.
   b. to come to the appointment with a full bladder.
   c. not to take any mediation for one day before the appointment.
   d. not to douche within 24 hours of the appointment.

4. An elderly client comes to the senior center for blood pressure screening. He says he feels lonely since he's retired and misses his family who lives in another state. A proper referral for this man would be:
   a. the local mental health agency.
   b. to call the family.
   c. a personal care home.
   d. the foster grandparent program.

5. A client is ordered furosemide (Lasix) 40 mg PO BID. What laboratory value should the nurse assess before administering the medication?
   a. Serum sodium.
   b. Serum iron.
   c. Serum hemoglobin.
   d. Serum CO_2.

6. The nurse is leading a smoking cessation group. A male client starts perspiring, breathing more rapidly and complains of chest pain. The nurse knows the client is wearing a nicotine patch. What other assessment data might be important?
   a. Blood pressure readings have been low this past month.
   b. Heart rate is 96 beats per minute.
   3. The client smoked a cigarette prior to the group session.
   4. The client was unusually silent for most of the group session.

7. A 17 year old male is brought to the emergency department by his mother. He is an insulin dependent diabetic and, according to his mother, has had polyuria, anorexia, nausea and abdominal pain that has gotten worse throughout the day. The nurse notices a fruity odor to his breath. Based on these findings the nurse should suspect which of the following?
   a. Hypoglycemia.
   b. Diabetic ketoacidosis.
   c. Hyperosmolar nonketotic syndrome.
   d. Hypoglycemic ketoacidotic syndrome.

8. The nurse discovered a 72 year old male client, two days post-operative after a transurethral resection of the prostate gland, lying next to his bed on the floor at 4 p.m. All four side rails on the bed were in the upright position at the time. Which entry should be included by the nurse when filling out the incident report?
   a. Client was disoriented, however this is not unusual for an elderly client who undergoes surgery.
   b. Client was found lying on floor next to his bed at 4 p.m. Four side rails on his bed in upright position.
   c. Client probably crawled out the bottom of his bed since all four side rails were in upright position.
   d. Client was confused at the time I found him and seemed to have forgotten about using the nurse call light.

9. A nursing student is practicing percussion with one of her classmates. Which of the following statements indicates a need for further learning?
   a. The purpose of percussion is to transmit vibrations through the bones of the joints.
   b. Movement should be at the wrist.
   c. Tympany is heard when there is a large pneumothorax.
   d. Flatness should be heard when percussing the liver.

10. A client with diabetes mellitus contacts the clinic stating she thinks there is something wrong because she has difficulty getting blood from her finger to use in the blood glucose machine. The best response by the nurse would be:
    a. "Come into the clinic and we'll do a regular blood glucose."
    b. "The blood glucoses may be inaccurate so your physician should be notified."
    c. "How do you prepare to get the drop of blood from your finger?"
    d. "Have you checked the machine for proper calibration?"

11. A nurse is working with a couple who have just lost their baby at delivery. The nurse knows that an intervention that is most helpful in establishing the reality of their loss is to:
    a. focus on other positive aspects of their lives.
    b. allow the parents to see and hold the infant.
    c. encourage the parents not to name the infant.
    d. encourage the parents to discuss their feelings as soon as possible.

12. A client comes to a busy emergency room for treatment and asks the triage nurse how long it will take. The nurse replies, "Oh, you aren't so bad as some of the others. You'll be here a long time yet." Which of the following is the best evaluation of the nurses's statement?
    a. The statement is a correct evaluation of the client's situation.
    b. It belittles the client's need and does little to reassure the client.
    c. It helps the client understand how priorities are made in the emergency room.
    d. The statement offers false reassurance of the client's chances for rapid treatment.

13. Randy, a 15 year old, was recently diagnosed with insulin dependent diabetes mellitus (IDDM). He has been following his diet and exercise program rigidly since his discharge. His glucose levels have been within normal limits. During his last visit to the diabetic clinic he complains to the nurse that he always feels left out. When his friends go out after the game for pizza, he goes home because he can't eat. Which of the following suggestions by the nurse would be most helpful?
    a. Discuss with Randy ways to adjust his insulin doses so he can eat the pizza.
    b. Introduce Randy to a group of teenagers with IDDM who have learned how to deal with situations like his.
    c. Plan a diet with Randy so that on days when he goes out with friends he can take substitute snacks.
    d. Ask Randy to talk more about how he feels when he is left out.

14. Leeann Bearsley, 20 years old, is about to deliver her first child. She states she is having some abdominal contractions and thinks she is in labor. The nurse would assess for which of the following signs of true labor?
    a. Irregular contractions and lightening.
    b. Cervical effacement and weight loss.
    c. Uterine contractions and bloody show.
    d. Ruptured membranes and backache.

15. The physician orders meperidine (Demerol) 75 mg IM with hydroxyzine (Vistaril) 50 mg IM STAT. The pharmacy supplies meperidine (Demerol) 100 mg/ml and hydroxyzine (Vistaril) 50 mg/ml. What will be the total amount of milliliters administered?
    a. 0.75 ml.
    b. 1 ml.
    c. 1.5 ml.
    d. 1.75 ml.

STOP You have now completed Practice Session: 3. Now take a few minutes and correct your answers. Calculate your accuracy rate by dividing the number of questions you completed correctly by the total number of questions you completed (15).

Correct answers ÷ total number of questions completed = accuracy rate.

_____ ÷ _____ = _____

PRACTICE SESSION: 3

ANSWERS AND RATIONALES

1. The question asks what would be appropriate for the care of a client with incontinence. Let's look at the answers. Offering the urinal every two hours (option a) might help with patterning. It doesn't violate any principles so this option is a possibility. Let's look to see if there is a better answer. Option (b) says to restrict fluids. This could cause problems for the client. Restricting fluids will promote fluid volume depletion which may help with incontinence but would also make the client more prone to dehydration. This option can be eliminated. Adult diapers (option c) will prevent changing bedclothes more often but will not assist the client to become continent and may cause other problems such as infection. Also some clients and family members view this as demeaning so this option can be eliminated. Keeping the urinal in place (option d) is a temporary measure that may lead to skin problems if used in the long term so this option can be eliminated. The correct answer is (a). Encouraging voiding every two hours will assist in bladder training and will empty the bladder before it becomes overly full. This would encourage continence and preserve the client's dignity (Lewis & Collier, 1992; p. 1209).

Nursing Process: Planning
Client Need: Physiological Integrity

2. The nurse is using some type of lift to help a client into a chair. The question asks for the initial position of the bed. The key word here is initial. If the nurse has some type of assistive device to help a client into a chair, what would be the first thing that would happen? Let's examine the options. If the bed is flat in the high position, (option a) that might make sense because that is where the nurse will be working with the client. The upright position will help prevent backstrain in the nurse. If the bed is in the low position, (option b) the nurse has to bend over and may hurt the back so we can eliminate this option. If the client is in a sitting position, (option c) the lift will be difficult to place under the client so we can eliminate this option. Option (d) could be correct. Client rolled away from the lift could be true to place the lift under the client. So between options (a) and (d), which would happen first? The correct answer is (a). When placing a client in a hoyer lift, the bed should be flat and in the high position. This position allows turning and positioning without backstrain of the staff. The client is rolled from side to side when positioning the canvas underneath the client. Once the canvas is positioned and the straps are secured to the lift, the client can be placed in the sitting position and placed in the bedside chair (Smith & Duell, 1993; p. 215).

Nursing Process: Implementation
Client Need: Safe, Effective Care Environment

3. This question asks what instructions should be given to a client who is coming for a routine gynecological examination and a pap smear. This can be determined by looking at the options to see if they would interfere in any way with an examination. Making an appointment during the menstrual period (option a) may interfere with visualization and a proper pap smear so the nurse would probably not tell the client to do that; therefore option (a) is eliminated. If the client has a full bladder (option b), this may interfere with a complete examination. The full bladder will make it difficult to palpate the abdomen properly so this option can be eliminated. Medication the day before the appointment (option c) should not interfere with an examination unless they are vaginal medications. However, the answer didn't stipulate the type of medication and all medications will not interfere with the examination so this option can be eliminated. Douching before the appointment (option d) may interfere with the exam because it may cause a change in the cells and will change the pH of the vaginal canal. Option (d) is the correct answer (Ford, 1987; pp. 458-461).

Nursing Process: Implementation
Client Need: Health Promotion & Maintenance

4. The client is lonely because he is retired and does not have work friends or family around him. What would help the client deal the most with his loneliness? Let's examine the options. The local mental health agency (option a) might be true if mental illness was present but there is no evidence of it. Loneliness in these circumstances is normal so this option can be eliminated. Calling the family (option b) would probably be a temporary solution. The client misses his distant family but did not state any problems in maintaining contact or that he wanted more contact so this option can be eliminated. A personal care home (option c) would be inappropriate because this client does not have difficulty in maintaining his home. He asked for some type of social contacts. Older adults need to keep their independence and there is no evidence to suggest he needs assistance for self care. Option (d), the foster grandparent program, would assist the client in meeting his social needs, family needs and give him a sense of purpose. Option (d) meets the client's need for meaningful activity and companionship (Spradley, 1990; pp. 605-607).

Nursing Process: Implementation
Client Need: Health Promotion & Maintenance

5. The question says there is a relationship between furosemide (Lasix) and one of the laboratory tests. Which one? Well, furosemide (Lasix) helps rid the body of fluids so this might be a clue to the answer. Also the medication is potassium wasting so that may be another clue. Let's examine the options. Serum sodium (option a) might be related to the medication since there is a relationship between sodium and fluid retention. The body would want to get rid of sodium so there would be less fluid retention but if the sodium is too low to begin with, the medication could cause extra problems; therefore this option is a possibility. Serum iron

doesn't seem to be related to fluid retention or potassium so option (b) can be eliminated. Serum hemoglobin (option c) deals mainly with the amount of blood in the system as well as oxygen transport and not fluid so this option could be eliminated. Serum carbon dioxide (option d) would be unrelated to fluid retention or potassium so this option can be eliminated. The correct answer is (a). The action of furosemide (Lasix) inhibits the absorption of sodium and chloride from the loop of Henle and the distal renal tubules. Furosemide (Lasix) increases renal excretion of water, sodium, chloride, magnesium, hydrogen, and calcium (Deglin, Vallerand & Russin, 1990; pp. 42, 503, 510, 787).

Nursing Process: Analysis
Client Need: Safe, Effective Care Environment

6. This client is showing certain symptoms, has a nicotine patch and the nurse is assessing him. There is one piece of assessment data that will be significant when combined with the data given in the situation so let's examine the options. Low blood pressure (option a) would not cause these symptoms nor would wearing a nicotine patch cause low blood pressure. Let's move on to the next option. Heart rate is fast (96 beats per minute) but not extremely high. The pulse is in line with the other symptoms the client is showing but does not really add any significant information so this option can be eliminated. Smoking a cigarette (option c) may cause problems if the client is already wearing a nicotine patch which introduces more nicotine into the system.

Lots of nicotine in the system may cause the symptoms being shown by the client so this may be a significant piece of information. Let's continue to see if option (d) is a better answer. The client was very quiet during the session (option d). This may happen if the client was feeling ill as some of the above symptoms started so this would not be more significant than option (c). The correct answer is (c). Smoking while wearing a nicotine patch increases the amount of nicotine in the blood-stream. Nicotine increases epinephrine and norepinephrine in the circulation which increases heart rate and blood pressure as well as causing vasoconstriction. Less oxygen may be circulating, causing pain and possible damage to the myocardium (heart muscle) (Lewis & Collier, 1992; p. 784).

Nursing Process: Analysis
Client Need: Physiological Integrity

7. The client is showing certain symptoms and the question asks the nurse to analyze the data. The client is diabetic so we can first look for the symptoms of low blood sugar and symptoms of high blood sugar. Polyuria (increased urine output), polydipsia (increased thirst), weakness and headache occur when there is too much glucose in the system. The body tries to get rid of the glucose (polyuria), the body craves water to decrease the concentration of the glucose in the system (polydipsia), glucose isn't being burned off and this creates feelings of weakness and headache. The correct answer is (b). Diabetic ketoacidosis (DKA) is caused by a severe insulin deficiency. The lack of insulin results in high glucose and burning of fat for

145

energy. The symptoms of DKA come from both the excess glucose as well as the breakdown of fat. Excess glucose results in polyuria, polydipsia, weakness and headache. The metabolism of fat results in acetone breath, anorexia, nausea, vomiting and abdominal pain. Hyperosmolar nonketotic syndrome (option c) occurs when enough insulin is present to avoid fat breakdown but not enough to prevent high blood glucose. Thus the abdominal, digestive symptoms and the acetone breath would not be present. The symptoms of hypo-glycemia (option a) are: sweating, tremor, tachycardia, nervousness and hunger. Option (d), hypoglycemic ketoacidotic syndrome, does not exist (Smeltzer & Bare, 1992; p. 1050).

Nursing Process: Analysis
Client Need: Physiological Integrity

8. This is a documentation question and asks what should be legally documented after a fall. With legal documentation the note should only include the facts as they were observed and should not include any conclusions, analysis or other insights or comments by the nurse. Let's look at the options. Option (a) draws a conclusion (client was disoriented) and a comment (this is not unusual in an elderly client who undergoes surgery). Actually if this is true then the nurse has just proven negligence because the client was not properly supervised after surgery. If this problem could have been predicted, then the nurse should have acted to prevent it. This option can be eliminated. Option (b) states exactly what was observed. It draws no con-clusions and gives no extra comments so

this option is a possibility. Option (c) states an observation (four side rails in the upright position) but also tries to write a story about what might have happened beforehand to the client. Since there is no evidence to support the conclusion, this option can be eliminated. Option (d) draws a conclusion about what went on but also what the client was probably thinking. Since the nurse has not been taught mindreading in school, this option can be eliminated. The correct answer is (b). Information contained in an incident report should be a factual account of the occurrence and should not offer opinions or conclusions (Ellis & Nowlis, 1989; p. 268; Taylor, Lillis & LeMone, 1989; p. 91).

Nursing Process: Evaluation
Client Need: Safe, Effective Care Environment

9. The question asks which option shows a need for further learning. In other words, one of the options is wrong. Let's look at the options. Is the purpose of percussion (option a) to transmit vibrations through the bones of the joints? Yes, this option is a correct statement and would indicate the learning had taken place so this option can be eliminated. Is it true that movement (option b) should be at the wrist? Yes, this option is a correct statement and would indicate learning had taken place so this option can be eliminated also. Is it true that tympany is heard (option c) when there is a large pneumothorax? Yes, so this is correct and can be eliminated. The last option is probably wrong but we still need to read it to make sure. Is it true that

flatness should be hear (option d) when percussing the liver? No, dullness is heard when percussing the liver. Flatness is heard when percussing the thigh. Option (d) would indicate a need for further learning so it is the correct answer (Bates, 1991; pp. 246-247).

Nursing Process: Evaluation
Client Need: Physiological Integrity

10. The client has problems getting blood from her finger. What should the nurse tell the client to do? Let's look at the options. Doing a regular blood glucose (option a) will get the glucose for the client but won't solve the problem if she can't get blood next time. Since this response does not address the issue, option (a) can be eliminated. There is no evidence to suggest that the blood glucoses are abnormal (option b). Again this does not address the issue so option (b) can be eliminated. Asking how the client gets the blood from her finger (option c) addresses the issue and asks what the client is presently doing. It assesses the situation so this may be a possible correct answer. Checking for proper calibration (option d) focuses on the machine and not on getting blood from the finger. Again, it does not address the issue so option (d) can be eliminated. The correct answer is (c). The client states she cannot obtain the blood to place on the test strip and that is where the intervention should start (Ignatavicius & Bayne, 1991; pp. 1602-1603).

Nursing Process: Implementation
Client Need: Physiological Integrity

11. The question asks which option will help present the reality of the death of the couple's newborn baby. Keep in mind that emotions often run high when reading a question concerning death, especially of a baby. Don't base your answer on what you think you would be able to do (as either the nurse or the client) in that situation but base it on which option will reinforce the reality of the death. Focusing on other aspects of their lives (option a) helps the couple avoid the death, not talk about its reality so option (a) can be eliminated. Allowing the couple to see and hold the dead baby (option b) might be difficult for both the nurse and the couple but it would show the reality of the death so option (b) is a possibility. Encouraging the couple not to name the infant (option c) keeps the death from being real so option (c) can be eliminated. Option (d) seems to force discussion of feelings rather than allowing it to take place naturally so option (d) can be eliminated. The correct answer is (b). When the nurse encourages the parents to see and touch the infant, it helps them accept reality of the infant's death. The parents should be encouraged to name the infant and should be given articles confirming the reality such as an identification bracelet and documentation of the infant's birth. The parents should be given the opportunity to discuss their feelings of loss and grief to promote healing and should not be encouraged to focus on other aspects of their lives which could promote delayed grieving. However, the most important intervention should be helping the parents accept the reality of the infant's

death (Johnson, 1993; p. 725).

Nursing Process: Implementation
Client Need: Health Promotion & Maintenance

12. The nurse makes a statement and the question asks you to evaluate it. This means that one of the evaluations is correct and the others are not. How can we evaluate the statement? Let's use communication theory. The first part of the statement belittles the client as if the client's illness is not important. The second part of the statement makes it seem as though the wait will be so long that something may happen to the client and that the nurse doesn't care since the problem isn't important anyway. This nurse's statement is definitely nontherapeutic. Let's look at the options. We've already determined that the nurse's statement was nontherapeutic so that eliminates option (a). Option (b) looks like it is close to what we decided about the nurse's statement so this is a possibility but let's see if the other options are better and says something we didn't think of. The nurse's statement doesn't really explain anything about priorities except that this client isn't one of them so that eliminates option (c). Reassurance means that the client will feel better and the statement doesn't make the client feel any better so option (d) can be eliminated. The correct answer is (b). The client believes her complaint is valid or would not be seeking treatment. Although the problem may not be very serious, the nurse should refrain from making judgmental statements and help the client understand why she may have to wait while others go ahead of her (Stuart &

Sundeen, 1991; pp. 116, 121).

Nursing Process: Evaluation
Client Need: Psychosocial Integrity

13. This teenage client is expressing his developmental need to be like his peers and also to go out with them. This can be a crucial issue for this client and the nurse because it may make a big difference in the compliance level of the client as well as his future health status. How can the nurse help this client adjust, meet his developmental needs and also stay healthy? Let's look at the options. Adjusting the insulin dose (option a) should be done by the physician. The nurse should not encourage clients to "play" with their medications or future problems could occur. This eliminates option (a). Introducing the client to a group of his peers with the same problems (option b) is a possibility since it would meet his social, developmental and treatment needs. Taking substitute snacks (option c) could draw attention to the fact the client is different and not help meet his needs. Compliance would probably be low. This would be unnecessary since dietary adjustments can be made to accommodate the client's lifestyle. Therefore, option (c) can be eliminated. Asking him to focus on why he feels left out (option d) will probably not further define the problem and may create more troublesome feelings. Now could be the time to take some action so option (d) would be eliminated. The correct answer is (b). Randy is feeling left out. Identification with a peer group who has experienced what he is going through will increase his ability to cope. The group will also help Randy find

ways of planning his diet so he can eat some pizza while out with his friends (Whaley & Wong, 1991; pp. 1821-1826).

Nursing Process: Implementation
Client Need: Health Promotion & Maintenance

14. This question asks which of the signs is true labor. The key word here is true. It means how do you absolutely know this woman is in labor. Let's look at the options. Irregular contractions (option a) may be Braxton Hicks contractions which may occur at any time throughout gestation but usually become more prominent four to six weeks before delivery. Lightening (option a) is when the presenting fetal part engages the pelvis and occurs two to three weeks before true labor begins in primigravidas. Since both parts of option (a) happen before a person goes into true labor then option (a) can be eliminated. Cervical effacement (thinning and shortening of the cervix) occurs late in the pregnancy and is considered a sign of impending labor. Weight loss from loss of body water may result from electrolyte changes late in pregnancy and are considered a sign of impending labor. Both parts of option (b) are signs of impending labor (we're getting closer) but not true labor so option (b) can be eliminated. Uterine contractions and bloody show (option c) are related to true labor so option (c) is a possibility. Ruptured membranes (option d) are also a sign of true labor. Backache (option d) may result from the hormone relaxin which is released to relax pelvic muscles. Lower back pain usually results from muscle strain and postural changes (option d) Since part of option (d) is wrong (backache), this option can be eliminated. The correct answer is (c). The true signs of labor include regular uterine contractions, bloody show, and spontaneous rupture of membranes. Other signs of impending labor include softening and dilation of the cervix, increased vaginal discharge from pelvic congestion and nesting behavior (May & Mahlmeister, 1994; pp. 460-461).

Nursing Process: Assessment
Client Need: Health Promotion & Maintenance

15. This question asks for a drug calculation. Let's take a minute to think this through before we calculate. Meperidine (Demerol) 75 mg is ordered and it comes in 100 mg/ml. That means we won't need a whole ml, we'll only need ¾ of the ml or .75 ml of the meperidine (Demerol). Hydroxyzine (Vistaril) 50 mg is ordered and it comes as 50 mg/ml so we'll need the whole ml for that. We need .75 ml of meperidine (Demerol) and 1 ml of hydroxyzine (Vistaril) which adds up to 1.75 ml or option (d). The calculation is:

$$\frac{\text{desired dose}}{\text{on hand dose}} \times \text{volume} = \text{dose to administer}$$

STEP ONE: meperidine (Demerol)

$$\frac{\text{desired dose}}{\text{on hand dose}} \times \text{volume} =$$

$$\frac{75 \text{ mg}}{100 \text{ mg}} \times 1 \text{ ml} = .75 \text{ ml}$$

STEP TWO: hydroxyzine (Vistaril)

$$\frac{\text{desired dose}}{\text{on hand dose}} \times \text{volume} =$$

$$\frac{50 \text{ mg}}{50 \text{ mg}} \times 1 \text{ ml} = 1 \text{ ml}$$

STEP THREE: Add STEPS ONE and TWO together for total dose to be administered.

$$.75 \text{ ml} + 1 \text{ ml} = \underline{1.75 \text{ ml}}$$

(Weaver & Koehler, 1992; p. 65)

Nursing Process: Implementation
Client Need: Health Promotion & Maintenance

PRACTICE SESSION: 4

Instructions:

Allow yourself 30 minutes to complete the following 30 practice questions. Use a timer to notify yourself when 30 minutes are over so that you are not constantly looking at your watch while completing the questions.

---

1. A 25 year old woman with a history of rheumatic fever is admitted with abdominal pain. The nurse understands that, prior to certain procedures of the diagnostic workup, which of the following medications would be administered to prevent bacterial endocarditis?
   a. Anticoagulant therapy.
   b. Antacid therapy.
   c. Antibiotic therapy.
   d. Antihypertensive therapy.

2. Mrs. Lisa Gabriel, 32 years old, has been newly diagnosed with multiple sclerosis. Mrs. Gabriel asks why the symptoms come and go. The nurse's answer is based on the understanding that multiple sclerosis:
   a. results from increased cholinesterase at the nerve-muscle junction which interferes with the impulse.
   b. is not a neurologic problem but results from atrophied voluntary muscles.
   c. is a degeneration of the brain characterized by plaques and impaired intellectual functioning.
   d. occurs due to demyelinization of the nerves which may slow or block the impulse.

3. The nurse has prepared a medication for a client. The nurse checks the client's identification bracelet, but the bracelet is smudged and is illegible. What action should the nurse take?
   a. Do not administer the medication and document in the nurses' notes.
   b. Hold the medication and notify the doctor immediately.
   c. Report situation to the charge nurse and follow her direction.
   d. Acquire a new identification bracelet and ask the client to state his full name.

SITUATION: Kim Grier, 6 months old, was referred for testing due to recurrent pulmonary infections. She is later diagnosed with cystic fibrosis. (The next two questions refer to this situation.)

4. The nurse is teaching the parents about chest physical therapy. The nurse explains that the purpose of the therapy is to:
   a. reduce the severity of lung infection.
   b. assist in removing mucopurulent drainage.
   c. encourage purse-lip breathing.
   d. provide expectorant therapy.

5. The parents should be taught that which of the following will be necessary as the child grows?
   a. Increased fat intake.
   b. Decreased caloric intake.
   c. Protein supplements.
   d. Pancreatic enzyme supplements.

6. A post-operative client currently on a general diet is discussing her nutritional needs with the nurse. Which of the following breakfast menus should the nurse recommend to optimize wound healing?
   a. Poached egg on toast, sausage, milk and orange juice.
   b. Pancakes with syrup, bacon, and decaffeinated coffee.
   c. Bagel with jelly, applesauce, and 2% milk.
   d. Cereal with milk, banana, and decaffeinated coffee.

7. Mr. Domenick Miller, 62 years old, has had surgery due to esophageal cancer. A percutaneous endoscopic gastrostomy (PEG) tube was inserted for feeding and he was discharged. The home care nurse visits Mr. Miller. He complains of diarrhea and abdominal cramping after feedings. The nurse should further assess:
   a. if blenderized feedings are used.
   b. the temperature of the feedings when taken.
   c. that the head is elevated during the feedings.
   d. if more than 1000 ml of water is given daily.

8. A 30 year old female is admitted to the dermatological unit for treatment of psoriasis. The physician orders tar baths and the nurse educates the client. Which of the following statements by the client indicates that teaching has been successful?
   a. "I should remove excess scales by scrubbing with a soft brush in the shower."
   b. "Tar preparations increase the speed at which normal skin proliferates."
   c. "Tar preparations cure psoriasis in about 30% of the cases."
   d. "Exposure to the sun in combination with tar therapy often improves results."

9. An appropriate nursing diagnosis for a client with a brain tumor is:
   a. cardiac output, increased related to ineffective stimulation.
   b. coping, ineffective individual related to crying and depression.
   c. skin integrity, impaired (actual) related to immobility.
   d. anxiety and fear related to diagnosis and surgery.

10. A manic client is moving and talking rapidly. She moves from one client to another quickly giving tidbits of advice as she goes. When another client turns on the radio, the manic client breaks into song. The priority nursing intervention at this time would be to:
    a. serve the client finger foods that she can carry around with her to prevent malnutrition.
    b. ignore the behavior as it provides secondary gain for the client.
    c. encourage the client to join in activities with other clients for distraction.
    d. decrease the client's environmental stimulation and remove the client from the general unit milieu.

11. A 24-hour urine collection for creatinine clearance was started this morning at 8 a.m. It is now 10:30 p.m. and a urine specimen was accidentally discarded. The best action of the nurse would be to:
    a. encourage the client to drink fluids to increase his urinary output.
    b. change the ending time to 10:30 a.m. the next morning.
    c. continue to collect urine until 8 a.m. the next morning.
    d. start the 24 urine collection over, and the beginning time will be 10:30 p.m.

12. While reviewing the client's chart prior to surgery, the nurse notes that the consent form signed by the client states the procedure to be performed as "open reduction, internal fixation of tibia, left leg." The chart contains an x-ray report which indicates a compound fracture of the right leg and the client currently has traction on her right leg. What should the action of the nurse be in this situation?
    a. Contact the radiology department to verify the x-ray report then correct the form.
    b. Communicate the discrepancy to the surgeon directly and allow him to correct the error.
    c. Notify the operating room so that the surgeon is aware of the discrepancy when the client arrives.
    d. Place a line through the word "left" on the consent form and above it write the word "right".

13. A gravida 1 para 0 client is admitted to the labor suite in active labor. Her vaginal exam reveals she is 6 cm dilated/40% effaced/-1 station with membranes intact. After placing her on the external fetal monitor, the nurse notices that uterine contractions are about every 45 seconds and lasting 2 minutes. The client is calling out very anxiously between uterine contractions, "Help, I just can't take this anymore." The nurse determines the client is in which stage of labor?
a. Stage I, Latent phase.
b. Stage I, Active phase.
c. Stage I, Transition phase.
d. Stage II.

14. A woman at a picnic site yells, "Please help me. I've been stung by a wasp on my arm. I'm allergic." The nurse determines the woman does not have an emergency kit with her. The next step would be to:
a. observe for laryngeal edema.
b. massage the area to dissipate the venom.
c. constrict venous flow with a tourniquet.
d. go to the nearest hospital.

15. A 51 year old male is admitted for a colonoscopy because of suspicious findings on a gastrointestinal series. All of the following steps were done prior to or during the procedure. Which step indicates that the test was done incorrectly?
a. He was premedicated with 10 mg of diazepam (Valium) orally.
b. He was placed in the left Sims position.
c. Air was insufflated into the colon to push mucous from the mucosa.
d. He was given a light supper the evening before the test and clear liquids after midnight.

16. A 75 year old man four days post-operative following a right total hip replacement has just had a massive hemorrhagic cerebral vascular accident (CVA). He is comatose and his respirations are shallow. The charge nurse observes on his chart that he is a Roman Catholic who has not received the sacrament, Anointing of the Sick, during this current hospitalization. In planning further action, the nurse is aware that this sacrament is commonly administered in which situation?
a. Only to clients whose death is imminent.
b. During periods of episodic illness.
c. In conjunction with daily Holy Communion.
d. Following expiration of the client.

154

17. A client is ordered 600 mg of a medication as a one-time dose. It is available in 2 grains (gr) per tablet. How many tablets should be administered?
    a. 3 tablets.
    b. 5 tablets.
    c. 6 tablets.
    d. 10 tablets.

SITUATION: Ms. Andrea Beland, 30 years old, visits her physician with complaints of increased vaginal discharge, perineal itching and dysuria. She is diagnosed with gonorrhea. (The next two questions refer to this situation.)

18. The nurse does health teaching about gonorrhea. The nurse would understand that further teaching is needed when Ms. Beland states:
    a. "I'll need to take this medicine for about a week."
    b. "I probably need to watch where I use the bathroom."
    c. "I should be tested for the AIDS virus."
    d. "I guess I should tell my boyfriend to see a physician."

19. Ms. Beland finds out that she is pregnant. She is worried about the effect of the gonorrhea on her unborn child. The nurse would tell Ms. Beland that:
    a. the fetus will probably be unharmed if the gonorrhea is treated.
    b. the fetus is also infected because gonorrhea passes through the placental barrier.
    c. the child will be healthy if the mother refrains from further sexual contact.
    d. the child will be born with an eye infection which is treated with silver nitrate.

20. Brandon is admitted to the pediatric unit following an emergency appendectomy. On his second day post-operatively, he develops a vesicular pruritic rash on his torso. His temperature is elevated. He has been diagnosed with varicella (chickenpox). After placing Brandon in strict isolation what should the nurse do first?
    a. Call the infection control physician so all the children on the unit can receive zoster immunoglobulin (ZIG).
    b. Determine what children, staff, and visitors have come in contact with Brandon since his admission.
    c. Restrict Brandon's visitors to his parents.
    d. Place the unit on strict respiratory quarantine.

SITUATION: Mr. Marshall Kingston, 40 years old, is admitted to the hospital with flank pain and hematuria. He states he has been unable to sleep due to the excruciating pain. Diagnostic tests indicate renal calculi. It is Mr. Kingston's third admission for removal of kidney stones. (The next two questions refer to this situation.)

21. The physician determines that the stone formation is due to increased uric acid. Prevention of further stone formation would include teaching the client to:
    a. limit dairy products.
    b. prevent urinary tract infections.
    c. take his thiazide diuretic as ordered.
    d. avoid excess protein intake.

22. Mr. Kingston undergoes percutaneous ultrasonic lithotripsy (PUL). The nurse evaluates that the procedure has been successful if:
    a. stone particles are strained from the urine.
    b. bright red blood is evident in the urine.
    c. the urine turns dark red in color.
    d. the client's pain subsides.

23. The nurse is working with a client who is experiencing suicidal ideation. The initial goal in caring for this client is:
    a. maintaining a totally safe hospital environment.
    b. planning specific interventions.
    c. performing a suicidal assessment.
    d. developing a therapeutic relationship.

24. A middle-aged businessman collapses at his office. An ambulance transports him to the emergency room and he is diagnosed as having a cerebrovascular accident (CVA) from unknown causes. Upon admission, the initial action of the nurse would be to:
    a. perform a complete neurological assessment.
    b. orient to surroundings and allay fear.
    c. administer pain medication as ordered.
    d. begin an intravenous infusion and oxygen.

25. A 55 year old female is given a diagnosis of rule out endometrial cancer. Given this diagnosis, the nurse should assess her for which of the following common signs?
    a. Post-menopausal bleeding.
    b. Endometrial cancer is almost always asymptomatic.
    c. Dry thickened skin on the vulva.
    d. Rectal fullness and urinary frequency.

26. When caring for a post-operative client who is receiving patient controlled anesthesia (PCA) via a PCA pump, the nurse understands that the intravenous analgesic is administered:
    a. each time the client consciously pushes the control button.
    b. in small predetermined amounts throughout the day.
    c. by the client in accordance with prescribed dosage limits.
    d. at predetermined dosage intervals throughout the day.

27. Karen Frank, a 2 year old, presents to the pediatric clinic for her annual physical. Mrs. Frank tells the nurse that, although Karen is very healthy and likes to play with her older siblings, she is concerned because all of her other children were talking by now and Karen is not. Which of the following nursing interventions would be most appropriate at this time?
    a. Assess Karen for signs and symptoms of autism.
    b. Tell Mrs. Frank that not all children speak at two years and she need not be concerned.
    c. Encourage the use of language and books at home.
    d. Refer Karen for a complete hearing evaluation.

28. A 22 year old male comes to the outpatient medical clinic for treatment of an upper respiratory infection. After the nurse takes a history, the client becomes embarrassed, looks at the floor and says, "I also want to know how to use a condom." The best action of the nurse would be to:
    a. suggest he come back with his partner for an appointment.
    b. instruct him how to leave a space at the end to catch the semen.
    c. explain condoms cannot be used during a woman's menses.
    d. inform him that condoms are only 50% effective against sexually transmitted diseases.

29. In planning care for a newly admitted chronic schizophrenic client, which factors should be considered by the nurse?
    a. Consistency and reassuring touch.
    b. Meetings with several other clients.
    c. Short meetings spaced throughout the day.
    d. Honesty and direct questioning.

30. A 50 year old female client is admitted to the hospital with a diagnosis of possible hypothyroidism. The nurse should assess her for symptoms of hypothyroidism which include:
    a. hair loss, constipation and bradycardia.
    b. exopthalamos, constipation and fatigue.
    c. weight loss, hair loss and bradycardia.
    d. goiter, bradycardia and nervousness.

STOP You have now completed Practice Session: 4. Now take a few minutes and correct your answers. Calculate your accuracy rate by dividing the number of questions you completed correctly by the total number of questions you completed (30).

Correct answers ÷ total number of questions completed = accuracy rate.

_____ ÷ _____ = _____

PRACTICE SESSION: 4

ANSWERS AND RATIONALES

1. **The correct answer is c.** Individuals with a history of rheumatic fever are susceptible to bacterial endocarditis. Therefore, they must receive prophylactic antibiotics before and after surgical or dental procedures to avoid cardiac complications as well as systemic organ and tissue involvement (options a, b and d) (Black & Matassarin-Jacobs, 1993; p. 1215; Ignatavicius & Bayne, 1991; pp. 2178-2179;).

   Nursing Process: Analysis
   Client Need: Physiological Integrity

2. **The correct answer is d.** Multiple sclerosis results from a demyelinization of the nerve tract in the brain and spinal cord. This creates slowing or blocking of the nerve impulse and what may appear to . be transient symptoms. Myasthenia gravis results from an increased cholinesterase or a decrease in acetylcholine at the muscle-nerve junction which results in interruption of the impulse across that junction (option a). Muscular dystrophy is an atrophy of the voluntary muscles resulting in increasing impairment. It is a muscle disease but does not involve the neural junctions or tracts (option b). Alzheimer's disease is characterized by plaques on the neural fibers of the brain as well as fibrillary tangles. It produces a progressive decline in intellectual, cognitive and physical functioning

(option c) (Phipps, Long, Woods & Cassmeyer, 1991; p. 1826).

Nursing Process: Analysis
Client Need: Physiological Integrity

3. **The correct answer is d.** If an identification bracelet becomes smudged or illegible, the nurse acquires a new one for the client. When asking the client's name, the nurse should not merely speak the name and assume that the client's response indicates that he is the right person. Instead, the nurse asks the client to state his full name. Options (a), (b) and (c) identify the problem, but do not take action to solve the problem (Potter & Perry, 1991; p. 560).

   Nursing Process: Implementation
   Client Need: Safe, Effective Care Environment

4. **The correct answer is b.** The goal of chest physical therapy or postural drainage is to assist in the removal of thick mucopurulent material from the lungs. The therapy includes percussion or cupping over the part of the lung to be drained and then vibrating over that same section while the child exhales. The treatment is used more frequently during pulmonary infection but does not, by itself, make the infection less severe (option a). Antibiotic therapy and inhalation therapy are used to lessen the infection. Purse-lip breathing (option c) is used during exhalation to prevent airway collapse and is part of chest physical therapy. Expectorant therapy

(option d) is often accomplished by use of systemic drugs. It's effects are controversial (Marlow & Redding, 1988; pp. 667-669).

Nursing Process: Implementation
Client Need: Health Promotion & Maintenance

5. **The correct answer is d.** Pancreatic enzyme supplements are necessary due to the viscid secretions of the pancreas and their reduced ability to reach the duodenum caused by the disease process. The usual diet includes increased dietary intake of protein rather than supplements (option c); increased caloric intake (option b) which is often doubled for age; and normal to decreased fat (option a) depending on the child's tolerance (Marlow & Redding, 1988; pp. 654, 669-670).

Nursing Process: Implementation
Client Need: Physiological Integrity

6. **The correct answer is a.** Optimal wound healing is dependent on adequate amounts of calories, proteins, vitamins, minerals, and water. The eggs and sausages are a protein source, while milk contains proteins, carbohydrates, and vitamins. Orange juice is an excellent source of vitamin C and bread is a source of iron and zinc. The other selections (options b, c and d) are deficient in the nutrients vital to wound healing (Ignatavicius & Bayne, 1991; pp. 1165-1168).

Nursing Process: Planning
Client Need: Physiological Integrity

7. **The correct answer is b.** The percutaneous endoscopic gastrostomy (PEG) tube feeding should be administered at room temperature orbody temperature to reduce the possibility of gastrointestinal complaints. Blenderized feedings (option a) may be used and are often pleasing to the client and usually promote good bowel functioning. The client's head should be elevated during the feeding (option c) but this is unrelated to the verbalized complaints. The client should have up to 2500 ml of water daily; less may be related to dehydration and constipation (option d) (Lewis & Collier, 1992; p. 1017).

Nursing Process: Assessment
Client Need: Physiological Integrity

8. **The correct answer is a.** The client should be instructed to remove excess scales in the shower. While tar preparations do not cure psoriasis (option b), they do retard the growth of psoriatic cells. They do not speed the growth of normal cells (option c). Coal tar preparations are photosensitizing and clients should be warned to avoid sun exposure (option d) (Smeltzer & Bare 1992; pp. 1474-1475).

Nursing Process: Evaluation
Client Need: Physiological Integrity

9. **The correct answer is d.** The client with a brain tumor experiences a great deal of fear and anxiety related to the outcome and treatment. Crying, depression and other expressions of emotion should be expected as normal

coping mechanisms (option b). If a brain tumor causes increased intracranial pressure, there may be decreased cardiac output from pressure on the brainstem (option a). If the client becomes unconscious, impaired skin integrity can be a problem (option c) (Ignatavicius & Bayne, 1991; pp. 950, 954; Smeltzer & Bare, 1992; pp. 1656, 1684).

Nursing Process: Analysis
Client Need: Psychosocial Integrity

10. **The correct answer is d.** The manic client is exceptionally vulnerable to a stimulating environment. This client needs a quiet space away from the noise and movements of the other clients. Manic clients' responses to even the slightest stimulus are exaggerated so decreasing stimulation is the first priority. Option (a) is also an important intervention but does not address the client's behavior in this question. Ignoring this behavior (option b) would not be appropriate because the client is not able to meet her own needs at this point and the nurse must provide the decreased environmental stimulus. Option (c) would only increase the already over-stimulated client (Townsend, 1993; p. 372).

Nursing Process: Implementation
Client Need: Psychosocial Integrity

11. **The correct answer is d.** The client's urine is collected for a 24-hour period. The urine is sent to the laboratory for measurement of volume and quantity of creatinine. The 24-hour collection begins after the client urinates. This indicates the time the urine collection begins. All specimens voided by the client during the next 24-hours are collected. Test results are calculated on the basis of the 24-hour output and results will be inaccurate if any specimen is missed. If one voided specimen is accidentally discarded, the 24-hour urine collection must start over again. Option (a) has nothing to do with the measurement of creatinine in the urine because you cannot increase the creatinine in urine by increasing urine volume. Options (b) and (c) will alter the results because results are calculated on the basis of a 24-hour urine output (Pagana & Pagana, 1994; pp. 231-232).

Nursing Process: Implementation
Client Need: Physiological Integrity

12. **The correct answer is b.** It is the responsibility of the physician to obtain informed consent from the client and correct errors on the consent form. The nurse should not alter the signed consent form (options a and d) and the error should be corrected before the client is sent to the operating room (option c) (Loeb, 1992; p. 53).

Nursing Process: Implementation
Client Need: Safe, Effective Care Environment

13. **The correct answer is b.** In stage I, active phase, the cervix dilates from 3 cm to 8 cm and fetal descent is progressive. The first stage, stage I latent phase, (option a) is defined by cervical dilatation from 0-3 cm, effacement begins and there is usually little or no fetal descent for a gravida 1 para 0 client. Stage I, transition phase, (option c), is defined as change in cervix from 8 to 10 cms. Fetal descent

progresses quickly and effacement is complete by the end of this stage. The client is also in a very anxious state and may begin to fear loss of control as the pressure changes in the uterus are great from fetal descent and the intensity of the uterine contraction is very forceful. In option (d), stage II is known as "the pushing stage." This stage is defined from where the cervix is completely dilated to the birth of the infant (Ladewig, London & Olds, 1990; p. 378).

Nursing Process: Analysis
Client Need: Health Promotion & Maintenance

14. **The correct answer is c.** If a person is allergic to insect stings and anaphylaxis is a possibility, this constitutes an emergency situation. If an emergency kit is available, the epinephrine should be administered. Massaging the site of the epinephrine injection will help to hasten absorption. The stinger should be removed but massaging or squeezing at the sting site may inject more of the venom (option b). The sting site should be cleansed and ice applied to slow the reaction time. Since the sting is on the arm, a tourniquet should be applied to constrict venous and lymphatic flow. The client should then be taken to the nearest emergency room for treatment and observation (option d). Laryngeal edema (option a) may occur, but immediate treatment could lessen the reaction (Smeltzer & Bare, 1992; pp. 1968-1969).

Nursing Process: Implementation
Client Need: Safe, Effective Care Environment

15. **The correct answer is d.** This indicates that the test was done incorrectly. Clients are usually NPO for at least 8 hours prior to the procedure. They usually are on clear liquids for only two days beforehand. It is usual to premedicate with diazepam (Valium) (option a). The left Sims position (option b) is normal. Air is used (option c) to push mucous away for better visualization (Black & Matassarin-Jacobs, 1993; pp. 1568-1569).

Nursing Process: Evaluation
Client Need: Physiological Integrity

16. **The correct answer is b.** This Roman Catholic sacrament may be administered more than once to an individual, but usually only once during each period of illness (option c). The sacrament is usually administered to the living (option d), and is not only administered to those who are about to die (option a) (Ellis & Nowlis, 1989; pp. 488-489).

Nursing Process: Planning
Client Need: Safe, Effective Care Environment

17. **The correct answer is b.**
First, convert the units into the same measurements:

$$1 \text{ gr} = 60 \text{ mg}$$

$$\frac{2 \text{ gr}}{X \text{ mg}} = \frac{1 \text{ gr}}{60 \text{ mg}}$$

$$X = 60 \times 2 = 120 \text{ mg}$$

Second, calculate the dosage by setting up the proportion:

$$\frac{600 \text{ mg}}{X \text{ tabs}} = \frac{120 \text{ mg}}{1 \text{ tab}}$$

$$120 \, X = 600$$

$$X = \frac{600}{120} = 5 \text{ tabs}$$

(D'Anqelo & Welsh, 1988; p. 55).

Nursing Process: Planning
Client Need: Physiological Integrity

18. **The correct answer is b.** Gonorrhea is a sexually transmitted disease and is not transmitted on inanimate objects. An antibiotic is usually given intramuscularly and followed up by antibiotic treatment for about a week (option a). Clients who have one sexually transmitted disease may have been exposed to other viruses such as HIV or syphilis and testing should be suggested as part of the health teaching (option c). Any sexual partners exposed within the last month should be informed and treated if needed (option d). Clients may find that difficult but the nurse should encourage expression of feelings and emphasize the complications if the infection is not treated. Clients should be given the needed psychosocial support and assured of confidentiality (Ignatavicius & Bayne, 1991; pp. 1783-1785).

Nursing Process: Evaluation
Client Need: Health Promotion & Maintenance

19. **The correct answer is a.** If the gonorrhea is treated appropriately, the baby should be born unharmed. If the mother remains untreated, the baby may be infected during the birth process, not in utero (option b). Most states have laws requiring that a newborn be promptly treated with silver nitrate or an antibiotic to prevent (not treat) eye infection which may be caused by the child passing through an infected vaginal canal (option d). The mother needs only refrain from sexual contact until the gonorrhea is cured unless otherwise contraindicated by complications of the pregnancy or another physical problem (option c) (Ignatavicius & Bayne, 1991; p. 1785).

Nursing Process: Implementation
Client Need: Health Promotion & Maintenance

20. **The correct answer is b.** It is important to find out who was exposed to Brandon since the period of communicability for chickenpox is one day before eruption of lesions to six days after the first crop of vesicles, when crusts have formed. Zoster immunoglobulin (ZIG) is only given to high risk (immunosuppressed) clients who have no history of varicella (option a). Brandon's visitors should be restricted to people who have had chickenpox. Others are susceptible and this may or may not include his parents (option c). There is no need to quarantine the unit for one child with chickenpox until more information is known concerning who was exposed and who is at high risk for infection

(option d)(Whaley & Wong, 1991; pp. 706-707).

Nursing Process: Implementation
Client Need: Physiological Integrity

21. **The correct answer is d.** Uric acid is related to increased protein intake. The client should be cautioned to reduce purines as found in such meats as sardines, venison and liver. Medications such as allopurinol may be used to decrease uric acid. Dairy products (option a) would be limited in treatment of calcium urinary stones. Urinary tract infections (option b) are known to be a factor in struvite urinary calculi and are more common in women than men. Thiazide diuretics (option c) are often used to reduce urinary calcium excretion to prevent renal calculi from calcium compounds (Lewis & Collier, 1992; pp. 1197-1199).

Nursing Process: Implementation
Client Need: Health Promotion & Maintenance

22. **The correct answer is a.** Ultrasonic waves will break up the stone(s). A saline irrigation is used to flush the particles which can then be found by straining the urine. Bright red bleeding (option b) and later dark red urine (option c) are expected after lithotripsy procedure but do not indicate the stone has been removed. Absence of pain (option d) may indicate that the stone has moved to where the stone is less irritating but not necessarily is removed (Lewis & Collier, 1992; pp. 1199-1200).

Nursing Process: Evaluation
Client Need: Physiological Integrity

23. **The correct answer is c.** Identification of suicidal clients is the initial goal of nursing care and is done by completing a suicidal assessment. Option (a) is incorrect because it is not a realistic goal; no environment can be totally safe. Options (b) and (d) are interventions that would be appropriate but not the initial goal (Johnson, 1993; p. 743).

Nursing Process: Planning
Client Need: Psychosocial Integrity

24. **The correct answer is a.** The nurse will assess the baseline neurological status (to detect changes) and identify actual and/or potential problems. Once the level of consciousness has been determined it may be necessary to orient the client to the surroundings (option b). Pain medication is usually not given (option c) until the neurological status has been determined because of the medication's effect on the level of consciousness and respiratory system. An intravenous infusion and oxygen may be included in the course of care under a physician's order (option d) (Ignatavicius & Bayne, 1991; p. 882).

Nursing Process: Implementation
Client Need: Physiological Integrity

25. **The correct answer is a.** About half of the women that experience post-menopausal bleeding have cancer of the endometrium. Endometrial cancer is usually not asymptomatic (option b). Cancer of the vulva may present as dry thickened skin (option c). Although rectal fullness and urinary frequency could represent advanced endometrial cancer (option d), they are not common signs (Smeltzer & Bare, 1992; pp. 1279-

1280).

Nursing Process: Assessment
Client Need: Physiological Integrity

26. **The correct answer is c.** The client self-administers small amounts of analgesic by pressing a button attached to the PCA pump. For a pre-set amount of time after the client presses the button, the pump will not release any analgesic (option a). Options (b) and (d) imply that the client does not have any input as to when the analgesic would be released (Black & Matassarin-Jacobs, 1993; pp. 436-438).

Nursing Process: Analysis
Client Need: Safe, Effective Care Environment

27. **The correct answer is d.** Sixty-five percent of a 2 year old's speech is intelligible. If children are not speaking by 2 years it is usually an indication of hearing loss and they need to be further evaluated. Children are able to use multiword sentences such as "Daddy go bye-bye." or "All gone." (option b). Impaired verbal communication is only one symptom of autism. Children with autism have an impairment in social interaction. Karen does not display this impairment (option a). While using language and books at home will increase language use, it is of no help if the child cannot hear (option c) (Whaley & Wong, 1991; pp. 633, 651, 1096-1099).

Nursing Process: Implementation
Client Need: Physiological Integrity

28. **The correct answer is b.** A condom is a thin rubber barrier to sperm. It is fitted along the erect penis with some extra slack left to catch ejaculated semen. Condoms are 85% effective and will form a barrier against sexually transmitted diseases including acquired immune deficiency syndrome (AIDS) (option d). Failure is related to slipping or tearing. Because a condom is thin, sharp objects such as fingernails may cause tearing. Slipping may occur upon withdrawal of penis. Men should be instructed to hold the condom in place during withdrawal. Condoms are not contraindicated during a woman's menses (option c); however, vaginal sponges should not be used during menses. Since the client is asking for information now, teaching would be & most effective at this time (option a) (Lewis & Collier, 1992; pp. 1418-1420).

Nursing Process: Implementation
Client Need: Health Promotion & Maintenance

29. **The correct answer is c.** Schizophrenic clients are often mistrustful and may be unable to tolerate prolonged interpersonal interaction with the nurse. It is usually more therapeutic for the client if the nurse schedules brief but frequent interactions throughout the day. Although a consistent approach is necessary, using touch may increase the client's feelings of mistrust (option a). The client will do better if he is assigned the same person with which to initiate interaction at first, and later gradually encouraging interaction with others (option c). Avoid the use of direct questioning as it may intimidate the client (option d) (Haber, Leach-

McMahon, Price-Hoskins & Sideleau 1992; pp. 533, 536).

Nursing Process: Planning
Client Need: Psychosocial Integrity

30. **The correct answer is a.** The thyroid is responsible for maintaining the body's metabolic rate. Hypothyroidism results in a slowing of body metabolism. Symptoms include: dry skin, hair loss, bradycardia, cold intolerance, weight gain and fatigue. Exopthalamos occurs in hyperthyroidism as does goiter, nervousness, and weight loss (options b, c and d) (Smeltzer & Bare, 1992, p. 1081).

Nursing Process: Assessment
Client Need: Physiological Integrity

PRACTICE SESSION: 5

Instructions:

Allow yourself 30 minutes to complete the following 30 practice questions. Use a timer to notify yourself when 30 minutes are over so that you are not constantly looking at your watch while completing the questions.

1. In morning shift report the charge nurse reports that Mrs. Elaine Manston has a superficial thrombophlebitis at the intravenous site on her arm. The nurse would expect to see what assessment data?
   a. Warm, red, tender area around the intravenous site.
   b. Temperature elevation of 38.3°C (101°F) and leukocytosis.
   c. Positive Homan's sign.
   d. Chest and back pain.

2. A 26 year old female is being treated with chemotherapy for metastatic ovarian cancer. She complains of having severe nausea the whole way in to the office to receive her treatment. Her mother, who drives her to treatment, says that it becomes worse the closer she gets to the office. She has thiethylperazine (Torecan) and lorazepam (Ativan) which she takes as needed at home. Which of the following suggestions by the nurse may help relieve anticipatory nausea?
   a. Instruct her to take thiethylperazine (Torecan) immediately after the treatment when she gets home.
   b. Instruct her to take nothing by mouth (NPO) for twelve hours prior to treatment.
   c. Instruct her to take her prescribed lorazepam (Ativan) prior to leaving the house.
   d. Explain that anticipatory nausea is common and, since it is psychological, no medications will help.

Situation:

Mrs. Rachel Garrett is an 82 year old woman admitted to the hospital because of worsening Alzheimer's Disease. The physician is placing Mrs. Garrett on medication to decrease her wandering behavior and to assist her to sleep at night. Mrs. Garrett is accompanied to the hospital by her husband and their daughter. (The next three questions refer to this situation.)

3. The night of admission, Mrs. Garrett gets out of bed and wanders down the hall. She walks into Mr. Morrison's room and climbs into the empty bed in the same room. Mr. Morrison becomes alarmed and rings for the nurse. The nurse walks into the room and gently wakens Mrs. Garrett. When the nurse attempts to redirect Mrs. Garrett to her room Mrs. Garrett says, "But nurse, why can't I sleep here with my husband?" The best reply by the nurse is:
   a. "It's hard to be in a different place, Mrs. Garrett, let me help you."
   b. "We don't allow men and women to sleep together in the hospital, Mrs. Garrett."
   c. "Mrs. Garrett, your husband is not here. This person is Mr. Morrison."
   d. "If you go back to your room, Mrs. Garrett, I'm sure your husband will visit you shortly."

4. While escorting Mrs. Garrett to her room she states, "Nurse, I don't want to go in there. I want to find my husband. He doesn't know where I am." The best action by the nurse would be to:
   a. orient Mrs. Garrett and ask her to talk about her husband.
   b. suggest that Mrs. Garrett sit up with you in the nurses' station.
   c. inform Mrs. Garrett she must stay in her room or she may be restrained.
   d. ask Mrs. Garrett if she understands the reasons for her admission to the hospital.

5. Fifteen minutes after the nurse sits with Mrs. Garrett, she falls asleep. The best action for the nurse would be to:
   a. place Mrs. Garrett in a soft restraint for the remainder of the night.
   b. check frequently on Mrs. Garrett during the night.
   c. leave the overhead light on so Mrs. Garrett stays oriented.
   d. ask a nursing assistant or family member to remain with Mrs. Garrett through the night.

6. A 56 year old female client diagnosed with congestive heart failure was scheduled to receive furosemide (Lasix) 80 mg intravenously, every other day. Although she had received her furosemide (Lasix) dose the previous day (Tuesday), the nurse mistakenly administered it again the next day (Wednesday). When she notifies the physician, which statement by the nurse best addresses the situation?
   a. "I will document the error in the client's nurse's note, however not the fact that I filed an incident report."
   b. "The incident report is in her chart since it is now part of the permanent record."
   c. "Since the client is stable, I would prefer not to file an incident report noting that I made a medication error."
   d. "I will document that error in the client's nurse's note, as well as the fact that an incident report was filed."

7. Mr. Joseph Cabrizzi, 57 years old, is admitted to the cardiac intensive care unit with a myocardial infarction. Which of the following nursing orders would assist the client to decrease vagal stimulation?
   a. Maintaining bedrest.
   b. Preventing constipation.
   c. Discussing a low cholesterol diet.
   d. Monitoring vital signs.

8. Mrs. Etta Harrison, 50 years old, has a history of emphysema related to cigarette smoking. She has come to the clinic to receive an influenza vaccine. The nurse should not administer the vaccine if Mrs. Harrison:
   a. has never had influenza.
   b. is taking amantadine hydrochloride (Symmetrel).
   c. is allergic to egg protein.
   d. has not been exposed to the influenza virus.

9. Amy, a 5 year old with pneumonia, is placed in a mist tent with oxygen. Which of the following nursing implementations is necessary in the care of Amy?
   a. Change Amy's pajamas and bed linens every twelve hours.
   b. Maintain the oxygen level at 80%.
   c. Open the tent every hour to monitor vital signs.
   d. Tuck the canopy under the mattress and place a folded sheet across the edge.

10. Mr. James Logan, 34 years old, has been ordered a unit of packed red blood cells to be infused today. He has an existing intravenous line. Use of the existing intravenous line would be contraindicated if:
   a. an 18 gauge needle had been originally inserted.
   b. an isotonic saline solution is being infused.
   c. a glucose solution is being infused.
   d. the blood has been chilled prior to use.

11. A 27 year old female comes to the emergency department stating she suddenly came down with chills, high fever, nausea and vomiting. Further assessment reveals palmar rash and third day of menses. Toxic shock syndrome is diagnosed. Upon recovery, the nurse should instruct the client to:
    a. continue using tampons if she desires as long as she alternates them with sanitary pads.
    b. use tampons at night and sanitary pads during the day.
    c. wash her hands thoroughly before inserting a tampon.
    d. discontinue use of tampons until staphylococcus aureus is no longer noted in the vagina.

12. Matthew Weaver, 14 years old, sustained a sprained ankle when he fell during a track meet three weeks ago. He comes to the clinic for a checkup. The nurse should now instruct him to:
    a. remain off his foot for the next three weeks.
    b. use ice to reduce swelling.
    c. keep the dislocated joint immobile.
    d. do warmup exercises to prevent injury.

13. After a ten day hospitalization, a client with schizophrenia is ready for discharge. Which of the following would be most important to include in his discharge teaching?
    a. Teach client and family to report signs such as difficulty sleeping, loss of interest and increased nervousness to the mental health care team.
    b. Teach the family that they are not responsible for the client's progress.
    c. Teach the client and family side effects of prescribed medication so they will be able to regulate drug holidays.
    d. Teach family members the phases of the illness so they will know exactly what to expect.

14. A client is receiving warfarin (Coumadin) 2.5 mg everyday. An increase in which of the following laboratory results would indicate to the nurse that the medication is effective?
    a. Partial thromboplastin time (PTT).
    b. Platelet count.
    c. Prothrombin time (PT)
    d. Fibrin split levels.

15. A woman with myasthenia gravis is admitted to the medical unit. The most common nursing diagnosis would be:
    a. altered nutrition: more than body requirements related to weak jaw muscles.
    b. impaired skin integrity related to immobility.
    c. potential for infection related to respiratory muscle weakness.
    d. impaired physical mobility related to muscle fatigue.

16. The nurse is teaching a client who has been prescribed an antibiotic for a respiratory infection. The most common side effect associated with tobramycin sulfate (Nebcin) administration is:
    a. abdominal cramping.
    b. nephrotoxicity.
    c. blurred vision.
    d. general muscle weakness.

17. A Native American woman and her husband have just been informed that she has a bowel mass which requires surgical intervention. Her husband tells the surgeon they will need additional time to discuss the matter prior to consenting to surgery. Several family members, including the client's parents who have been in the waiting room, see the surgeon leave the room. Based on customary behavior of many in this cultural group, the nurse would expect that:
    a. the couple will be receptive to family consultation regarding the surgery.
    b. family members will want to speak privately to the surgeon.
    c. the nurse will be included in discussions between the couple and their family.
    d. the client and her husband will spend time in quiet meditation together.

18. A psychiatric client tells the nurse that he is really the king of a small country that very few people know about. When the nurse tells the client it's time to go to the dining room for lunch, the client refuses to go stating, "Have my food brought to me. I do not eat with peasants!" An appropriate response by the nurse would be:
    a. "Even kings must eat in the dining room."
    b. "You are not a king and will get no special privileges."
    c. "Alright, your majesty, you may eat in your room for lunch but will have to go to the dining room for dinner."
    d. "Believing that you are a king must help you feel more powerful."

19. The physician ordered 40 mEq of potassium chloride orally, every two hours, times four doses, for an 80 year old client with end stage renal disease. The nurse should:
    a. dilute each dose of potassium chloride in two ounces of water.
    b. administer potassium chloride as ordered, one hour before meals.
    c. prepare parenteral solution of potassium chloride and administer slowly.
    d. hold potassium chloride and clarify the order with the physician.

Situation:

Mr. Phillip Castner, 34 years old, has been complaining of paresthesia of the lower extremities. Further assessment shows beginning paralysis. He is diagnosed with Guillian-Barré Syndrome. (The next two questions refer to this situation.)

20. Which of the following data would be related to the onset of Guillian-Barré Syndrome?
    a. Recently quit cigarette smoking.
    b. History of cardiac problems.
    c. Respiratory infection two weeks ago.
    d. Rheumatic fever as a child.

21. Mr. Castner says to the nurse, "This isn't happening to me! I'll never be able to walk again. It just isn't fair!" The best reply of the nurse would be:
    a. "All of your muscle function will eventually come back."
    b. "Maybe you could talk to someone else who has paralyzed legs."
    c. "Anger won't help you get better. Let's play cards to take your mind off of the problem."
    d. "You have a right to feel angry. How will this affect your life right now?"

22. A 50 year old client is given a diagnosis of hypothyroidism secondary to autoimmune thyroiditis. Because of this diagnosis, which of the following actions should not be a priority in the client's care?
    a. Provide extra blankets.
    b. Provide food high in protein.
    c. Explain the rationale for thyroid replacement therapy.
    d. Provide food high in fiber.

23. Mrs. Sonya Hill, 20 years old, has an infant who was diagnosed with phenylketonuria (PKU). Mrs. Hill states she doesn't think she can follow the diet restrictions and wants to know what will happen if she doesn't. The nurse replies that this will result in:
    a. increased tyrosine levels.
    b. mental retardation.
    c. brown eyes and fair skin.
    d. an acetone breath odor.

24. All of the following medications are ordered for a client. The client has difficulty breathing and the physician requests that the bronchodilator be given immediately. The nurse would administer:
    a. ipratropium (Atrovent).
    b. isoniazid (Isotamine).
    c. isosorbide dinitrate (Isorbid).
    d. isotretinoin (Accutane).

25. A 17 year old is admitted to the inpatient psychiatric unit after the death of her friend related to gang violence. She admits to trying to leave the gang several times but doesn't know what she'll do if she does leave it. The best nursing diagnosis related to this problem is:
    a. fear related to inability to form consistent life values.
    b. impaired social interaction related to social anxiety.
    c. self-esteem disturbance related to gang dependent relationship.
    d. fear related to denial of mortality.

26. A 75 year old man with emphysema is extremely dyspneic. Which of the following positions should the nurse suggest to enhance effective breathing patterns?
    a. Sitting in a recliner chair leaning slightly backward.
    b. Standing while supporting his chest against the wall.
    c. Sitting on edge of bed, arms folded over pillows placed on a nightstand.
    d. Semi-Fowlers position in bed, with knees slightly flexed.

27. The nurse is assisting with debridement of a large contaminated wound. What protective barriers are indicated?
    a. Apron, head wear, gloves if in direct contact with secretions.
    b. Gloves only.
    c. Mask, goggles, gloves, gown.
    d. Shoe covers, mask if within six inches of contaminated area.

28. A 44 year old client becomes quite anxious when he awakens to find himself hospitalized after a car accident. The nurse works to decrease his anxiety level and he becomes calmer. The best nursing strategy to maintain his reduced level of anxiety while hospitalized is to:
    a. provide diversionary activities.
    b. assign personnel to sit with him.
    c. offer him progressive relaxation tapes.
    d. refer him to a social worker for counseling.

29. Mrs. James is one day post-vaginal delivery and is suspected of having a puerperal infection of the episiotomy. The nurse would expect to assess what symptoms?
    a. Skin edges are well approximated, coloration shows bruising on each side of the incision to 0.25 cm bilaterally. The discharge is serum in nature, and edema is localized to the perineal area.
    b. Skin edges are separated and subcutaneous fat visible, minimal serosanguinous drainage noted, coloration shows redness within 0.5 cm of the incision bilaterally with minimal bruising and edema in the perineal area.
    c. Skin edges are separated, coloration shows it's reddened to 0.5 cm of incision bilaterally, edematous from vulva to perineum, draining an odorous sanguinous liquid with musculature visible.
    d. The nurse can't locate the episiotomy on the perineum as the edges are well approximated, and there is no redness or bruising noted.

30. A 28 year old white female was referred to the oncology outpatient services for evaluation of a suspicious area on the lower leg. If the area is cancerous, the nurse would expect to find:
    a. an area of dry, scaly, pruritic skin.
    b. a raised, brown, lesion 2 mm in diameter.
    c. a 3 mm circular, flat lesion that blanches to pressure.
    d. a 3 mm black and brown lesion, irregular borders.

STOP You have now completed Practice Session: 5. Now take a few minutes and correct your answers. Calculate your accuracy rate by dividing the number of questions you completed correctly by the total number of questions you completed (30).

Correct answers ÷ total number of questions completed = accuracy rate.

_____ ÷ _____ = _____

PRACTICE SESSION: 5

ANSWERS AND RATIONALES

1. **The correct answer is a.** The most common cause of superficial thrombophlebitis in the arms is intravenous therapy. Superficial thrombophlebitis is manifested by palpating a hard cord-like vein and a warm red and painful area surrounding the intravenous site. Leukocytosis and a slight temperature elevation may occur. Temperature elevations over 38.3°C (101°F) accompanied by edema, pain and leg warmth at the site generally indicate a deep vein thrombophlebitis (option b). A positive Homan's sign (option c) is indicated by calf pain when the foot is dorsiflexed and may indicate a deep vein thrombophlebitis. Chest and/or back pain (option d) may indicate a pulmonary embolus from a dislodged clot (Lewis & Collier, 1992; pp. 934-935).

   Nursing Process: Assessment
   Client Need: Physiological Integrity

2. **The correct answer is c.** Anticipatory nausea is an association between getting chemotherapy and remembering that it caused nausea. While antiemetics will help the nausea afterward (option a), lorazepam (Ativan) will have a somewhat amnesic effect and may help to suppress it (option d). She should not be NPO (option b) but should drink plenty of fluid to help dilute the drugs (Smeltzer & Bare, 1992; p. 364).

   Nursing Process: Implementation
   Client Need: Physiological Integrity

3. **The correct answer is c.** This response gently reorients Mrs. Garrett and helps preserve her personal integrity. Wandering behavior is often caused in response to a stressful situation. Hospitalization, being in a different environment with unfamiliar people and new routines, is stressful for most clients but particularly stressful for clients with a cognitive impairment who may not have the reasoning skills to cope with the new situation. Option (a) demonstrates therapeutic communication skill but is not specific as to the help Mrs. Garrett needs. Mrs. Garrett believes the male client is her husband. Orientation assists Mrs. Garrett more specifically in the direction of her need. Option (b) implies that the male client may be her husband but Mrs. Garrett can't stay with him. This will cause more anxiety through perceived forced separation from a source of comfort and security. Option (d) is inappropriate because it encourages Mrs. Garrett in her disorientation and promises something that cannot be delivered (Stuart & Sundeen, 1991; pp. 586-590).

   Nursing Process: Implementation
   Client Need: Psychosocial Integrity

4. **The correct answer is a.** Mrs. Garrett should be gently reoriented that she is in the hospital and that her husband is aware of her whereabouts. Mrs. Garrett is probably missing someone who is familiar to her. Asking her to talk about her husband will have a calming effect on Mrs. Garrett, help her to feel closer to him and more secure, and help the nurse show empathy toward the client so that the therapeutic relationship is enhanced. Option (b) will not help Mrs. Garrett get needed rest and conserve physiological integrity. It is often done for the observational convenience of the nurse rather than the client. Option (c) is nontherapeutic because it threatens a client who is already anxious. Option (d) is inappropriate because she is not expressing a misunderstanding of why she was admitted. This approach of repeating reasons for admission may be valid as part of an every day orientation routine but does not address the problem this client is demonstrating (Stuart & Sundeen, 1991; pp. 586-590).

Nursing Process: Implementation
Client Need: Psychosocial Integrity

5. **The correct answer is b.** Checking on Mrs. Garrett frequently during the night will ensure her safety and allow adequate rest without using personnel inappropriately. Option (a), placing Mrs. Garrett in restraints, is inappropriate because she has not demonstrated unsafe behavior. However, if Mrs. Garrett awakens to find herself restrained, she may become agitated and injure herself. Option (c), an overhead light, will cause her to stay wakeful. Lights should be low to promote rest yet retain the ability to distinguish objects so she stays

oriented and does not fall. Option (d), asking a nursing assistant or family member to stay with her is inappropriate use of personnel because Mrs. Garrett's condition does not warrant constant supervision. Asking a family member to stay may imply that the nurses cannot perform their duties (Stuart & Sundeen, 1991; pp. 589-590).

Nursing Process: Implementation
Client Need: Psychosocial Integrity

6. **The correct answer is a.** The nurse should document the medication error in the nurse's note and an incident report should be initiated. Incident reports are documentation that an unusual situation has occurred and can be a valuable source of information to risk management if trends are developing, or if subsequent legal action is taken. They are not part of a client's permanent record (option b), nor an admission of guilt (option c). It is not advisable to note in the client's record that an incident report was filed (option d) (Craven & Hirnle, 1992; p. 587; Taylor, Lillis, & LeMone, 1989; pp. 91-92).

Nursing Process: Implementation
Client Need: Safe, Effective Care Environment

7. **The correct answer is b.** Constipation may result from bedrest and narcotic administration. If the client strains due to constipation, vagal stimulation may result in serious dysrhythmias. Maintaining bedrest (option a) decreases cardiac workload. Low cholesterol diet (option c) may be ordered but is unrelated to vagal stimulation. Vital signs are monitored (option d) as a

175

reflection of cardiac workload (Lewis & Collier, 1992; p. 806).

Nursing Process: Planning
Client Need: Physiological Integrity

8. **The correct answer is c.** The influenza vaccine includes egg protein and may produce allergic reactions including anaphylaxis if administered to clients allergic to eggs. Since vaccines are a preventive measure, they should be given before the client has been exposed to or has symptoms of the disease (options a and d). Amantadine hydro-chloride (Symmetrel) is used to prevent infection by the influenza virus (Lewis & Collier, 1992; pp. 472-473).

Nursing Process: Planning
Client Need: Health Promotion & Maintenance

9. **The correct answer is d.** This keeps the mist in the tent and maintains the cool humidified environment. Bed linens and pajamas become damp and chilling occurs if they are not changed more often than every 12 hours (option a). Oxygen levels should not exceed 60% (option b). Opening the tent every hour decreases the effectiveness and frequent vital signs are not necessary (option c) (Mott, Sperhac & James, 1990; p. 991; Whaley & Wong, 1991; p. 1446).

Nursing Process: Implementation
Client Need: Physiological Integrity

10. **The correct answer is c.** A glucose solution may cause red blood cell agglutination which causes clotting and plugging of the filter and intravenous line. It may also cause red blood cell hemolysis. Lactated ringer's solution may also cause cell agglutination. If glucose or lactated ringer's solutions are being infused, isotonic saline solution (option b) should be used to flush the tubing before and after blood administration. An 18 gauge needle (option a) is sufficient for blood administration. Blood should be chilled (option d) before it is given to maintain its viability. Blood would be warmed only if it is to be administered rapidly or in large quantities such as with shock (Lewis & Collier, 1992; pp. 709-710).

Nursing Process: Planning
Client Need: Safe, Effective Care Environment

11. **The correct answer is d.** Toxic shock syndrome (TSS) is believed to be the result of staphylococcus aureus toxins which enter the bloodstream through abrasions in the vaginal wall. TSS is most often found in women who use tampons while menstruating or have chronic vaginitis. Upon recovery, clients should be told to discontinue use of tampons until no signs of staphylococcus aureus are present so toxins cannot be reintroduced into the circulatory system. As a means of prevention, women using tampons should avoid using the superabsorbent type which holds more menstrual flow and provides a medium for germ growth. As further prevention, women should alternate tampons with sanitary pads (option a) but should not wear tampons at night (option b). Good handwashing should be taught to avoid

germ introduction (option c) (Lewis & Collier, 1992; p. 1431).

Nursing Process: Implementation
Client Need: Physiological Integrity

12. **The correct answer is d.** Warmup exercises stretch muscles and ligaments which increases nerve transmissions to respond to the demands of sports. Ice is used to reduce swelling (option b) for the acute phase of injury which is the first 24 to 48 hours. After that period, warm moist heat is used to promote healing. Given the correct support, the client should use the ankle (option a). This increases circulation which helps with nutrition and absorption of the hematoma. A sprain indicates muscle and ligament tearing but does not include dislocation (option d) (Lewis & Collier, 1992; p. 1644).

Nursing Process: Implementation
Client Need: Health Promotion & Maintenance

13. **The correct answer is a.** Difficulty sleeping, loss of interest and increased nervousness are signs of exacerbation of the illness. Early identification of these signs is needed to prevent relapse. Although there is a shift from blaming families for causing the schizophrenia, family members are seen as active partners in successful home management of the client (option b). Health teaching conducted with the client and family should be individualized to the particular client. There are no specific stages that the client will go through when discharged. It is important to give families realistic expectations about the client based on the client's capabilities (option d). While it is important for client and family to understand side effects of the client's medications, the physician will regulate medication dosages and the need for drug holidays (option c) (Haber, Leach-McMahon, Price-Hoskins & Sideleau, 1992; pp. 545-546).

Nursing Process: Planning
Client Need: Psychosocial Integrity

14. **The correct answer is c.** Prothrombin time (PT) evaluates the effectiveness of the extrinsic coagulation cascade and is used to determine warfarin (Coumadin) therapy. Warfarin (Coumadin) therapy, when the appropriate dose is administered, will prolong the prothrombin time by 1.5 to 2 times normal. Partial thromboplastin time (PTT) (option a) is increased with heparin therapy. An increase in platelets (option b) and fibrin split levels (option d) would be present when clotting occurs. A decrease in either level may result in bleeding (Ignatavicius & Bayne, 1991; pp. 1233, 2249).

Nursing Process: Evaluation
Client Need: Physiological Integrity

15. **The correct answer is d.** A common nursing diagnosis for a client with myasthenia gravis is impaired physical mobility related to the muscle weakness due to the decreased amount of acetylcholine receptors at the neural junctions. Muscular weakness is the major symptom of the disease. The weakness increases when the client is fatigued. Some other important nursing diagnoses related to muscular weakness include ineffective airway clearance, ineffective

breathing pattern, impaired gas exchange and potential for injury. Altered nutrition (option a) should be less than, not greater than, body requirements. Weakened jaw muscles lead to less intake. Impaired skin integrity related to immobility (option b) and potential for infection related to muscle weakness (option c) may be true of some clients but are less common (Ignatavicius & Bayne, 1991; pp. 971-973).

Nursing Process: Analysis
Client Need: Physiological Integrity

16. **The correct answer is b.** The most frequent side effect of tobramycin sulfate (Nebcin) is nephrotoxicity. A nursing intervention when administering tobramycin sulfate (Nebcin) is to monitor daily input and output and daily weight of the client to assess hydration status and renal function. General muscle weakness (option d) and blurred vision (option c) are not associated with this medication. Tobramycin sulfate (Nebcin) is administered intravenously or intramuscularly, and abdominal cramping (option a) is not a side effect since it bypasses the gastrointestinal tract (Deglin, Vallerand & Russin, 1991; pp. 1120-1121).

Nursing Process: Analysis
Client Need: Physiological Integrity

17. **The correct answer is a.** Because family is very important to the Native American, the client and her husband may wish to consult with them before consenting to surgery. Therefore, neither the surgeon (option b) nor the nurse (option c) is likely to be included in the discussion. Since family members are present, it is unlikely the client and her husband would discuss the matter privately (option d) (Ellis & Nowlis, 1989; pp. 413-415).

Nursing Process: Planning
Client Need: Psychosocial Integrity

18. **The correct answer is d.** This response focuses on what the client feels and communicates empathy as well as how much the nurse is trying to understand the client. Options (a) and (d) feed the client's delusion by agreeing or calling the client by the delusional name. Option (b) is punitive. Delusions of grandeur (believing you are someone important) usually result from feelings of insecurity and inadequacy. Delusions are used as a way to cope with the stress of life. One form of coping should not be removed until the client has a more constructive way of coping (Cook & Fontaine, 1991; pp. 534-535).

Nursing Process: Implementation
Client Need: Psychosocial Integrity

19. **The correct answer is d.** The prescribed dosage of potassium chloride is too large over a short time period. Recommended dosage of potassium chloride to treat hypokalemia is 20 mEq daily, up to four times per day. The dosage was especially too large for the client with end stage renal disease. The kidneys are unable to excrete this large dosage due to previous impairment. All oral forms of potassium chloride must be administered with 120 to 240 ml of fluid to minimize gastrointestinal irritation. Two ounces (60 ml) of water (option a) is too small of a dilutant for administering potassium chloride. Oral

potassium chloride should be administered with or after meals to minimize gastrointestinal symptoms (option b). Option (c) is the incorrect route. The ordered dose is for oral administration, not intravenous (Baer & Williams, 1992; pp. 801-803).

Nursing Process: Implementation
Client Need: Physiological Integrity

20. **The correct answer is c.** Paresthesia and paralysis may begin to develop within three weeks of viral illness, trauma, surgery or vaccination. It is a type of polyneuritis which creates a loss of myelin from parts of the peripheral nervous system. Inflammation and edema result in a decreased transmission of impulses especially to the periphery. Cigarette smoking (option a), cardiac problems (option b) and childhood rheumatic fever (option d) are unrelated (Lewis & Collier, 1992; p. 1620).

Nursing Process: Analysis
Client Need: Physiological Integrity

21. **The correct answer is d.** This response gives credence to his feelings and assists him to verbalize his most pressing concerns. Telling him that all of his muscle function will return (option a) is false reassurance since the amount of residual dysfunction cannot be predicted. Suggesting he talk to others with paralysis (option b) gives advice which is nontherapeutic and is also premature since total dysfunction is unknown. Mr. Castner is also between the denial and anger stages of grief and is not ready to take action to further deal with possible longer term effects. Telling Mr. Castner

that anger is not helpful then diverting his attention (option c) belittles his feelings and blocks expression of concerns and is nontherapeutic (Cook & Fontaine, 1991; pp. 62, 218, 417; Lewis & Collier, 1992; p. 1620).

Nursing Process: Implementation
Client Need: Psychosocial Integrity

22. **The correct answer is b.** Providing a diet high in protein is not a priority for this client. This client will have weight gain and a normal appetite and this should not be a concern. Symptoms of hypothyroidism include cold intolerance and constipation, so blankets (option a) and foods high in fiber (option d) should be provided. The treatment for hypothyroidism from any cause (thyroiditis is the number one cause) is thyroid replacement (option c) and this should be explained to the client (Smeltzer & Bare, 1992; pp. 1081-1082).

Nursing Process: Implementation
Client Need: Physiological Integrity

23. **The correct answer is b.** Phenylketonuria (PKU) is caused by a genetic inability to convert phenylalanine to tyrosine resulting in low tyrosine levels (option a). The phenylalanine stays in the bloodstream and creates abnormal brain and central nervous system development resulting in mental retardation. Since tyrosine is needed for melanin, children with PKU are often blond haired and blue eyed and have fair skin (option c). Phenylalanine metabolites create a musty odor to breath and perspiration (option d). Acetone breath often indicates

179

hyperglycemia (Lewis & Collier, 1992; pp. 1060, 1300; Wong, 1993; pp. 258-260).

Nursing Process: Implementation
Client Need: Physiological Integrity

24. **The correct answer is a.** Ipratropium (Atrovent) is a bronchodilator. It inhibits cholinergic receptors in the bronchial smooth muscle. Option (b), isoniazid (Isotamine), is used as a first-line anti-tubercular in combination with other agents in the treatment of active disease. Option (c), isosorbide dinitrate (Isorbid), is a vasodilator and is used for acute treatment of anginal attacks. Option (d), isotretinoin (Accutane), is an anti-acne agent used for the management of cystic acne (Deglin, Vallerand & Russin, 1991; pp. 603, 610, 615, 617).

Nursing Process: Implementation
Client Need: Physiological Integrity

25. **The correct answer is c.** The main problem facing teenagers during this period of growth is forming a separate identity. This adolescent is having difficulty in separating from her gang and becoming independent. A consistent life value (option a) is not substantiated by the data presented. Values are learned during this stage but there is no data that states the client has not formed these values. In fact, the client may be trying to act on these newly found values by leaving the gang and needs help to do so. There is also no data to suggest social anxiety (option b). The client was an accepted member of a gang and is socially competent within that group. The problem is related to personal goals

after leaving the gang, not social interaction. The client does not appear to be denying mortality (option d) but has recently had to face it due to the death of her friend (Cook & Fontaine, 1991; pp. 221-222).

Nursing Process: Analysis
Client Need: Psychosocial Integrity

26. **The correct answer is c.** Sitting on the edge of a bed leaning over a nightstand propped up with pillows facilitates full chest expansion and conserves energy. If the client were in a recliner (option a), he should lean forward, not backward. If the client is standing (option b), his back and hips should be against the wall. Semi-Fowlers position (option d) does not allow for optimal use of accessory muscles for breathing (Ignatavicius & Bayne, 1991; pp. 2031-2033).

Nursing Process: Planning
Client Need: Physiological Integrity

27. **The correct answer is c.** All are protective barriers recommended by the Center for Disease Control (C.D.C.). The C.D.C. mandates health care professionals follow universal precautions when in direct or indirect contact with blood and body fluids. An apron and gloves are indicated during invasive procedures; however, headwear is not listed in the C.D.C.'s guidelines for universal precautions (option a). Gloves alone (option b) are not sufficient protection during an invasive procedure. Splashing and soiling of mucous membranes and clothing are possible requiring additional protective barriers. Shoe covers will protect from soiling with blood and body fluids. However,

masks should be worn regardless of proximity to contaminated blood and body fluids if splashing is possible (option d) (Ignatavicius & Bayne, 1991; p. 615; Phipps, Long, Woods & Cassmeyer, 1991; p. 294).

Nursing Process: Planning
Client Need: Safe, Effective Care Environment

28. **The correct answer is a.** Once the client's anxiety is reduced, the nurse can assist with problem-solving and offer diversional activities to keep the anxiety down. The activities assist the client by channelling the energy into more productive outlets. Once anxiety is decreased, personnel no longer have to stay with the client (option b). The nurse must continue to assess the client. If the client's anxiety increases, the nurse's presence will help the client feel more secure. Relaxation tapes may assist the client to maintain a lowered level of anxiety. However, clients must be taught how to use them appropriately as a method of decreasing anxiety. Merely offering the tapes (option c) without proper health teaching would not benefit the client. Referral to a social worker (option d) would be unnecessary since counseling the client in ways to maintain a decreased anxiety level is within the practice domain of the nurse (Varcarolis, 1990; pp. 181-184).

Nursing Process: Implementation
Client Need: Psychosocial Integrity

29. **The correct answer is c.** In using the REEDA scale to evaluate healing, the 5 areas evaluated are Redness, Edema, Ecchymosis, Discharge, and Approximation. Points are awarded 0-3, based on severity. Using this scale, option (a) has a total score of 4. Option (b) has a total score of 7. Option (c) has a total score of greater than 8. Option (d) has a total score of 0, indicating there is no infection (Ladewig, London & Olds, 1990; p. 802).

Nursing Process: Assessment
Client Need: Physiological Integrity

30. **The correct answer is d.** Some of the cardinal signs of a cancerous melanoma include asymmetry, irregular borders, combination of colors and diameter greater than 5 mm (option b). Dry pruritic skin can have many causes and does not usually indicate melanoma (option a). A circular lesion (regular borders) that blanches is often derived from a venous malfunction (option c) (Smeltzer & Bare, 1992; pp. 1486-1487).

Nursing Process: Assessment
Client Need: Physiological Integrity

181

PRACTICE SESSION: 6

Instructions:

Allow yourself 30 minutes to complete the following 30 practice questions. Use a timer to notify yourself when 30 minutes are over so that you are not constantly looking at your watch while completing the questions.

Situation:

Stephen Kaczmerak, 9 years old, is taken by his mother to the pediatrician due to a throat infection. The physician notes that Stephen has had multiple throat infections and episodes of tonsillitis. He is scheduled for a tonsillectomy. (The next three questions pertain to this situation.)

1. The morning of surgery, Stephen is admitted and helped into hospital pajamas. What should Stephen be told about the surgery?
    a. Nothing unless he asks questions.
    b. While he sleeps two doctors will make his tonsils disappear.
    c. He'll have a little sore throat and eat lots of popsicles.
    d. Only what his parents choose to tell him about it.

2. The surgery is completed and Stephen is placed in the recovery room. The best position for Stephen is:
    a. on his back with head elevated on a pillow.
    b. prone with his head turned to the side.
    c. semi-Fowler's position.
    d. reverse Trendelenburg.

3. Stephen is discharged to home. Stephen's mother wants to know how she can best keep her usually active 9 year old entertained. Which of the following would be the best type of activity for Stephen?
    a. Playing with hand puppets to act out the surgery.
    b. Playing a board game with his 6 year old brother.
    c. Collecting model cars or airplanes to make.
    d. Having visits from boys and girls from his school class.

4. A 68 year old client with bone metastasis from prostate cancer is placed on morphine sulfate (Morphine) 20 mg every 4 hours. He should be observed for side effects of this medication which include:
    a. peripheral neuropathy.
    b. nasal congestion and blurred vision.
    c. heartburn and tinnitus.
    d. constipation and dry mouth.

5. A client has been started on total parenteral nutrition (TPN). During the evening shift, the nurse notices that the TPN is not infusing as quickly as it should and it will not be finished on time. The best action of the nurse would be to:
   a. speed up the rate so that the solution will finish on time.
   b. allow the solution to infuse until it is finished, then hang the next bag.
   c. hang the next bag when it is due even if the other bag has not fully infused.
   d. slow the present rate until the physician is notified to change the order for infusion.

6. A 24 year old female client is admitted to the surgical unit. She had burn grafts done to her right wrist and forearm. The nurse should encourage the client to eat a diet rich in:
   a. vitamin B complex and caffeine.
   b. vitamin A and protein.
   c. vitamin C and calcium.
   d. zinc and low density lipoproteins.

7. A client is brought to the emergency room by his friend who tells the nurse he's "acting funny". The client is agitated, flushed, diaphoretic and has rapid pulse and respirations. Upon questioning the client admits to smoking "crack" cocaine. The nurse should assess for which signs of impending lethal complications?
   a. Lethargy and increased blood pressure.
   b. Increased body temperature and chest pain.
   c. Constricted pupils and flaccid reflexes.
   d. Euphoria and cold bluish skin.

8. A nurse is in the grocery store shopping when someone yells, "HELP, this lady is having a baby!" On quick assessment the nurse notes that the woman's membranes are ruptured and the fetus is crowning. The nurse provides privacy as best as possible and instructs a crowd member to call the ambulance. However, the infant's birth is imminent. The correct action of the nurse would be to:
   a. ask the mother to pant so the baby is not delivered until paramedics have arrived.
   b. assist with extension, then external rotation, followed by expulsion, place infant on mother's abdomen with cord attached and keep baby warm.
   c. assist with descent, internal rotation, flexion and then expulsion of fetus, place the infant on mother's abdomen with cord attached and keep baby warm.
   d. move the mother to the doorway to enable quick transport to the closest hospital.

9. A 42 year old woman with insulin dependent diabetes mellitus (type I) is admitted to the hospital for evaluation of numbness and tingling in her extremities. The physician orders her to receive isophane (NPH) insulin 32 units and regular insulin 6 units each morning before breakfast. Prior to administering the injection, the nurse informs her of the insulin type and dosage. The client states: "I've been taking Humulin for some time now, but apparently he's changed my insulin." The proper action of the nurse would be to:
   a. administer the insulin as prescribed and note the client's comments in your nurse's note.
   b. administer the insulin as prescribed because the responsibility ultimately rests with the physician.
   c. do not administer the insulin and note this in the medication record.
   d. consult with the physician prior to insulin administration regarding he client's concern.

10. A 48 year old male client is being admitted to the hospital with the diagnosis of multiple myeloma. Considering this diagnosis, the client is most likely to have which of these symptoms?
   a. Fever and hypercalcemia.
   b. Hypocalcemia and rectal bleeding.
   c. An irregular shaped black mole.
   d. Alopecia and blurred vision.

11. A client with increased intracranial pressure is ordered each of the following tests. The nurse would clarify which test with the physician?
    a. Magnetic resonance imaging (MRI).
    b. Lumbar puncture (LP).
    c. Electrocardiogram (ECG).
    d. Arterial blood gases (ABG's).

12. The physician orders a vaginal irrigation for a client. After preparation, the douche bag should be hung at a maximum of how far above the client?
    a. 2 feet (60 cm)
    b. 5 feet (152 cm)
    c. 6 inches (15 cm)
    d. 2 inches (5 cm)

13. The nurse identifies a knowledge deficit regarding contraceptive methods. A correct nursing intervention would be:
    a. that the client will choose a contraceptive method that the client and partner will feel comfortable using.
    b. to assess communication patterns between the client and partner.
    c. that the client selected using condoms as a contraceptive method.
    d. to teach the effectiveness and possible side effects of each contraceptive method.

14. A client with a C_4 fracture complains of blurred vision, headache and nausea. His blood pressure is 210/92 and apical heart rate is 46 beats per minute. Based on these findings, the nurse suspects the client has:
    a. trigeminal neuralgia.
    b. spinal shock.
    c. autonomic dysreflexia.
    d. a cerebrovascular accident.

15. A client with degenerative joint disease is being discharged. The nurse evaluates that further teaching is needed if the client says:
    a. "I should take my aspirin with food."
    b. "I'll put cold packs on my joint every day."
    c. "I'll try to take a nap every afternoon."
    d. "My ultrasound treatments will help my joint stiffness."

16. A 56 year old male client is admitted to the neurosurgical floor following craniotomy for partial resection of a glioma. One of the nursing goals identified is to prevent intracerebral edema. Which of the following nursing actions should be included in his plan of care?
    a. Turn his head to one side to prevent aspiration of saliva.
    b. Report immediately an intracranial pressure reading of 10 mm Hg.
    c. Elevate the head of his bed 30 degrees.
    d. Report immediately a $PaCO_2$ of 33 mm Hg.

17. A client is scheduled for an electroencephalogram (EEG) in the morning. What would the nurse include in client education?
    a. The client should shampoo her hair the night before the test.
    b. The procedure is painful, but it will only last for 5 minutes.
    c. Hold all anticonvulsants the day of the test, and administer the anticonvulsants after the EEG is completed.
    d. The client will be NPO after midnight for the EEG.

18. A client with a history of bronchiectasis is admitted to the medical unit. The nurse should expect to find which predisposing factor related to bronchiectasis?
    a. High number of respiratory infections in childhood.
    b. History of cigarette smoking starting in the teenage years.
    c. Family history of chronic obstructive pulmonary disease (COPD).
    d. Childhood heart murmurs.

19. A 27 year old woman is diagnosed with pre-menstrual syndrome (PMS). A treatment related goal would be that the client will:
    a. keep a record of symptoms to aid in diagnosis.
    b. verbalize when to use sick time during severe syndrome times.
    c. report violent reactions.
    d. demonstrate coping skills during problem times.

20. The nurse is providing discharge instructions for a client with new onset seizure activity receiving phenytoin (Dilantin) therapy. Which of the following instructions would be appropriate?
    a. Take phenytoin (Dilantin) when aura is experienced.
    b. Alcohol may be consumed as desired.
    c. Frequent oral hygiene.
    d. Unrestricted activity level.

21. A client is admitted with expressive aphasia following a cerebral vascular accident. Communication can best be facilitated by which statement?
    a. "Tell me about your family."
    b. "Don't cry, we'll work to get you better."
    c. "Can you point to the word you want to say on the picture board?"
    d. "It's difficult to talk with you when you're angry."

22. The circulating nurse is to place a client in the lithotomy position. The nurse would also:
    a. support the legs on a pillow.
    b. place the arms on arm boards.
    c. secure the knees with a strap.
    d. drape the legs to preserve dignity.

23. The major goal for a client with Parkinson's disease is to:
    a. adjust to changes in body image.
    b. maintain proper bowel elimination.
    c. maintain the highest level of independence possible.
    d. demonstrate less pain related to rigidity and immobility.

24. A 60 year old coal miner has suffered with chronic obstructive pulmonary disease (COPD) for 15 years. Which of these goals would be appropriate? The client will:
   a. maintain a breathing pattern that is not tiring.
   b. maintain a normal forced expiratory volume (FEV).
   c. maintain a carbon dioxide level of less than 45 mm Hg.
   d. not use accessory muscles to breathe.

25. When assessing a 52 year old woman with a history of right ventricular failure secondary to mitral stenosis, physical findings would include:
   a. mild dyspnea and a nonproductive cough.
   b. dyspnea on exertion and bilateral crackles.
   c. dependent edema and hepatomegaly.
   d. paroxysmal nocturnal dyspnea and arrhythmias.

26. A client is twelve hours post-operative craniotomy. The nurse observes an increased urine output from 60 cc per hour to 220 cc per hour by foley catheter for the past two hours. An increased urine output in this client would be indicative of:
   a. improved renal function.
   b. hypovolemic shock.
   c. a normal response post-craniotomy.
   d. diabetes insipidus.

27. A 50 year old female client presents in the outpatient breast clinic for evaluation of a self-found lump. She asks the nurse what her risk factors for breast cancer are. Of all of the following data, which finding does not place her at higher risk for the development of breast cancer?
   a. Onset of menarche at age 9 years.
   b. Breast fed both of her children for 8 months each.
   c. She delivered her first child at age 35.
   d. At age 43 she had removal of an early cancerous colon lesion.

28. A male client states he does not know how he contracted genital herpes. "After all," he says, "she had no genital lesions." Could the client be telling the truth?
   a. No, open genital lesions would need to be present for disease transmission.
   b. No, he probably had another sexual partner who infected him.
   c. Yes, it is unusual for the virus to be transmitted without sexual contact.
   d. Yes, if oral-genital contact occurred when she had a cold sore.

29. Jenna, a 5 year old, has been diagnosed with a bilateral Wilm's tumor. Which of the following actions by the graduate nurse caring for Jenna would necessitate intervention by the team leader?
    a. Discussing the upcoming surgery with Jenna, without her parents present.
    b. Palpating Jenna's abdomen to determine location of the mass.
    c. Assessing for absence of Jenna's iris and ambiguous genitalia.
    d. Answering the parents' questions concerning the need for a bone marrow aspiration.

30. A 62 year old male client comes into the oncology outpatient unit for a check up. He is status post-deep resection and radiation for squamous cell carcinoma of the lateral margin of the tongue. Which one of the following symptoms should be reported?
    a. Reddened oral mucosa and xerostomia.
    b. Reddened dry skin at area of radiation.
    c. An enlarged non-tender anterior cervical node.
    d. Frequent periods of fatigue.

STOP You have now completed **Practice Session: 6. Now take a few minutes and correct your answers. Calculate your accuracy rate by dividing the number of questions you completed correctly by the total number of questions you completed (30).**

Correct answers ÷ total number of questions completed = accuracy rate.

_____ ÷ _____ = _____

PRACTICE SESSION: 6

ANSWERS AND RATIONALES

1. **The correct answer is c.** Nine year olds often fear the operative procedure and what will happen afterwards. Children should be told the truth about what will happen to them and what to expect afterwards (option a). Stephen is old enough to be told the truth rather than a fairy story. This may cause more apprehension and mistrust (option b). The nurse has the responsibilities for teaching both Stephen and parents (option d) (Wong, 1993; pp. 640, 651).

    Nursing Process: Implementation
    Client Need: Physiological Integrity

2. **The correct answer is b.** The best position post-tonsillectomy is prone with head turned to the side which facilitates drainage and lessens the chance of aspiration. Lying on the back with head elevated (option a) does not promote sufficient drainage but may cause blood to be swallowed or aspirated. Semi-Fowler's position would be contraindicated due to post-anesthesia state and drainage being swallowed or aspirated (option c). Reverse Trendelenburg (option d) would be unnecessary unless the child was in shock (Smeltzer & Bare, 1992; p. 485-486).

    Nursing Process: Planning
    Client Need: Safe, Effective Care Environment

3. **The correct answer is c.** School age children enjoy hands on experiences as well as collecting and organizing objects. Collecting model cars or airplanes would be a quiet activity to promote restful recovery yet keep his attention. Playing with hand puppets (option a) is a more dramatic and imaginary type of play which usually occurs in pre-school children. Playing a game with a six year old (option b) might be difficult. Six year olds are more prone to breaking the game rules in order to win. Nine year olds are more rigid and fanatical about game rules and ensuing friction might result in shouting and rough-housing. Visits from boys in his class, if properly supervised, can meet a need for preserving peer relationships. Visits from girls may not be welcomed until adolescence when girls become more important and relationships more open (option d). A nine year old may like girls but often won't acknowledge it (Wong, 1993; pp. 428-430, 434, 450-451).

    Nursing Process: Planning
    Client Need: Health Promotion and Maintenance

4. **The correct answer is d.** The common side effects of morphine sulfate (Morphine) include: respiratory depression, hypotension, constipation, nausea, vomiting, sedation, dry mouth and sweating. The others listed (options a, b and c) are not expected side effects

189

(Smeltzer & Bare, 1992; p. 427).

Nursing Process: Analysis
Client Need: Physiological Integrity

5. **The correct answer is c.** If the infusion is behind, allow the present bag to infuse until time for the next bag to be hung. The next bag should be hung on time even if the solution is left in the bag (option b). Since total parental nutrition (TPN) contains a large amount of glucose, the solution is an excellent growth medium for bacteria. If left to infuse for a long time, bacterial growth may occur and cause intravenous site and possible systemic infection (option d). TPN infusions should be neither speeded up nor slowed down. Increasing the infusion rate (option a) may cause a rise in the glucose entering the system. Bodily insulin cannot handle the influx. The renal system may be unable to handle this large amount of glucose and the increased glucose spills into the urine. If the infusion rate is decreased, hypoglycemia may result (Lewis & Collier, 1992; p. 1023).

Nursing Process: Implementation
Client Need: Physiological Integrity

6. **The correct answer is b.** Protein is necessary for healing because collagen is a protein. Vitamin A promotes growth of epithelial cells. Although vitamin B-complex is helpful for wound healing, caffeine is not needed and may be detrimental to health especially if taken in large quantities (option a). Vitamin C is very important in wound healing because it helps form collagen and provides structure to the walls of capillaries supplying the wound area.

However, calcium could cause problems such as kidney stones (option c). Zinc is helpful in wound healing but low density lipoproteins may inhibit circulation and are linked to cardiovascular disease (option d). Other substances which promote wound healing include magnesium and copper (Phipps, Long, Woods & Cassmeyer, 1991; pp. 430, 496, 618-619).

Nursing Process: Implementation
Client Need: Physiological Integrity

7. **The correct answer is b.** Chest pain is a sign of overdose and, if left untreated, hyperpyrexia, convulsions and cardio-vascular collapse may occur resulting in death. Cocaine is a type of stimulant. Increased blood pressure occurs soon after taking the cocaine, probably due to its vasoconstrictor effects. Lethargy is a sign that the effects of the cocaine are subsiding (option a). Pupils are dilated and reflexes are brisk with cocaine use. Constricted pupils may be present with opiate use (option c). Euphoria may be present as this is usually the desired effect of cocaine use although not a sign of overdose or complications. However, cold bluish skin occurs with opiate use (option d) (Lewis & Collier, 1992; pp. 1789, 1802-1803).

Nursing Process: Assessment
Client Need: Physiological Integrity

8. **The correct answer is b.** The cardinal movements of labor are (in order) descent into the pelvic inlet, flexion of the head, internal rotation of the head into the pelvic cavity, extension of the head as it passes under the symphysis pubis and starts to emerge from the

vagina, restitution where the head and shoulders become aligned with the back in the birth canal, external rotation as the shoulders and head are turned further to one side, followed finally by expulsion of the rest of the body. Option (a) is incorrect as the fetus may suffer harm if delivery is not allowed to progress. Option (c) is incorrect as descent, flexion and internal rotation are movements done by fetus without intervention on behalf of a caregiver if it is an uncomplicated vaginal delivery which most spontaneous emergency deliveries are. The cardinal movements are out of order in option (c). Option (d) is incorrect as it does nothing to assist mother or fetus through the delivery process (Ladewig, London & Olds, 1990; p. 386).

Nursing Process: Implementation
Client Need: Safe, Effective Care Environment

9. **The correct answer is d.** The knowledgeable nurse understands the basis for various therapies ordered by the physician, especially in regard to medication actions and side effects. The nurse should notify the physician and discuss the discrepancy in insulin types as stated by the client. It could be detrimental to the client if the nurse administers the wrong type of insulin (option a), and the physician and nurse share responsibility when the nurse carries out physician orders (option b). Not administering the insulin (option c) without notifying the physician is negligence by the act of omission, in that failure to act may cause harm to the client (Ellis & Nowlis, 1989; p. 68,

266-267).

Nursing Process: Implementation
Client Need: Safe, Effective Care Environment

10. **The correct answer is a.** Because of malignant infiltration into the bone marrow, bone destruction takes place. This results in hypercalcemia (option b) and pathological fractures. In addition, neutropenia occurs which causes increased risk for infection. An irregular shaped mole (option c) is a classical sign of melanoma. Alopecia (option d) does not occur primarily but can be a result of treatment; therefore, he should not have this treatment at this time. Rectal bleeding (option b) and blurred vision (option d) are not related to the diagnosis (Smeltzer & Bare, 1992; p. 806).

Nursing Process: Analysis
Client Need: Physiological Integrity

11. **The correct answer is b.** A lumbar puncture is contraindicated in the client with increased intracranial pressure. Insertion of a needle in the subarachnoid space causes a rapid reduction of pressure in the spinal column. This may induce cerebral or cerebellar herniation through the foramen magna. Magnetic resonance imaging is a noninvasive diagnostic scanning device frequently ordered to diagnose increased intracranial pressure due to cerebral lesions, infarctions, vascular disruptions and edema (option a). The electrocardiogram is not contraindicated in the client with increased intracranial pressure (option c). The test is non-

invasive, involves minimal client preparation and can be performed in less than five minutes at the bedside. The electrocardiogram is frequently ordered to detect arrhythmias induced by increased intracranial pressure. Arterial blood oxygen saturation (option d) may be impaired secondary to compression on cerebral vasculature from increased intracranial pressure. Decreased oxygenation leads to impaired respiratory status (Pagana & Pagana, 1992; pp.287, 481, 500-503, 537).

Nursing Process: Analysis
Client Need: Physiological Integrity

12. **The correct answer is a.** The douche bag should be hung no higher than 2 feet (60 cm) above the client (option b). If the fluid is instilled too rapidly or with too much pressure, reflux to the tubes and uterus will occur and the treatment will no longer be therapeutic. Options (c) and (d) would take too long for the fluid to be instilled (Smeltzer & Bare, 1992; p. 1239).

Nursing Process: Planning
Client Need: Physiological Integrity

13. **The correct answer is d.** Option (a) is a nursing process goal. Option (b) is a nursing process assessment. Option (c) is a nursing process evaluation statement (Taylor, Lillis, & LeMone, 1989; pp. 1090-1091).

Nursing Process: Implementation
Client Need: Health Promotion & Maintenance

14. **The correct answer is c.** Autonomic dysreflexia occurs when impulses along the sympathetic nervous system are disrupted and no longer are influenced by the cerebral cortex. Stool impaction and urinary retention are the major causes of autonomic dysreflexia. Trigeminal neuralgia (option a) is a neurological condition of the trigeminal nerve, the fifth cranial nerve, resulting in facial pain. Spinal shock (option b) is a complication of cervical fractures and may precede autonomic dysreflexia. A cerebrovascular accident (option d) would not be related to a C_4 fracture (Ignatavicius & Bayne, 1991; p. 937).

Nursing Process: Analysis
Client Need: Physiological Integrity

15. **The correct answer is b.** Cold packs are only used for acute inflammation in the joints. For chronic inflammation, heat such as warm compresses and ultrasound (option d) will help to decrease pain, swelling and stiffness in joints. Sleep is important and naps during the day (option c) help rest the joints. If aspirin is ordered, it should be taken with food (option a) to prevent gastrointestinal side effects (Ignatavicius & Bayne, 1991; pp. 678-679).

Nursing Process: Evaluation
Client Need: Physiological Integrity

16. **The correct answer is c.** Elevate the head of the bed 30 degrees. This is done to promote venous drainage from the head. Turning the head to one side (option a) can obstruct venous drainage and should be avoided routinely. The $PaCO_2$ is normally 30-35 mm Hg (option d). Normal intracranial pressure (ICP) is 0-10 mm Hg (option b), same parameters as central venous pressure.

Small fluctuations do occur and coughing or other valsalva type activities will normally cause brief elevations (Smeltzer & Bare, 1992, p.1681).

Nursing Process: Implementation
Client Need: Physiological Integrity

17. **The correct answer is a.** The client is instructed to shampoo his or her hair the night before the study. Oils, sprays, or lotions may be not used. The electro-encephalogram (EEG) procedure is not painful (option b) and there is no need to fast before the test (option d). Anti-convulsants are not usually discontinued before the study (option c) because of the risk of precipitating seizures (Pagana & Pagana, 1994; p. 185).

Nursing Process: Implementation
Client Need: Safe, Effective Care Environment

18. **The correct answer is a.** Bronchiectasis is a chronic respiratory disease which permanently dilates bronchi in the lungs. Although it is often thought to be part of the chronic pulmonary disease (COPD) group starting in adults, it is really the result of a high number of infections as a child. A history of cigarette smoking (option b) and a family history of COPD (option c) are related to adult onset COPD. Although cardiac dysrhythmias may occur due to hypoxemia, childhood cardiac murmurs (option d) are unrelated to bronchiectasis (Ignatavicius & Bayne, 1991; pp. 1992-1993).

Nursing Process: Analysis
Client Need: Physiological Integrity

19. **The correct answer is d.** Treatment for premenstrual syndrome (PMS) is aimed at reducing symptoms and increasing coping skills. A record of symptoms may be kept prior to diagnosis to assist with the diagnostic process. In this case, diagnosis has already been made (option a). The record may still be kept to look for correlation and treatment of symptoms. Work load may need to be flexible if possible when severe symptoms occur but the client should not be encouraged to take days off work indiscriminately (option b). Violent reactions (option c) should be decreased if treatment is successful (Smeltzer & Bare, 1992; pp. 1242-1243).

Nursing Process: Planning
Client Need: Health Promotion and Maintenance

20. **The correct answer is c.** Good mouth care is necessary to prevent gingival hyperplasia, a common side effect of long term phenytoin (Dilantin) therapy. All anticonvulsants should be administered on a regular basis to maintain therapeutic blood levels (option a). The client is taught that the medication must not be stopped because the seizures stopped. This could lead to seizure activity and possibly status epilepticus. Extra doses of anticonvulsants should not be taken unless prescribed by the physician, since phenytoin (Dilantin) toxicity is possible. Alcohol consumption should be avoided by all clients with seizure activity. Alcohol lowers the seizure threshold, thus, increasing the risk of injury (option b). Adequate rest is necessary in preventing seizures (option d). The

client with a new onset of seizure activity should avoid fatigue, stress and excessive excitement which may trigger a seizure. Once seizures are controlled with medication and adherence to prevention principles, activity level may be increased (Phipps, Long, Woods & Cassmeyer, 1991; pp 1823-1825).

Nursing Process: Implementation
Client Need: Health Promotion & Maintenance

21. **The correct answer is c.** Expressive aphasia occurs when Brocca's area, located in the frontal lobe, is damaged. The client experiences a motor speech deficit in which speaking, writing and gestures are disturbed. The picture board improves communication by allowing the client to express self through words and objects. Open questions requiring lengthy statements are very difficult for the client with expressive aphasia (option a). Asking yes/no questions and encouraging speech in short phrases allows the client to have control when communicating. Crying and anger are two common emotions expressed by the aphasic client (options b and d). Both are expressions of frustration from the inability to communicate. The nurse should acknowledge frustration and support the client's needs at this time (Carpenito, 1992; pp. 253, 259-262).

Nursing Process: Implementation
Client Need: Physiological Integrity

22. **The correct answer is d.** The client is supine with legs elevated in stirrups when positioned in the lithotomy position. To maintain dignity, the

client's legs should be draped to avoid exposure of genitalia. When the client is supine it may be necessary to support the legs on a pillow (option a) and use a strap (option c) to prevent a fall. Arms are secured on arm boards (option b) when they are extended from the table (Ignatavicius & Bayne, 1991; pp. 468, 469).

Nursing Process: Implementation
Client Need: Safe, Effective Care Environment

23. **The correct answer is c.** Parkinson's disease is a progressive neuromuscular disease related to a decrease in dopamine. It is characterized by muscular rigidity, tremors, a mask-like facial affect, stooped posture and gait problems. Muscular problems and tremors may lead to an inability to care for self requiring more dependence. The nurse's role is to time medications and schedule activities so that the client may keep as much independence as possible. Body image (option a), bowel elimination (option b) and decreased pain (option d) would relate to independence and are important, but the primary goal is independence (Ignatavicius & Bayne, 1991; pp. 911-913).

Nursing Process: Planning
Client Need: Physiological Integrity

24. **The correct answer is a.** A main goal of treatment of the chronic obstructive pulmonary disease (COPD) client is to conserve energy through an effective breathing pattern. Fatigue and weakness from respiratory efforts hamper daily activities. A normal forced expiratory volume (FEV) is unrealistic (option b).

FEV is the amount of air exhaled during a specified time and decreases with the progression of the COPD. COPD clients will rarely have a normal PCO_2 (option c). Their bodies have adjusted to high levels of carbon dioxide and no longer respond accordingly. COPD clients are stimulated to breathe by a lowered PO_2 level rather than an elevated PCO_2. COPD clients need to use accessory muscles to maintain adequate respirations (option d) and are instructed on how to use them when taught alternate breathing techniques. (Ignatavicius & Bayne, 1991; pp. 1995, 1996, 2003).

Nursing Process: Planning
Client Need: Physiological Integrity

25. **The correct answer is c.** Dependent edema and hepatomegaly are signs of right ventricular failure associated with increased systemic venous pressures. Signs of left ventricular failure (options a, b and d) are associated with elevated pulmonary venous pressure and decreased cardiac output (Ignatavicius & Bayne, 1991; p. 2166).

Nursing Process: Assessment
Client Need: Physiological Integrity

26. **The correct answer is d.** Diabetes insipidus is the result of decreased production and/or release of antidiuretic hormone (ADH) from the pituitary gland. Antidiuretic hormone facilitates the reabsorption of water in the body by acting upon the kidney tubules. The lack of ADH or ineffective kidney response results in excessive water loss from the body. Urine output in a 24-hour period may vary from 4 to 30 liters a day. Common causes of diabetes insipidus include neurosurgery and cerebral trauma. Edema and/or damage to the hypothalamus influences production and release of ADH. A significant increase in urine output, exceeding 200 cc/hr following neurosurgery should always be evaluated for diabetes insipidus (option c). Hourly urine output monitoring is essential to detect changes. Improvement in renal function is possible due to a variety of reasons such as diuretics or intravenous fluids; however, this information was not provided in the question (option a). Hypovolemic shock causes a decreased urine output due to inadequate fluid volume (option b) (Hickey, 1986; pp. 287-290; Ignatavicius & Bayne, 1991; pp. 1539-1540; Pagana & Pagana, 1992; pp. 51-52; Phipps, Long, Woods & Cassmeyer, 1991; pp. 1034-1035).

Nursing Process: Analysis
Client Need: Physiological Integrity

27. **The correct answer is b.** Breast feeding does not increase the risk of breast cancer. Some factors that are known to place women at higher risk include: early menarche (option a) late menopause, first birth after age 30 (option c) nulliparous and previous cancers (option d). (Phipps, Long, Woods & Cassmeyer, 1991; p. 1658; Smeltzer & Bare, 1992; p. 1297).

Nursing Process: Analysis
Client Need: Health Promotion & Maintenance

28. **The correct answer is d.** Genital herpes can be transmitted by oral-genital contact through an oral herpes lesion (option a). Clients are usually instructed not to have sexual contact while lesions are present (options b and c). Clients are also advised to use condoms even though lesions are not present since viral shedding can still occur while the virus is dormant (Ignatavicius & Bayne, 1991; pp. 1779-1781).

Nursing Process: Analysis
Client Need: Physiological Integrity

29. **The correct answer is b.** Palpation of a known Wilm's tumor may cause dissemination of cancer cells to adjacent and distant sites. A school-aged child is focused on developing a sense of industry. This is done through an interest of acquiring knowledge. The nurse can facilitate this developmental need by discussing the upcoming surgery. The parents do not need to be involved in order for the child to accomplish this task (option a). Wilm's tumor is associated with aniridia (absence of the iris) and ambiguous genitalia (option c). Bone marrow aspiration is electively performed to rule out metastasis. This can cause parental anxiety which can be decreased by the nurse's availability to answer questions (option d) (Whaley & Wong, 1991; pp.1190, 1703-1705).

Nursing Process: Implementation
Client Need: Physiological Integrity

30. **The correct answer is c.** An enlarged lymph node should be reported because of the risk of metastasis from the disease. Reddened oral mucosa and xerostomia (dry mouth), reddened dry skin at area of radiation and frequent periods of fatigue are expected side effects of surgical excision and radiation that require nursing intervention (options a, b, and d) (Smeltzer & Bare, 1992, p. 852-854).

Nursing Process: Analysis
Client Need: Physiological Integrity

PRACTICE SESSION: 7

Instructions:

Allow yourself 30 minutes to complete the following 30 practice questions. Use a timer to notify yourself when 30 minutes are over so that you are not constantly looking at your watch while completing the questions.

Situation:
Mrs. Julia Moore, 75 years old, is admitted for management of her rheumatoid arthritis. She has had increasing difficulty managing self-care tasks. (The next three questions refer to this situation.)

1. The priority nursing diagnosis would be:
   a. impaired physical mobility.
   b. activity intolerance.
   c. altered home health maintenance.
   d. self-esteem disturbance.

2. Mrs. Moore has a nursing diagnosis of chronic pain related to joint deformity. The appropriate long term goal would be:
   a. reduced chronic pain through non-surgical means.
   b. weight loss to reduce joint stress.
   c. knowledge of drug therapy to lower pain.
   d. importance of splinting to rest the affected joints.

3. Mrs. Moore is to be discharged on prednisone (Deltasone). The nurse would evaluate that Mrs. Moore understands her medication regimen when she states:
   a. "I have to check my urine for protein."
   b. "I'll need to return for periodic bloodwork."
   c. "Mouth ulcers may occur and I should report them immediately."
   d. "Bruising or bleeding of my gums may occur and it will be normal."

4. A 35 year old female client is scheduled for a hysterosalpingography, an infertility study to test for tubal patency. The nurse should:
   a. administer an enema prior to the test.
   b. schedule the test during ovulation.
   c. ask the client to keep a basal body temperature record.
   d. instruct the client not to bathe or douche before the test.

5. A 22 year old male client is seen in the physician's office. In teaching him about testicular self-exam, which of the following responses indicates the client needs further teaching?
   a. "I would be at greater risk if I were sexually active."
   b. "If it is detected early, there's a 90-100% chance for cure."
   c. "The epididymis feels like a cord on the top and back of the testicle."
   d. "I should check myself monthly, while in the shower."

6. The best approach of a community health nurse in initial contact with the family should be that of:
   a. participant observer.
   b. firm assistant.
   c. family therapist.
   d. supportive change agent.

7. A 16 year old male client fractured his foot playing basketball. A cast is applied and the nurse is reviewing crutch walking with the client. The nurse should instruct the client to:
   a. use a three point gait.
   b. use a four point gait.
   c. walk with the affected extremity pointed toward the back with knee flexed.
   d. swing the affected and non-affected extremities forward at the same time.

8. The physician orders an intravenous solution of 1000 cc lactated ringers over 8 hours. The drip factor is 10. How many drops (gtts) per minute will the nurse regulate the intravenous solution?
   a. 25 gtts/minute.
   b. 125 gtts/minute.
   c. 21 gtts/minute.
   d. 167 gtts/minute.

9. A 2 day old baby boy has just been circumcised using the Gomco clamp. He is diapered after applying a petroleum jelly gauze strip to the circumcised area. What should the nurse tell the parents regarding his care?
   a. "Because this is a fresh surgical site, the baby probably won't be able to void for a few hours."
   b. "The gauze is put on to prevent infection to the fresh excision site."
   c. "The gauze is put on to help control bleeding and to prevent the diaper from adhering to the site."
   d. "The infant should not have a complete bath as the circumcised area should not get wet."

10. A 27 year old female client was admitted to the hospital two days ago following a motor vehicle accident in which she sustained multiple trauma. She has subsequently developed guaiac positive stools and is complaining of epigastric pain. Which of the following actions by the nurse indicates a complete knowledge base about peptic ulcers?
    a. Explains to the nursing student that the goal of antacid therapy is to maintain a pH above 2.0.
    b. Explains to the client that peptic ulcers can occur anywhere from the esophagus to the duodenum.
    c. Explains to the client that sucralfate (Carafate) acts by blocking the production of stomach acid.
    d. Explains to the client that famotidine (Pepcid) should be taken one hour after meals.

11. A 28 year old male client is admitted with injuries after an accident on the ski slopes. He is paralyzed from the waist down. The client is approaching discharge. The nurse would expect the client's chief concern to be:
a. whether he intends to finish his college degree.
b. if his fiancee will still marry him.
c. his marketability in the work force.
d. how he will best contribute to society.

12. A 51 year old female client has just been told by her physician that she must have open heart surgery. She tells the nurse, "I'll die. I won't make it through the surgery." The best reply of the nurse would be:
a. "A positive attitude is very important for your recovery."
b. "Many people are shocked by the thought of surgery at first. Let's talk about it."
c. "I don't believe that. Tell me how you feel about the upcoming surgery."
d. "Maybe we can talk about what you think is happening with this surgery."

13. A 41 year old female client has been diagnosed with a middle ear infection. The physician orders amoxicillin trihydrate (Amoxil). The most important information the nurse should assess about the client is:
a. history of gastrointestinal disturbances.
b. allergies to penicillin.
c. presence of fever.
d. if she is diabetic.

14. A client has received instructions for a scheduled exercise electro-cardiography (Stress Test). Which of these comments by the client indicates the need for further teaching?
a. "The last cigarette I had was last night."
b. "These shoes are comfortable and easy to walk in."
c. "All I had for breakfast was a cup of coffee."
d. "I have not eaten for at least three hours."

15. A 12 year old boy suffers a C_7 fracture resulting from a diving accident. The nurse determines that the priority goal is to:
a. immobilize the neck and maintain proper body alignment.
b. prevent contractures by performing range of motion to all extremities.
c. maintain accurate intake and output to avoid dehydration.
d. provide a stimulating environment to enhance recovery.

16. The physician has ordered irondextran (Inferon) for a client. The intramuscular injection is to be given by Z-track. What is the purpose of administering a medication by Z-track?
a. Diagnose individuals who have developed antibodies against specific pathogens.
b. Make sure the medication is deposited in the muscle.
c. Provide the client with medication that cannot be absorbed by the oral route.
d. Avoid depositing irritating medication through superficial layers of tissue.

17. A 66 year old Puerto Rican woman is newly admitted to the hospital for evaluation of osteoarthritis. The nurse arrives, introduces herself, and prepares to obtain baseline data on the client. Based on her cultural background, how might the nurse expect the woman to react during the interview assessment?
   a. She may avoid sustained eye contact during the interview.
   b. She may be extremely modest during the physical exam.
   c. She may be hesitant to answer personal questions.
   d. She may extend her hand to greet the nurse.

18. A 26 year old male client with leukemia is considering a bone marrow transplant. After client teaching is completed, he makes the following statements. Which of the following responses indicates that he has sufficient knowledge about the procedure?
   a. "Almost any blood relative is a probable donor for the transplant."
   b. "During the treatment, my visitors will have to wear gowns and masks."
   c. "After the transplant, I won't need drugs to suppress my immune system."
   d. "I'll look forward to having a roommate while I recover from the transplant."

19. The nurse returns from witnessing a 52 year old female client sign a consent form for a coronary angiography procedure. At the desk, the nurse meets her charge nurse and states, "Although this woman said she understood the procedure, its risks, and complications following the physician's explanation, she still seems doubtful." The appropriate response of the charge nurse would be:
   a. "The nurse's signature on the consent form validates the client's informed consent."
   b. "You and the physician share equal responsibility when obtaining informed consent."
   c. "Since you've already witnessed the consent, document your concerns on the client's chart."
   d. "Your signature on the consent form verifies the client's signature only; however, you have a moral and ethical obligation to notify the physician."

20. John, a 9 year old, is admitted to the pediatric trauma unit with a gunshot wound to the abdomen. John and his best friend, Todd, had made a suicide pact and shot each other from close distance. Todd died instantly, but John is now in stable condition. The day after the accident the nurse is changing John's dressing while he is watching television. The news announces the suicide pact of John and Todd. Which of the following actions would be most appropriate at this time?
    a. Turn off the television and distract John by playing a board game.
    b. Watch the announcement with John and tell him not to worry about anything, he is safe now.
    c. Watch the news with John and ask him if he would like to talk about what happened.
    d. Continue to change the dressing and tell John that the wounds are healing and he should be ready to go home in a week.

21. Saundra Kelsey, 32 years old, is the mother of three preschool children. She is tired much of the time and complains of feeling nervous. Mrs. Kelsey describes a situation where her husband complained to her that dinner is always late. She then yelled at her husband stating it was his fault dinner was late because he never gets home from work on time. This is an example of:
    a. reaction formation.
    b. displacement.
    c. projection.
    d. introjection.

22. A 2 year old boy is hospitalized for extensive testing and treatment. His mother is a single parent and must return to work. She explains this to the boy who starts to cry and then becomes quiet. He says, "Mommy go." and begins to play with his trucks. The best analysis of the interaction is that:
    a. the boy understands why his mother can't stay with him.
    b. the boy is responding with a despair reaction.
    c. the boy has adjusted to being hospitalized.
    d. the boy's mother feels guilty about leaving her son.

23. A 65 year old female client is receiving 5-fluorouracil treatments for metastatic breast cancer. She reports to the nurse that she just has no appetite and has not been eating. To meet the goal of maintaining nutritional status, which of the following interventions is appropriate?
    a. Encourage her to drink low calorie ginger ale with meals.
    b. Instruct her to avoid taking her pain medications for three hours prior to meals.
    c. Instruct her to limit foods high in protein until the end of the meal.
    d. Encourage her to drink a small glass of wine just before a meal.

24. A 21 year old female client has come to the outpatient gynecology clinic for treatment of a vaginal infection. The nurse will know that the client understands the teaching when she states:
   a. how urinary infections occur and are spread.
   b. how sexual activity and infections may be related.
   c. how to practice "safe sex".
   d. how to communicate more effectively with her partner.

25. A 55 year old female client who is newly diagnosed with type II diabetes mellitus comes into the outpatient clinic for teaching. Which of the following statements indicates that this teaching has been successful?
   a. "Once I start insulin injections, they will never be discontinued."
   b. "If my insulin dose has to be adjusted upward it probably means my disease is getting worse."
   c. "Urine and blood glucose testing should not be used inter-changeably."
   d. "Type II diabetes is caused by eating too much sugar."

26. The nurse is giving discharge instructions to a 55 year old man who has had an anterior myocardial infarction (MI). Guidelines for sexual intercourse should include which of the following?
   a. Foreplay should be prolonged.
   b. Intercourse after heavy meals is recommended.
   c. Morning intercourse should be avoided.
   d. Place pressure on arms during intercourse.

27. A client is ordered two compatible pre-operative medications to be given intramuscularly. One medication is in a multi-dose vial and one medication is in a single-dose vial. The current procedure for administration should be to:
   a. draw up the medication from the multi-dose vial then draw it up from the single-dose vial.
   b. draw up the medication from the single-dose vial and then draw it up from the multi-dose vial.
   c. draw up the medication from the single-dose vial then change needles before drawing up the medication from the multi-dose vial.
   d. draw up the medication in two separate syringes.

28. A client delivered a healthy boy 2½ days ago. She is breast feeding her son. Today she complains of feeling breast engorgement and is having difficulty breast feeding. Which of the following comments by the client would indicate a need for further health teaching?
   a. "I should wear a well-fitting supportive bra."
   b. "I should apply ice to nipples to improve nipple erection."
   c. "I can take a prescribed mild analgesic 20 minutes before feeding if I'm too uncomfortable."
   d. "I can breast feed frequently."

29. A 74 year old client is brought to the hospital by her daughter for tests relating to sudden changes in cardiac status. During admission she seems nervous and glances quickly around the room stating she doesn't know why she is here and she'd feel more comfortable at home. An appropriate short term goal would be that the client will:
   a. be oriented to time, place and person by the end of the shift.
   b. be cooperative with hospital routine by the end of the day.
   c. demonstrate less anxiety by the end of two hours.
   d. state the reason for her hospitalization by the end of one hour.

30. A 60 year old female client is given a diagnosis of hyperthyroidism. Considering this diagnosis, the client is most likely to exhibit:
   a. myxedema, goiter and diaphoresis.
   b. exopthalamos, fatigue and weight loss.
   c. weight gain, increased appetite and tachycardia.
   d. goiter, weight loss and increased appetite.

STOP You have now completed Practice Session: 7. Now take a few minutes and correct your answers. Calculate your accuracy rate by dividing the number of questions you completed correctly by the total number of questions you completed (30).

Correct answers ÷ total number of questions completed = accuracy rate.

_____ ÷ _____ = _____

ANSWERS AND RATIONALES

1. **The correct answer is a.** Impaired physical mobility takes into account her difficulty with self-care, pain and physical deformities which accompany severe rheumatoid arthritis, including the complications. Activity intolerance (option b), altered home health maintenance (option c), and self-esteem disturbance (option d) are also possible nursing diagnoses related to the pain and immobility but are secondary to impaired physical mobility due to its consequences and may improve if physical mobility improves (Ignatavicius & Bayne, 1991; p. 678).

   Nursing Process: Analysis
   Client Need: Safe, Effective Care Environment

2. **The correct answer is a.** The diagnosis deals with chronic pain so the long term goal should address this area. Weight loss to reduce joint stress (option b), drug therapy (option c) and splinting (option d) are all methods to reduce pain and may be used as areas for short term goals (Ignatavicius & Bayne, 1991; p.678).

   Nursing Process: Planning
   Client Need: Physiological Integrity

3. **The correct answer is b.** Clients on prednisone (Deltasone) will have periodic bloodwork done for glucose and electrolytes. Effects of the steroids on the system may result in sodium and fluid retention, lowered potassium levels or increased glucose. These complications have serious consequences which would necessitate treatment. Checking for urinary protein (option a) and mouth ulcers (option c) may be complications of gold therapy. Bruising or bleeding gums (option d) would not be considered normal since they represent a decreasing ability for clotting. They are often complications of salicylate therapy (Ignatavicius & Bayne, 1991; pp. 678-680).

   Nursing Process: Evaluation
   Client Need: Health Promotion & Maintenance

4. **The correct answer is a.** A hysterosalpingography is a test commonly used to assess problems related to infertility. A radiopaque dye is injected through the cervix and x-rays are taken to check for abnormalities of the tubes or endometrial cavity. An enema is given to enhance visualization. The test is unrelated to the occurrence of ovulation (option b). A basal body temperature record (option c) is another type of infertility study to determine if regular ovulation is occurring. Bathing or douching would not affect a hysterosalpingography but would be avoided prior to a postcoital examination for sperm count and motility (option d) (Lewis & Collier, 1992; pp. 1422-1423).

   Nursing Process: Implementation
   Client Need: Physiological Integrity

5. **The correct answer is a.** Being sexually active doesn't protect one from testicular cancer. When testicular cancer is detected early it has a very high rate of cure (option b). The epididymis is the cordlike structure on the top and back of the testis (option c). Testicular self-exam should be performed monthly and during or after a warm bath or shower when the scrotum is more relaxed (option d) (Smeltzer & Bare, 1992; pp. 1338-1339).

Nursing Process: Evaluation
Client Need: Health Promotion & Maintenance

6. **The correct answer is a.** The initial approach of the nurse to a family should be as participant observer. The nurse should observe family interactions and then participate by joining with the family. Identifying the family members, accepting cultural norms and validating communications are also important tasks during early visits. Assisting families (option b) and being a supportive change agent (option d) would be true later in treatment. Family therapy (option c) is practiced only after graduate education (Danielson, Hamel-Bissell & Winstead-Fry, 1993; pp. 197-199).

Nursing Process: Implementation
Client Need: Psychosocial Integrity

7. **The correct answer is a.** The usual gait taught to clients with musculoskeletal injuries is a three-point gait. The client is taught to point the affected foot forward (option c) then swing the crutches and affected extremity forward at the same time. The unaffected leg is then advanced forward to meet the crutches (option d). A four-point gait (option b) may be used for partial weight-bearing (Ignatavicius & Bayne, 1991; p. 801).

Nursing Process: Implementation
Client Need: Safe, Effective Care Environment

8. **The correct answer is C.**
Step One:
Total volume ÷ hours to infuse = cc/per hour
$$1000 \text{ cc} \div 8 = 125 \text{cc/hour}$$

Step Two:
$$\frac{\text{Total cc} \times \text{drop factor}}{\text{minutes}} = \text{drops/minute}$$

$$\frac{125 \text{ cc} \times 10}{60} = 20.8 \text{ (round up)} = 21 \text{ gtts/minute}$$

(Weaver & Koehler, 1992; pp. 96-98).

Nursing Process: Implementation
Client Need: Safe, Effective Care Environment

9. **The correct answer is c.** The petroleum gauze facilitates healing by applying light pressure to the site and by preventing the clot formation from adhering to the diaper. Option (a) is incorrect as it may frighten the parents. The nurse does need to assess the baby's voiding for amount, adequacy of stream and bleeding. Option (b) is incorrect as there is not any antimicrobial in petroleum jelly to affect potential infection. Option (d) is incorrect as there is no contraindication to wetting the penis to keep it clean, however, neonates should not have complete baths

until the cord stump has fallen off (Ladewig, London & Olds, 1990; p. 634).

Nursing Process: Implementation
Client Need: Health Promotion & Maintenance

10. **The correct answer is b.** Peptic ulcers can occur anywhere along the gastro-intestinal tract where the lining comes in contact with stomach acid. The goal of antacid therapy is to keep the pH above 3.5. A pH of 2 would still be very acidic (option a). Sucralfate (Carafate) forms a protective coating directly on the lining of the stomach (option c). Famotidine (Pepcid) is absorbed and blocks the production of acid by the parietal cells. There is no advantage to giving it after meals (option d) (Smeltzer & Bare, 1992; pp. 898-899).

Nursing Process: Implementation
Client Need: Physiological Integrity

11. **The correct answer is b.** The client is 28 years old and the usual developmental stage for him would be intimacy versus isolation according to Erikson. Relationships are important in this stage and the injury introduces a new variable. The client would be concerned that his fiancee would accept him with the injury (intimacy) and continue in the relationship or abandon him (isolation). Option (a), follow-through of plans, deals more with the industry versus inferiority stage. Option (c), work force concerns, deals more with the generativity versus stagnation stage. Option (d), contributing to society, deals more with the integrity versus despair

stage (Johnson, 1993; pp. 307-308).

Nursing Process: Analysis
Client Need: Health Promotion & Maintenance.

12. **The correct answer is d.** This response suggests collaboration in dealing with the problem. It also follows most crisis theories which start by dealing with misperceptions of the problem. Option (a) gives false reassurance since there is some possibility of death with all surgeries. This will decrease trust in the nurse for giving needed information. Option (b) does not take the client seriously. It belittles the fear expressed by lumping her with "many people". Option (c) blocks communication by disagreeing with the client. The nurse conveys to the client an unwillingness to be open to what the client needs (Cook & Fontaine, 1991; pp. 60-61, 221-224).

Nursing Process: Implementation
Client Need: Psychosocial Integrity

13. **The correct answer is b.** If the client is allergic to penicillin, a similar allergy reaction to amoxicillin trihydrate (Amoxil) may occur. This could result in severe reactions including anaphylaxis. The medication should be given with food to prevent gastrointestinal disturbance (option a). Fever would be present with an infection (option c). However, if temperature returns to normal then fever returns while the client is taking the antibiotic, the physician should be notified since this may indicate super-infection or hypersensitivity. If a client is diabetic (option d) she would need to be

instructed that a false positive glycosuria may occur with copper sulfate test strips (Loeb, 1990; pp. 69-70).

Nursing Process: Assessment
Client Need: Physiological Integrity

14. **The correct answer is c.** The client should be instructed to avoid smoking, alcohol, or caffeine containing beverages the day of the test (option a). These activities can interfere with test results. A client may eat breakfast if it is not within two hours of the test (option d). The client should dress comfortably (option b) in clothes which allow easy movement while testing (Ignatavicius & Bayne, 1991; p. 2105).

Nursing Process: Evaluation
Client Need: Safe, Effective Care Environment

15. **The correct answer is a.** The major nursing goal is to avoid any further neurological insult thus stabilizing the fracture is essential. Range of motion (ROM) (option b), intake and output (option c) and environmental stimulation (option d) may be included in the nursing care plan through the course of treatment (Ignatavicius & Bayne, 1991, p. 944).

Nursing Process: Planning
Client Need: Physiological Integrity

16. **The correct answer is d.** Other purposes for administering solutions by Z-track include sealing the medication in the muscle so it cannot leak back through the upper layers of tissue and to prevent bruising or staining of the superficial layers of tissue. Option (a) is

the purpose of administering an intradermal injection. An example of a specific pathogen would be tubercle bacillus. Option (b) is the purpose of administering an intramuscular injection. Option (c) is the purpose of administering a subcutaneous injection (Timby, 1989; pp. 160, 165, 171, 177).

Nursing Process: Analysis
Client Need: Physiological Integrity

17. **The correct answer is d.** The Hispanic culture is traditionally not very territorial. The client will be most likely to extend her hand, and the touch of the nurse's hand would be welcome. Eye contact would not be avoided (option a). It would be unlikely for the Hispanic client to be extremely modest (option b) or hesitate to give information (option c), as they are usually trusting (Ellis & Nowlis, 1989; pp. 420-422).

Nursing Process: Analysis
Client Need: Safe, Effective Care Environment

18. **The correct answer is b.** The client will be in isolation during the transplant process (because of being immuno-suppressed) to reduce the risk of infection and graft versus host reaction (options c and d). Donor for a bone marrow recipient must be human leukocytic antigen (HLA) compatible or histocompatible (option a) (Smeltzer & Bare, 1992; p. 816).

Nursing Process: Evaluation
Client Need: Safe, Effective Care Environment

19. **The correct answer is d.** It is the physician's responsibility to obtain informed consent from the client, however, the nurse may clarify items of information for the client and family. The nurse's responsibility is to insure that the consent form is signed and, although she may witness the client's signature, the nurse's signature does not verify the client's informed consent (options a and b). As a client advocate, however, the nurse does have a responsibility to contact the surgeon if she believes the client has not been adequately instructed regarding the procedure (option c) (Ellis & Nowlis, 1989; p. 69; Ignatavicius & Bayne, 1991; p. 439).

Nursing Process: Implementation
Client Need: Safe, Effective Care Environment

20. **The correct answer is c.** This response allows expression of feelings and opens communication between the nurse and John. One-on-one talk therapy has been found to be helpful for the older child. While distraction is sometimes helpful in working through feelings, turning off the television sends a message of avoidance of the issue; a nontherapeutic approach (option a). Telling John not to worry and that he is safe now is false reassurance and does not encourage expression of feelings (option b). Changing the dressing without allowing John a chance to express his feelings is avoidance; a nontherapeutic technique (option d) (Clunn, 1991; pp. 363-364).

Nursing Process: Implementation
Client Need: Physiological Integrity

21. **The correct answer is c.** Projection occurs when a person disowns her true feelings about something and attributes the feelings to someone or something else. In this case, Mrs. Kelsey cannot emotionally accept the blame for the late dinner so she states it is her husband's fault. Blaming is a prominent feature of projection. Reaction formation (option a) occurs when feelings are acted out in an opposite way. For this situation, Mrs. Kelsey would have fixed her husband's favorite meals and told him what a wonderful husband he is. Displacement (option b) occurs when feelings are taken out on someone or something else rather than on the object of the feelings. For example, Mrs. Kelsey would have yelled at her children if angry with her husband. Introjection (option d) occurs when a value is identified in another and the value becomes a part of the person's lifestyle. For example, if Mrs. Kelsey decided that having dinner on time was a sign of respect, she may make timeliness a part of her lifestyle (Varcarolis, 1990; pp. 178-180).

Nursing Process: Analysis
Client Need: Psychosocial Integrity

22. **The correct answer is b.** Toddlers react to hospitalization in three stages. The protest stage is characterized by restlessness, crying, and calling parents constantly. The second stage is despair where crying may occur and then the child becomes quiet and withdrawn and clings to familiar objects. Regression may occur. The third stage, detachment, occurs when the child may not acknowledge the parents' coming or

going as well as signs of depression. Although these reactions were believed to show adjustment to hospitalization in the past (options a and c), continued study showed that this was a type of grief reaction. The parent may feel guilty at leaving the child (option d) but the question refers to the child's reaction (Marlow & Redding, 1988; pp. 759-760).

Nursing Process: Analysis
Client Need: Psychosocial Integrity

23. **The correct answer is d.** Wine tends to stimulate the appetite. It also provides calories and may decrease anxiety that she has developed about eating and becoming nauseated. Drinking low calorie fluids (option a) or water will decrease the appetite. Pain is an appetite suppressant, and unless a specific pain medication is causing nausea, it should not be avoided (option b). Foods high in protein (option c) and calories should be eaten when she is hungry (Smeltzer & Bare, 1992; p. 365).

Nursing Process: Implementation
Client Need: Physiological Integrity

24. **The correct answer is b.** When a client has a vaginal infection, it is important to teach the client and partner how infections occur and are spread as well as how they can be prevented. Urinary infections are important to prevent but vaginal infections would be the discussion topic since that was the reason for the clinic visit (option a). "Safe sex" (option c) and effective communications (option d) are also important but teaching regarding vaginal infections is the primary outcome criteria for this client (Phipps, Long, Woods & Cassmeyer, 1991; p. 1611).

Nursing Process: Evaluation
Client Need: Health Promotion & Maintenance

25. **The correct answer is c.** Directly testing the blood is the only accurate means of determining the blood sugar. The urine only provides useful information when the blood sugar is above about 200 mg/dl. It will not provide knowledge below the point of glucose being spilled into the urine. It also will not detect a low blood sugar. All other responses are misconceptions about diabetes. Often weight loss reduces or eliminates the requirement for insulin (option a). Insulin dose may need to be adjusted during times of stress (option b). Diabetes is caused by the pancreas not producing sufficient insulin (option d) (Smeltzer & Bare, 1992; p. 1046).

Nursing Process: Evaluation
Client Need: Physiological Integrity

26. **The correct answer is a.** Prolonging foreplay allows for the heart rate to increase gradually. Sexual intercourse is not recommended after a heavy meal (option b). Morning intercourse is recommended (option c) as the heart is rested, and sexual positions that place increased pressure on the arms (option d) are not advisable (Lewis & Collier, 1992; p. 814).

Nursing Process: Planning
Client Need: Physiological Integrity

27. **The correct answer is a.** Medication should first be drawn up from the multi-dose vial and then from the single-dose vial. This procedure keeps the medication in the multi-dose vial from becoming contaminated by the medication in the single-dose vial (option b). Changing the needle (option c) will not prevent contamination. Medication from the multi-dose vial would begin to mix with the medication from the single-dose vial as soon as the plunger is pulled back. If any adjustment is needed in the amount of medication being drawn from the multi-dose vial then the mixed medication will be drawn back into the multidose vial, contaminating that vial's medication. As long as the two medications are compatible, they may be given in the same syringe (option d). Two injections cause unnecessary discomfort to the client (D'Angelo & Welsh, 1988; p. 73).

Nursing Process: Implementation
Client Need: Physiological Integrity

28. **The correct answer is b.** A client with engorgement needs to have warm compresses applied or to take a warm shower just prior to feeding to facilitate triggering the let-down reflex. Option (b) is correct as ice is contraindicated in engorgement if one wishes to continue breast feeding. Ice may be applied to the nipples if there is a nipple inversion noted. Option (a) is indicated to provide support to the mammary musculature during lactation. Option (c) is indicated to assist the mother to relax and encourage the let-down reflex. Option (d) is indicated until mother and infant establish a balance between milk production and amount of milk the infant consumes (Ladewig, London & Olds, 1990; p. 652).

Nursing Process: Implementation
Client Need: Health Promotion & Maintenance

29. **The correct answer is d.** This client demonstrates signs of anxiety and states she does not understand why she has been hospitalized. Therefore, the short term goal should reflect that need. Although it is desirable to decrease the anxiety level (option c), the words "less anxiety" are not measurable. A nurse on the next shift would find that goal difficult to evaluate since it is not stated in behavioral terms. There is no assessment data to suggest that the client is disoriented since she knows she is in the hospital (option a). The client has not demonstrated signs of being uncooperative (option b) (Varcarolis, 1990; pp. 181-182).

Nursing Process: Planning
Client Need: Psychosocial Integrity

30. **The correct answer is d.** Since the thyroid hormones have a stimulatory effect on metabolism, hyperthyroidism is associated with an increase in metabolic rate. The gland also enlarges and has an increased blood flow. Symptoms of increased metabolic rate include: tachycardia, weight loss despite increased appetite, diaphoresis, heat intolerance and nervousness. Exopthalamos is also associated with hyperthyroidism. Myxedema (a thickening of the skin), fatigue and weight gain are associated with hypothyroidism (options a, b and c)

(Smeltzer & Bare, 1992; p. 1083).

Nursing Process: Assessment
Client Need: Physiological Integrity

PRACTICE SESSION: 8

Instructions:

Allow yourself 30 minutes to complete the following 30 practice questions. Use a timer to notify yourself when 30 minutes are over so that you are not constantly looking at your watch while completing the questions.

1. A 64 year old male client is scheduled for a cholecystectomy. When asked to sign a surgical consent form for the procedure, he states, "The surgeon and I discussed the surgery earlier today, but I've thought of a few more questions for him." The nurse's responsibility in this case is to:
   a. obtain the client's signature on the consent form, witness it, then notify the surgeon.
   b. contact the surgeon, informing him that the client does not have informed consent.
   c. explain the procedure, its risks and complications, and validate the client's informed consent.
   d. notify the nursing supervisor that the client does not have informed consent.

2. A 52 year old female comes to the gynecology clinic for a normal checkup. When the nurse asks if there are any problems, the client states she sometimes voids involuntarily when she laughs or coughs. The nurse should prepare to:
   a. suggest the client urinate every two hours.
   b. explain the Credé maneuver to the client.
   c. place the client on a urinary training schedule.
   d. teach the client to do Kegel's exercises.

3. An acid-fast bacilli sputum is to be collected on a client. Which of the following nursing actions would be indicated?
   a. Collect an early afternoon specimen.
   b. Administer mouth care before collecting sputum specimen.
   c. Collect sputum specimen early in the morning in a clean sputum container.
   d. Wear a mask when collecting sputum.

Situation:

Mr. Donald Silas, 78 years old, is admitted to the hospital for control of depression and behavioral problems associated with Alzheimer's disease. (The next four questions pertain to this situation.)

4. Mr. Silas is sitting in the lounge near the door. Another client with family members comes into the lounge and turns on the television. The other client offers Mr. Silas a snack. Mr. Silas shouts, "Get away from me. You're trying to hurt me. I don't know you people." The best response by the nurse should be:
   a. "Stop shouting, Mr. Silas, you're scaring the other people in the lounge."
   b. "You're in the hospital, Mr. Silas, I'll take you back to your room."
   c. "Mr. Silas, come back to your room with me and we'll talk."
   d. "I won't let anyone hurt you while you're in the hospital, Mr. Silas."

5. The nurse would document the incident as:
   a. an outburst of temper.
   b. an alteration in thought process.
   c. an episode of disorientation.
   d. a disturbance in self-concept.

6. Mr. Silas becomes agitated. He is pacing in his room, repeating "I don't know them, why are they bothering me?" Considering his behavior, the best response by the nurse would be:
   a. "Come sit in this chair and do some leather work with me, Mr. Silas."
   b. "I can see how this would be so upsetting to you, Mr. Silas."
   c. "I know I don't understand, Mr. Silas. Please try to explain it to me."
   d. "It's hard not to know the people around you. Maybe in a little while I'll introduce you to some other people."

7. The nurse is writing a plan of care for Mr. Silas. The best type of nursing care would be to:
   a. assign Mr. Silas to several groups to promote adaptability.
   b. increase environmental stimuli to prevent increased organic symptoms.
   c. limit the amount of time given for self-care activity so there is less distractibility.
   d. assist the client to maintain contact with family so respect is maintained.

8. An occupational health nurse is starting a preventive health program at the company. The nurse would plan what type of program?
   a. Weight reduction.
   b. Smoking cessation.
   c. Back strengthening.
   d. Stress reduction.

9. A 66 year old male with metastatic lung cancer is admitted to the hospital for his chemotherapy administration. One of his nursing diagnoses is: potential for bleeding secondary to low platelet count ($50,000/mm^3$). Because of this diagnosis, which of the following should be included in his plan of care?
   a. Instruct him to avoid his daily flossing routine.
   b. Catheterize intermittently to avoid renal infection.
   c. Recognize a platelet count of $90,000/mm^3$ as normal.
   d. Use fleet enema for constipation.

10. Following a liver biopsy the nurse should place the client in which position?
   a. Supine position.
   b. Left lateral position.
   c. Right side with pillow under costal margin.
   d. May ambulate one hour after procedure.

11. The nurse educates a client with pernicious anemia to increase intake of:
   a. animal proteins, eggs, and dairy products.
   b. green leafy vegetables, citrus fruits, and eggs.
   c. breads, pasta, and citrus fruits.
   d. fresh fruits, vegetables, and pasta.

12. A 53 year old client was admitted to the hospital after an automobile accident. Due to physical problems, an emergency tracheostomy was performed. When caring for the tracheostomy, the nurse should:
   a. inflate the cuff while the client speaks.
   b. remove the inner cannula before suctioning the client.
   c. remove the inner cannula before cleaning it.
   d. deflate the cuff while the client is eating.

13. A 27 year old client is hospitalized with a gastrointestinal disturbance resulting in dehydration. The physician orders 1000 cc D_5W with 20 mEq KCl to run over six hours followed by another 2000 cc to run over the next sixteen hours. Considering a drop factor of 15, what would be the rate of the intravenous solution in drops per minute?
   a. 42 gtts/minute; 31 gtts/minute.
   b. 28 gtts/minute; 21 gtts/minute.
   c. 17 gtts/minute; 12 gtts/minute.
   d. 40 gtts/minute; 53 gtts/minute.

14. A 25 year old female is admitted to the hospital for a diagnostic work-up for Meniere's disease. The results of her testing confirm this diagnosis. The nurse teaches her about the disease. Which of the following statements indicate that further teaching is needed?
   a. "Meniere's disease is caused by a benign tumor near the brainstem."
   b. "I should try to limit salt intake."
   c. "I should try to identify an aura that occurs before my attack of vertigo."
   d. "I will probably have some permanent hearing loss."

15. A post-operative client in the post-anesthesia care unit has just extubated. The client becomes dyspneic and is experiencing stridor. Based on these findings the nurse suspects which of these conditions?
    a. Laryngeal edema.
    b. Hypoxemia.
    c. Atelectasis.
    d. Pneumothorax.

16. A 24 year old female has come to the clinic for genetic counseling. She has one child who has been diagnosed with Duchenne's muscular dystrophy. Since this disease is the result of a sex linked recessive genetic trait, the nurse informs the client that:
    a. the trait is linked to her husband and he must come in for testing.
    b. only the female offspring will contract the disease.
    c. her sons will have a 50% chance of contracting the disease.
    d. only 50% of her children will have the disease; the other 50% will be carriers.

17. A client undergoing home peritoneal dialysis presents in the emergency room with fever, abdominal pain, and cloudy dialysate outflow. Based on these findings the nurse suspects:
    a. nephritis.
    b. bowel obstruction.
    c. strangulated hernia.
    d. peritonitis.

18. A baby girl is admitted to the newborn nursery after a normal delivery. Prior to discharge the nurse is to perform a Guthrie test to screen for phenyl-ketonuria. Which preparation would the nurse use for accurate results?
    a. The infant should have nothing by mouth 24 hours prior to the test.
    b. The infant should have received formula 72 hours prior to the test.
    c. The infant needs to receive a 10% glucose solution prior to the test.
    d. The infant should have voided 10 times prior to administration of the test.

19. A client is admitted to the cardiac care unit and placed on lanoxin (Digoxin) therapy. Which drug when given with lanoxin (Digoxin) may predispose a client to digitalis toxicity?
    a. Warfarin sodium (Coumadin).
    b. Furosemide (Lasix).
    c. Meperidine (Demerol).
    d. Mylanta.

20. The nurse should monitor clients receiving total parenteral nutrition (TPN) for which of these symptoms?
    a. Diarrhea.
    b. Elevated glucose.
    c. Abdominal distension.
    d. Thrombocytopenia.

21. A ten year old boy has surgery to repair a left tibial fracture with cast application. One hour post-operatively, the boy complains of severe pain and tightness in the affected area. The best action of the nurse would be to:
    a. explain that post-operative pain is common; reposition and evaluate in one hour.
    b. medicate with prescribed analgesic and document.
    c. remove cast and notify the physician immediately.
    d. assess neurovascular status of left leg and notify physician immediately.

22. A six year old post-tonsillectomy client vomits approximately 400 cc of bloody discharge. The best action of the nurse would be to:
    a. take the client's vital signs.
    b. place the client in shock position.
    c. continue to monitor the client for further emesis.
    d. notify the physician immediately.

23. In working with depressed clients, the nurse utilizes which of the following approaches?
    a. Reassuring and accepting.
    b. Optimistic and expressive.
    c. Non-judgmental and energetic.
    d. Empathic and firm.

24. Dana, an 18 month old, is believed to have roseola. Which of the following symptoms would the nurse assess?
    a. Axillary lymphadenopathy.
    b. Pruritic maculopapules on extremities.
    c. Koplik spots on the buccal mucosa.
    d. Rash that fades on pressure.

25. The charge nurse on a very busy unit tells a student nurse to give a newly ordered drug to her client. The student nurse giving the medication says she doesn't know the drug but will look it up later. The best action of the charge nurse would be to:
    a. tell her to give it but you'll ask her about the drug later.
    b. tell her what the drug is for.
    c. give the drug yourself.
    d. offer for the two of you to look up the drug now.

26. A 36 year old woman has recently discovered that her husband is involved in an extra-marital affair. She comes to the outpatient clinic because she is fearful and has difficulty functioning. She says, "Why does this have to happen to me?" The best response by the nurse is:
    a. "You believe bad things always happen to you?"
    b. "You believe your husband will leave you?"
    c. "Tell me more about what happened."
    d. "I don't think I understand what you mean."

27. Two student nurses are having a discussion and ask the charge nurse the difference between hemoptysis and hematemesis. The charge nurse replies that:
    a. hemoptysis is never sanguinous.
    b. hemoptysis requires cauterization with gastric endoscopy.
    c. hematemesis is acidic, erythemic vomitus.
    d. hematemesis is alkaline and frothy.

28. A client is in status epilepticus. The priority action of the nurse would be to:
    a. pad side rails with pillows.
    b. administer antiarrhythmics.
    c. restrain all extremities.
    d. prepare for intubation and assisted ventilation.

29. A client has just delivered a baby girl by spontaneous delivery six hours ago. The client is requesting assistance to the bathroom for the first time. When she stands, the client notes a gush of blood pouring down her leg and becomes alarmed. The best response by the nurse should be:
    a. "We must put you back to bed as you are hemorrhaging. I'll call the physician immediately."
    b. "This is lochia that has pooled in the vagina while you were lying down."
    c. "You have some retained placental fragments. We'll have to take you back to the delivery room."
    d. "I'll call the physician and he will probably prescribe medication to stop this bleeding."

30. A 16 year old female client with severe acne vulgaris is about to receive a prescription for oral tetracycline. Before the client is started on the tetracycline, a creatinine clearance is ordered by her physician. The client asks the nurse why she needs the test. The nurse explains that the purpose is to:
    a. prevent the possible side effect of glucosuria.
    b. monitor for a secondary urinary tract infection.
    c. confirm that there is no pregnancy.
    d. indicate a possible renal dysfunction.

STOP You have now completed Practice Session: 8. Now take a few minutes and correct your answers. Calculate your accuracy rate by dividing the number of questions you completed correctly by the total number of questions you completed (30).

Correct answers ÷ total number of questions completed = accuracy rate.

_____ ÷ _____ = _____

PRACTICE SESSION: 8

ANSWERS AND RATIONALES

1. **The correct answer is b.** The nurse should contact the surgeon to inform him of the problem. It is the physician's responsibility to obtain informed consent from the client (option a). The client should not sign the consent form until he receives informed consent. The nurse may clarify items of information, but it is not her responsibility to give detailed information regarding the surgical procedure (option c). The nursing supervisor may be made aware of the situation (option d), however the responsibility of informed consent rests primarily with the surgeon (Ignatavicius & Bayne, 1991; p. 439).

   Nursing Process: Implementation
   Client Need: Safe, Effective Care Environment

2. **The correct answer is d.** The client has described the symptoms of stress incontinence. This condition is often related to multiple pregnancies or obstetrical complications which results in relaxed pelvic muscles. Treatment is then aimed at strengthening pelvic muscles with exercises such as Kegel's exercises. Other treatments include estrogen cream prescriptions to help strengthen atrophied muscles and use of vaginal pessaries. Suggesting more frequent urination or scheduling (options a and c) is related to urge incontinence when little warning is given before

urination begins. The Credé maneuver (option b) is used to express urine from the bladder through pressured strokes and may be used in treatment of overflow incontinence (Lewis & Collier, 1992; pp. 1207-1208).

   Nursing Process: Planning
   Client Need: Psychosocial Integrity

3. **The correct answer is d.** An acid-fast bacilli specimen is usually ordered when tuberculosis is suspected. A mask protects a nurse from inhaling microorganisms from the client's respiratory tract. Obtaining a sputum specimen first thing in the morning (option a) is best because secretions pool and collect in the lungs during sleep. Mouthcare such as toothpaste or mouthwash (option b) can affect the viability of microorganisms in the sputum specimen. Sputum specimens should be collected in a sterile container (option c) so microorganisms can be easily identified (Pagana & Pagana, 1992; p. 137; Potter & Perry, 1991; p. 525).

   Nursing Process: Implementation
   Client Need: Physiological Integrity

4. **The correct answer is c.** When a client becomes upset, it is best to move the client away from the extra stimuli then talk to the client to deal with the matter. Option (a) is a reprimand and usually increases the client's anxiety because the client is scared for his safety and afraid the nurse doesn't understand. Option (b)

218

is incorrect because there is no evidence to suggest the client is disoriented. Option (d) is incorrect because it may be false reassurance (Johnson, 1993; p. 640).

Nursing Process: Implementation
Client Need: Psychosocial Integrity

5. **The correct answer is b.** Mr. Silas misperceives the verbal contact of the other client and believes he is in danger. This is often related to difficulty interpreting the actions of others and is an alteration in thought process. Option (a) is incorrect because the outburst relates to the fear of safety rather than to anger. Option (c) is incorrect because Mr. Silas does not show signs that he does not know who or where he is but his inability to deal with the added external stimuli of another client and his family talking to him. Option (d) is incorrect because there is no evidence to suggest there is a problem with his self-concept (Johnson, 1993; p. 640).

Nursing Process: Analysis
Client Need: Physiological Integrity

6. **The correct answer is d.** This statement first empathizes with the client then deals with the problem by waiting until Mr. Silas is calmer then promoting socialization in a less threatening way. Option (a) is incorrect because Mr. Silas first needs some time to rest and feel more in control. Then some distraction or other activity may be in order. A second activity occurring when a client already feels unsafe and vulnerable may lead to sensory overload and more agitation. Option (b) is incorrect. Having his own television set will

promote withdrawal rather than socialization. Option (c) is incorrect because the problem stems from over-stimulation which becomes worse as the client continues to dwell on it (Johnson, 1993; pp. 640-641).

Nursing Process: Implementation
Client Need: Psychosocial Integrity

7. **The correct answer is d.** This plan will serve to preserve the family unit and the dignity and self-worth of the client. Options (a) and (b) are incorrect because too much stimulation will cause sensory overload. Adaptability or ability to deal with change lessens in a client with an organic disorder. Changes must be made slowly. Therefore many groups would be too much stimuli. Option (c) is incorrect because it is advisable to give ample time and privacy for completing tasks to promote independent functioning (Johnson, 1993; pp. 641).

Nursing Process: Analysis
Client Need: Physiological Integrity

8. **The correct answer is c.** A back strengthening exercise program would prevent potential injuries. Weight reduction (option a), stress reduction (option d) and smoking cessation (option b) presume the problem is already present and corrective action is taking place (Spradley, 1990; p. 554).

Nursing Process: Implementation
Client Need: Physiological Integrity

9. **The correct answer is a.** Flossing could induce gingival bleeding. Catheterization (option b) should be avoided if possible as it causes trauma.

A normal platelet count (option c) is 200,000 - 350,000/mm^3. Stool softeners and increased fluid intake are encouraged to assist with regular bowel elimination. Avoidance of invasive procedures (option d) will decrease trauma and risk for bleeding (Smeltzer & Bare, 1992; pp. 360-361, 374).

Nursing Process: Planning
Client Need: Physiological Integrity

10. **The correct answer is c.** The client is maintained on bedrest for 24 hours after the procedure with pressure applied to the biopsy site. Pressure is necessary to prevent hemorrhage since the liver is highly vascular. The client is placed on the right side with a pillow under the costal margin for one to two hours. This position facilitates compression of the liver capsule against the chest wall; therefore, decreasing the risk of hemorrhage or bile leakage. The client is placed in the flat supine or left lateral position during the procedure (options a and b). Ambulation (option d) is contra-indicated for 24 hours following a liver biopsy due to the risk of hemorrhage (Pagana & Pagana, 1992; pp. 468-469; Phipps, Longs, Woods & Cassmeyer, 1991; pp. 1148-1149).

Nursing Process: Implementation
Client Need: Safe, Effective Care Environment

11. **The correct answer is a.** Pernicious anemia is caused by a deficiency of an intrinsic factor necessary for vitamin B_{12} absorption. Treatment is aimed at increasing the intake of foods high in vitamin B_{12} which include animal proteins, eggs, and dairy products. In option (b) only one food (eggs) contains vitamin B_{12}. Options (c) and (d) do not contain any vitamin B_{12} (Ignatavicius & Bayne, 1991; p. 254).

Nursing Process: Implementation
Client Need: Physiological Integrity

12. **The correct answer is c.** The inner cannula is removed in order to clean it. When the cuff is inflated, no air can pass through the trachea so the client is unable to speak (option a). Clients are often given magic slates or other means of communication. There is no reason to remove the inner cannula when the client is suctioned (option b). The cuff should remain inflated while the client is eating (option d) to prevent aspiration (Lewis & Collier, 1992; pp. 485-486, 489).

Nursing Process: Implementation
Client Need: Physiological Integrity

13. **The correct answer is a.**
$$\frac{1000 \text{ cc}}{(6 \text{ hrs})} \times \frac{1 \text{ hr}}{(60 \text{ min})} \times \frac{15 \text{ gtts}}{(cc)} =$$

$$\frac{15000 \text{ gtts}}{(360 \text{ min})} = 41.6 = 42 \text{ gtts/min}$$

$$\frac{1000 \text{ cc}}{(8 \text{ hrs})} \times \frac{1 \text{ hr}}{(60 \text{ min})} \times \frac{15 \text{ gtts}}{(cc)} =$$

$$\frac{15000 \text{ gtts}}{(480 \text{ min})} = 31.25 = 31 \text{ gtts/min}$$

(D'Angelo & Welsh, 1988; p. 182).

Nursing Process: Planning
Client Need: Physiological Integrity

14. **The correct answer is a.** This is an untrue statement. Meniere's disease often mimics a tumor at the cerebellopontine angle so part of the diagnostic workup is done to rule this out. Limiting salt intake (option b) is thought to help reduce symptoms. Learning to recognize an aura (option c) may help the client to take action to minimize an attack. There is usually at least some permanent hearing loss (option d) associated with Meniere's disease (Smeltzer & Bare, 1992; pp. 1609-1611).

Nursing Process: Evaluation
Client Need: Health Promotion & Maintenance

15. **The correct answer is a.** Laryngeal edema or spasm is a medical emergency that can occur when an endotracheal tube is removed and the larynx is stimulated. The spasming larynx can cause upper airway obstruction leading to hypoxemia (option b), a lowered blood oxygen level. Atelectasis (option c) is collapsed alveoli and can occur post-operatively necessitating coughing and deep breathing. Pneumothorax (option d) is an accumulation of air in the pleural space resulting in a collapsed lung (Ignatavicius & Bayne, 1991; pp. 474, 1963).

Nursing Process: Analysis
Client Need: Physiological Integrity

16. **The correct answer is c.** There is a 50% chance that the sons will be affected by the genetic trait. The affected male transmits the genetic trait to daughters but not to sons. Therefore,

females are the carriers and there is a 50% probability that the sons will be affected (options a, b and d) (Martin & Reeder, 1991; pp. 79-80).

Nursing Process: Implementation
Client Need: Health Promotion & Maintenance

17. **The correct answer is d.** Peritonitis is an infection of the peritoneum (lining in the abdomen) and is the major complication of peritoneal dialysis. Cloudy dialysate outflow should be checked since it indicates an infection. Nephritis, inflammation of the kidney (option a), bowel obstruction (option b) and strangulated hernia (option c) may cause fever and abdominal pain but would not affect dialysate. Dialysate outflow should be clear and yellow (Ignatavicius & Bayne, 1991; p. 1909).

Nursing Process: Analysis
Client Need: Physiological Integrity

18. **The correct answer is b.** Because phenylalanine is found in milk, its metabolites begin to build up for the baby who has phenylketonuria (PKU) once milk feedings are initiated. For best results the infant should have been on feedings 48 to 72 hours (option a). However, if discharge is done the following day, the test may be done on the infant and follow-up is indicated in 10 to 14 days if phenylalanine blood level is 4 to 6 mb/dl or greater. Option (c) is incorrect. If an infant is receiving 10% glucose solutions such as hyper-alimentation, the test should be deferred for at least 48 hours. Option (d) is incorrect as phenylalanine builds up in the blood and voiding won't decrease

levels (Ladewig, London & Olds, 1990; p. 740).

Nursing Process: Planning
Client Need: Health Promotion & Maintenance

19. **The correct answer is b.** Furosemide (Lasix) is a loop diuretic that enhances excretion of potassium. Hypokalemia potentiates the effects of digitalis. The heart becomes more excitable and dysrhythmias may occur when potassium is depleted in the body. Diuretics are commonly used in treatment of edema associated with congestive heart failure. Furosemide (Lasix) and lanoxin (Digoxin) are often administered together. Warfarin sodium (Coumadin) and meperidine (Demerol) (options a and c) do not interact with lanoxin (Digoxin). Warfarin sodium (Coumadin) enhances hypopro-thrombinemia. Meperidine (Demerol) is a narcotic analgesic. Antacids decrease the digitalis effect (option d). Higher digitalis doses may be required if antacids are given for an extended period of time (Baer & Williams, 1992; pp. 350, 353-354, 474-475, 631-633).

Nursing Process: Analysis
Client Need: Physiological Integrity

20. **The correct answer is b.** Total parental nutrition solution is hyperosmolar, consisting of 25-35% dextrose and 3-5% amino acids, electrolytes, minerals and vitamins. Intravenous fats may also be administered; therefore, increasing osmolarity and caloric intake. The high dextrose content increases the risk of hyperglycemia. Insulin may be required as coverage or added to the TPN solution. Hyperglycemia is enhanced by inadequate insulin coverage, rapid TPN infusion, hyponatremia and hypokalemia. Hyperglycemia produces a state of osmotic diuresis leading to sodium and potassium depletion. The nurse should monitor serial glucose and electrolyte levels in clients receiving TPN. Diarrhea and abdominal distension are associated with enteral feedings (options a and c) Thrombocytopenia is not directly associated with TPN administration (option d) but may be a side effect of other medications the client is receiving (Ignatavicius & Bayne, 1991; pp. 323-325; Pagana & Pagana, 1992; pp. 563-565; Phipps, Long, Woods & Cassmeyer, 1991; pp. 1095, 1259, 1262-1263).

Nursing Process: Assessment
Client Need: Physiological Integrity

21. **The correct answer is d.** Following a fracture and cast application, the client is at risk for developing compartment syndrome. Compartment syndrome is an emergency situation in which there is increased pressure within one or more muscle compartments of the extremity. Circulation is compromised which may lead to loss of limb if not treated immediately. Signs and symptoms of compartment syndrome include pain, pallor, absence of pulse, paresthesia and paresis of the affected extremity. Frequent neurovascular assessments are necessary to identify signs and symptoms of compartment syndrome. The physician must be notified immediately of changes in the client's neurovascular status for emergency intervention. Post-operative pain is common to all surgical procedures (option a). However, clients

with injuries to the distal portions of the upper and lower extremities are at risk for developing pain associated with compartment syndrome. Pain is associated with external and internal sources of pressure. The nurse evaluates for external (casts, dressings) and internal (bleeding, fluid accumulations) sources of pressure. Muscle ischemia due to vasodilation and edema cause severe pain. Analgesics may mask pain characteristic of compartment syndrome (option b). Repositioning and evaluating in one hour (option a) does not facilitate early assessment and intervention. Irreversible neuromuscular damage may occur four to six hours after onset of compartment syndrome. The nurse is not permitted to remove the cast without a physician's order (option c). This is outside the scope of nursing practice (Ignatavicius & Bayne, 1991; pp. 782-783).

Nursing Process: Implementation
Client Need: Safe, Effective Care Environment

22. **The correct answer is d.** When a post-tonsillectomy client vomits a significant amount of blood or spits blood frequently, danger of hemorrhage exists and the physician should be notified immediately so the client can be examined. Vital signs (option a) may or may not be altered at that point and the physician would need to be notified regardless of the results. Shock position (option b) or reverse Trendelenburg would not be necessary unless actual signs of shock are present. Action should be immediate so that the danger of shock, hemorrhage, and airway

compromise can be prevented (option c) (Smeltzer & Bare, 1992; p. 485).

Nursing Process: Implementation
Client Need: Safe, Effective Care Environment

23. **The correct answer is d.** In working with depressed clients the nurse utilizes an empathic but firm approach. She is nonjudgemental and accepting, but should avoid a cheerful optimistic attitude (options a and c). It is important to understand that the nurse can not talk the client out of his depression (option b). Too much expressiveness or reassurance from the nurse will cause the client to retreat in isolation (Haber, Leach-McMahon, Price-Hoskins & Sideleau, 1992; p. 569).

Nursing Process: Implementation
Client Need: Psychosocial Integrity

24. **The correct answer is d.** Roseola is found in 6 month to 24 month old children. It begins with a high fever that lasts 3 to 4 days. When the fever drops, a maculopapular nonpruritic rash appears on the trunk (option b) that fades with pressure. It is accompanied by cervical and postauricular lymphadenopathy (option a). Koplik spots are seen in rubeola (option c) (Whaley & Wong, 1991; pp. 708-709).

Nursing Process: Assessment
Client Need: Physiological Integrity

25. **The correct answer is d.** Even though the unit is busy, the nurse giving the medication and caring for the client

should understand the drug's actions and side effects to give the drug safely. Telling her to give the drug and ask about it later is an unsafe practice (option a). The student nurse will not be able to check for adverse reactions, side effects or expected actions. If the charge nurse tells the student nurse what the drug is for, the student will not learn other essential information nor responsibility for self-initiated learning and professional behavior (option b). If the charge nurse gives the drug herself, this takes her away from her duties and may cause the student to feel unable to do the job herself plus, the student will not know actions and side effects to check (D'Angelo & Welsh, 1988; pp. 12, 60).

Nursing Process: Implementation
Client Need: Safe, Effective Care Environment

26. **The correct answer is c.** This statement focuses on the event and her perceptions of it. Expression of facts and feelings is often the first constructive step toward coping with the problem. The nurse will also obtain necessary assessment data. Option (a) overgeneralizes and gives more meaning to the statement than is there. Option (b) does not address the concerns of the client and is a misinterpretation of the client's question which involves how unfair this is to her. Option (d) seeks clarification where none is needed. The client needs to continue expression of her problem (Cook & Fontaine, 1991; pp. 192-194, 221-224).

Nursing Process: Implementation
Client Need: Psychosocial Integrity

27. **The correct answer is c.** The nurse must differentiate between hemoptysis and hematemesis in order to assess the appropriate body system. Hematemesis is sanguinous, acidic vomitus which is never frothy. Hemoptysis is sanguinous, alkaline sputum which is usually frothy (options a and d). Surgical intervention is usually not indicated to treat hemoptysis. If bleeding does not subside, bronchoscopy with endo-bronchial tamponade or removal of bronchiectic lobe may be necessary. Hematemesis may require gastric endoscopy to cauterize a bleeding vessel or ulcer (option b) (Phipps, Long, Woods, & Cassmeyer, 1991; pp. 823, 938-939).

Nursing Process: Implementation
Client Need: Physiological Integrity

28. **The correct answer is d.** The first priority during a seizure is ensuring the client's airway and promoting oxygenation. During a seizure the tongue may obstruct the oropharynx and the glottis may not close completely, increasing the risk of aspiration. Side rails should be padded to prevent injury during a seizure. However, pillows should be avoided due to the danger of suffocation (option a). Antiarrhythmic medications are not the drugs of choice during a seizure (option b). Anticon-vulsants are the first line drugs used to treat seizures. The client should not be restrained during seizure activity (option c). Restraining increases the risk of the injury due to excessive motor activity. The client should be in constant view and protected against injury during the seizure (Phipps, Long, Woods & Cassmeyer, 1991; p. 1824).

Nursing Process: Implementation
Client Need: Safe, Effective Care Environment

29. **The correct answer is b.** Lochia is the discharge of blood and mucous from within the uterus after the birth of the infant. It should never exceed a moderate flow. Since the client has not been out of bed yet, the blood pooled in the vaginal vault. Upon standing, with the help of gravity, the lochia flows out and down her leg. For options (a), (c) and (d), further assessment is indicated before any of these conclusions could be reached. To do so, the nurse would assist the client to the bathroom so she may empty her bladder and place a clean peripad on the client and recheck it within one hour. If the client is saturating a pad in less than an hour, suspect uterine atony, for which fundal massage is the first response. If this does not correct a heavy flow, notify the physician (Ladewig, London & Olds, 1990; p. 763).

Nursing Process: Implementation
Client Need: Health Promotion & Maintenance

30. **The correct answer is d.** One of the side effects of tetracycline is the inability to concentrate urine. Therefore, adolescents with renal problems should not be given the tetracycline. Glucosuria is neither a side effect of tetracycline, nor can a creatinine clearance test prevent it (option a). Urinary tract infections are ruled out by routine urinalysis, not a creatinine clearance (option b). Chorionic gonadotropin is the test used to rule out a possible pregnancy (option c) (Mott,

Sperhac & James, 1990; p. 1162).

Nursing Process: Assessment
Client Need: Physiological Integrity

PRACTICE SESSION: 9

Instructions:

Allow yourself 30 minutes to complete the following 30 practice questions. Use a timer to notify yourself when 30 minutes are over so that you are not constantly looking at your watch while completing the questions.

1. A client is admitted to the psychiatric unit after being brought to the emergency room by the police who state she is known to be homeless. The client is dressed in three layers of clothes and has two garbage bags of belongings which she clings to vehemently. When the nurse introduces herself the client yells, "Dirty Gerty, Dirty Gerty. Stay away from my things." and runs to a corner of the room. The best action of the nurse would be to:
   a. leave the client alone until she becomes familiar with her surroundings and calms down.
   b. tell the client you'll be glad to place her things in the safe so no one takes them.
   c. escort the client to her room so she won't disturb others.
   d. explain that you won't touch her things and just want to talk to her.

2. The immediate goal of treatment for a client with open angle glaucoma is to:
   a. reduce intraocular pressure.
   b. increase lost peripheral vision.
   c. increase tonometry reading to 35 mm Hg.
   d. decrease episodes of blurred vision.

3. The nurse is instilling eye drops into a client's eyes. The correct placement of the eye drops is:
   a. on the eyeball.
   b. in the conjunctival sac.
   c. at the inner canthus.
   d. under the eyelid.

4. A 54 year old male is scheduled for femoral percutaneous cardiac catheterization with angiography. Which of the following instructions should the nurse give to the client?
   a. "Following the procedure we will have to limit your fluid intake for about 12 hours."
   b. "We will be in to check the incision site every 30 minutes for 2 hours."
   c. "It is normal to experience an occasional thudding sensation in the chest during the procedure."
   d. "You will have to remain on flat bedrest for 12 hours after the procedure."

5. A client presents with rupture of membranes. She is 32 weeks gestation by dates. The physician evaluates her and diagnoses her with premature rupture of membranes (PROM). The nurse would also expect to find:
   a. incompetent cervix.
   b. excessive weight gain.
   c. hypertension.
   d. nulliparity.

6. A 42 year old client being treated for arthritis refuses the medication offered by the student nurse. The student nurse documents: "Client refused medication. Medication not given." The staff nurse covering the client would evaluate this documentation as:
   a. not within the scope of the student's ability to chart.
   b. miscommunication about the medication incident.
   c. sufficient charting about the client's medication refusal.
   d. insufficient charting about the medication incident.

7. A 64 year old client is admitted to the emergency room with chest pain, shortness of breath and apprehension. The electrocardiograph strip demonstrates the following: an underlying normal sinus rhythm with a rate of 76. However, there are several irregular beats that lack a P wave and have a QRS complex 0.14-0.16 seconds long. The nurse would analyze this strip as indicative of:
   a. premature ventricular contractions (PVC).
   b. ventricular tachycardia.
   c. premature atrial contractions (PAC).
   d. paroxysmal atrial tachycardia.

8. A client with chronic renal failure (CRF) is starting peritoneal dialysis. The nurse explains to the client that peritoneal dialysis works by:
   a. increasing fluid intake to increase kidney perfusion.
   b. drawing fluid and metabolic by-products into the peritoneum.
   c. increasing electrolytes available for reabsorption by the kidneys.
   d. replacing fluid and glucose that has been lost with CRF.

9. A 26 year old male client is admitted to the orthopedic unit for total hip replacement secondary to avascular necrosis. Documentation in the progress notes by the physician states, "needs to see anesthesia prior to surgery to rule out malignant hyperthermia." Which of the information given to the nurse during the assessment indicates that the client is at risk for malignant hyperthermia?
   a. A brother who died after an appendectomy.
   b. Frequent night sweats.
   c. History of untreated hypertension.
   d. History of frequent cocaine use.

10. A 22 year old female has come to the medical clinic complaining of fatigue, palpitations and exertional dyspnea. After laboratory tests, she is diagnosed with iron-deficiency anemia. The nurse would use which nursing diagnosis to plan teaching?
    a. Sensory-perceptual deficit related to organic brain tissue damage.
    b. Activity intolerance related to imbalance between oxygen supply and demand.
    c. High risk for infection related to decreased resistance to pathogens.
    d. Fatigue related to impaired physical mobility.

11. The nurse should assess the client in halo traction for:
    a. erythema and drainage at pin sites.
    b. pain under cast site.
    c. proper alignment of belt encircling iliac crests.
    d. equal pulses in lower extremities.

12. A pregnant female comes to the hospital for delivery at 30 weeks gestation. She delivers an infant boy by spontaneous vaginal delivery. She has had no prenatal care. She states she is exhausted because she has been caring for her sister this past week who has German measles (rubella). Titers drawn on the mother indicate she is immune. What special precautions, if any, need to be done for the neonate?
    a. The neonate is infectious and needs to be isolated.
    b. No special care needs to be initiated for the neonate as the mother is rubella immune.
    c. A direct Coomb's test needs to be done on the neonate immediately.
    d. The neonate needs to be prepared for immediate surgery.

13. Betty, age 5, is admitted to the burn center after a car accident. Betty becomes confused and starts to pull on her tubes. The nurse also notes that respirations have increased significantly. The initial action of the nurse would be to:
    a. assess for further signs and symptoms.
    b. give a sedative to calm her and ease respirations.
    c. administer oxygen by nasal cannula.
    d. notify the physician and suggest that more fluids be ordered.

14. The physician orders diphenhydramine hydrochloride (Benadryl) 50 mg intramuscularly one hour prior to a pulmonary angiography. Which observation by the nurse would indicate the effectiveness of the medication?
    a. Increased oxygen to peripheral vessels.
    b. Decreased blood pressure and cardiac output following the procedure.
    c. Absence of angioedema and urticarial eruptions following procedure.
    d. Ability to cough up excess sputum.

15. A student nurse reports taking a central venous pressure (CVP) reading of 8. The nurse evaluates the student's reading was probably correct when the student reports:
    a. the reading was taken during the inspiratory phase of the respiratory cycle.
    b. the head of the bed was elevated to the same degree as the manometer.
    c. the zero on the manometer is at the level of the right atrium.
    d. there were no fluctuations of the fluid in the manometer.

16. Health teaching regarding possible lithium toxicity is completed prior to client discharge. The nurse knows that the health teaching has been effective if the client reports:
    a. dry mouth.
    b. macular rash, abdominal distention.
    c. diarrhea lasting over 24 hours.
    d. flu-like symptoms.

17. A client has been receiving chemotherapy for lung cancer. His white blood cell count (WBC) is $800/mm^3$. Because of his diagnosis of increased risk for infection, which of the following actions should be included in his plan of care?
    a. Instruct him to avoid fresh fruits.
    b. Keep his intravenous site clean and avoid changing it as long as possible.
    c. Instruct the family to bring cut flowers only, no potted plants.
    d. Administer packed red blood cells (PRBC's) replacement as ordered.

18. A 56 year old female has had her first mammogram at the outpatient breast center. The client has been given instructions about mammograms and recommendations specifically for her age group. Which of these comments by the client indicates that she understands the instructions?
    a. "Next time I'll use the clear deodorant."
    b. "I'll be back next year, even if my doctor's examination is normal."
    c. "Since my mammogram was negative, I know I don't have to be back for two years."
    d. "Since mammograms are done by ultrasound, I know there isn't any radiation exposure."

19. Matthew is eight months old and has been admitted with possible intussusception. Which of the following data would the nurse expect to find during the history and physical?
   a. Constipation and currant jelly stools.
   b. Diarrhea and gray stools.
   c. Abdominal cramping and fatty, foul smelling stools.
   d. Vomiting and tarry black stools.

20. A client with hepatitis B is admitted to a medical unit. What type of isolation should be maintained?
   a. Blood and body fluid precautions.
   b. Respiratory isolation.
   c. Enteric precautions.
   d. Good handwashing only.

21. A 35 year old female is admitted to the post-anesthesia care unit (PACU) from the operating room following a craniotomy for drainage of a hematoma. The client is snoring loudly and has diminished breath sounds bilaterally. Which of the following actions should the nurse take immediately?
   a. Place the client on oxygen and raise the head of the bed.
   b. Place the client on oxygen and call the anesthesiologist.
   c. Tilt the client's head back and move her jaw forward.
   d. Insert a nasal airway into the client.

22. A client is a gravida 2 para 1 at 28 weeks gestation. The mother's blood type is A negative, the father's blood type is O positive. Testing reveals a negative indirect Coomb's testing and negative antibody titers. Which of these statements is most appropriate to teach the mother at this time?
   a. "These results indicate that you are not sensitized and the fetus is not at risk so, as a prophylactic measure, you will receive your Rhogam now and after delivery."
   b. "These results indicate you are sensitized so the doctor will be in to talk with you regarding potential consequences to the baby and further actions."
   c. "These results indicate the fetus is definitely at risk so the doctor will most likely want to do an ultrasound test to determine the extent of hydrops fetalis."
   d. "These results indicate that a condition known as erythroblastosis fetalis is present and a fetal exchange transfusion is warranted."

23. Ms. Ruth Romano, R.N. answers her door to find a neighbor child sent by her mother. The child asks for assistance for her 3 month old baby sister who is ill and has stopped breathing. Ms. Romano wants to take some action but is unsure if she is covered under the Good Samaritan Law. What is the most action she could take and stay within the area of the law? The nurse could:
   a. inform the child that her mother should call her physician.
   b. assess the infant and start cardiopulmonary resuscitation, if needed.
   c. tell the child you'll call an ambulance immediately.
   d. instruct the mother in how to do cardiopulmonary resuscitation on the infant.

24. A 59 year old Orthodox Jewish man is admitted for evaluation of his right flank pain. He is on a general diet. In assisting him with his dinner selection for the next day, what foods would be appropriate to accompany lamb chops?
   a. Fruit salad with cottage cheese.
   b. A potato with sour cream.
   c. Vegetable soup in clear broth.
   d. Buttered sweet pecan rolls.

25. A 54 year old man is brought to the emergency room after collapsing in the supermarket. He refuses treatment saying, "I can't stay here. I have no insurance. My company went out of business." The initial approach by the nurse should be to:
   a. discuss health alternatives and consequences with the client.
   b. allow the client to leave the emergency room.
   c. listen to the client talk without interrupting until he becomes calm.
   d. change the subject to one that is less anxiety-producing.

26. A 45 year old male client comes to the outpatient clinic for symptoms related to an ear infection. To aid in health promotion, the nurse should also:
   a. teach about screening for prostate cancer.
   b. ask about decreasing sexual libido in this age group.
   c. teach the client about bi-monthly testicular self-examination.
   d. screen him for hearing loss.

27. A client received epidural anesthesia prior to delivery. The nurse would be alert for which common side effect?
   a. Headache.
   b. Hypotension.
   c. Tachycardia.
   d. Seizures.

28. Clients who have been taking neuroleptic medications are frequently taken off these medications for brief periods of time (drug holidays). The purpose of this practice is to:
    a. decrease the risk of tardive dyskinesia.
    b. treat neuroleptic malignant syndrome.
    c. slowly decrease client's dependence on the drug.
    d. decrease photosensitivity that frequently occurs with neuroleptic medication.

29. A 57 year old client is learning to use a metered dose aerosol inhaler. The nurse evaluates that the teaching has been successful if the client demonstrates which of the following?
    a. The client synchronizes dose delivery with inspiration.
    b. The client holds his breath while pumping the aerosol.
    c. A fine white powder residue is seen in the inhaler.
    d. A small tablet is first placed in the inhaler.

30. The nurse is teaching a client with newly diagnosed cluster headaches. What instructions would be advisable for this client?
    a. Visual and speech disturbances may occur prior to the headaches.
    b. Ipsilateral lacrimation may occur during the headaches.
    c. It may be comforting to lie still during the headaches.
    d. The headaches rarely occur during deep sleep or napping.

STOP **You have now completed Practice Session: 9. Now take a few minutes and correct your answers. Calculate your accuracy rate by dividing the number of questions you completed correctly by the total number of questions you completed (30).**

Correct answers ÷ total number of questions completed = accuracy rate.

_____ ÷ _____ = _____

PRACTICE SESSION: 9

ANSWERS AND RATIONALES

1. **The correct answer is d.** This response addresses the immediate needs of the client while maintaining contact. Option (a) deserts the client in a new and unfamiliar place and asks her to do what the nurse should be doing which is assisting the client to lower her anxiety level. Option (b) would be threatening to the client by stripping her of her belongings thus increasing her anxiety which may result in destructive behavior. Option (c) would be very threatening to a frightened client. Since the client shows no present danger to others, this option is unnecessary. Respecting the client's privacy and approaching the client calmly fosters trust which is of primary concern here (Wilson & Kneisl, 1992; pp. 270-273).

Nursing Process: Implementation
Client Need: Psychosocial Integrity

2. **The correct answer is a.** In glaucoma, intraocular pressure increases because the eye does not release aqueous humor as fast as it is made. This leads to increased pressure on the retina and that sensitive tissue is destroyed. Peripheral vision is usually destroyed first resulting in tunnel vision. The tissues cannot be repaired and any lost vision remains unrecoverable (option b). Normal tonometry readings are 12-22 mm Hg (option c) and treatment is aimed towards normal range. Decreasing

episodes of blurred vision (option d) will be a secondary effect of decreasing intraocular pressure. The blurred vision is a symptom of glaucoma (Lewis & Collier, 1992; p. 344).

Nursing Process: Planning
Client Need: Physiological Integrity

3. **The correct answer is b.** First, the eye should be cleansed with a sterile pad or cotton ball with warm water or saline to remove any old medication or encrusted matter in the eye. Then ask the client to tilt and turn the head back slightly toward where the eye drop is being instilled and to look up and away. The nurse should place her hand on the cheek and use fingers to pull skin away from the eye which exposes the conjunctival sac. With the other hand, the nurse should position the bottle above the sac and squeeze for the number of drops to fall into the conjunctival sac (options a, c and d). The nurse should release the eye so the client may blink to distribute the medication across the eye. Extra medication should be blotted away with a tissue (D'Angelo & Welsh, 1988; p. 130).

Nursing Process: Implementation
Client Need: Safe, Effective Care Environment

4. **The correct answer is c.** Clients often complain of palpitations during the procedure caused by extra beats from the catheter touching the heart. Fluid

233

should be encouraged following angiography (option a) to help flush the dye from the system. Usual post-catheterization care includes bedrest with the head of the bed no higher than 30 degrees and the affected leg straight and incision checks every 15 minutes for 2 hours then every hour for 2 hours (options b and d) (Smeltzer & Bare 1992; p. 635).

Nursing Process: Implementation
Client Need: Physiological Integrity

5. **The correct answer is a.** Premature rupture of membranes (PROM) is associated with an incompetent cervix. Other signs of incompetent cervix include painless cervical softening, effacement and dilatation and history of spontaneous abortion. Excessive weight gain (option b) is unrelated to PROM but may be related to hypertension (option c), gestational diabetes or thrombophlebitis. Nulliparity (option d) by definition means never having been pregnant, hence if one has never been pregnant one can not have premature rupture of membranes (Ladewig, London, and Olds, 1990; p. 482; Martin & Reeder, 1991; pp. 185, 611).

Nursing Process: Assessment
Client Need: Physiological Integrity

6. **The correct answer is d.** If a medication is not given, the reason should be explored with the client and documented along with the refusal. Often clients refuse medications because they don't understand why they're receiving the drugs or because they are experiencing side effects. Any time a routine order is not able to be carried out, the reason should be documented. The student nurse administered the medication and should be the person to document it (option a). The medication incident was not miscommunicated (option b) but more data is needed (option c) for complete charting (Perry & Potter, 1990; p. 454).

Nursing Process: Evaluation
Client Need: Safe, Effective Care Environment

7. **The correct answer is a.** Premature ventricular contractions are characterized by the absence of P waves and wide QRS complex (longer than 0.10 seconds). Any rhythm can be the underlying rhythm including normal sinus rhythm (NSR). Ventricular tachycardia (option b) differs by a regular rhythm that is more rapid (150-200 beats per minute). Premature atrial contractions (option c) are different from premature ventricular contractions in that they originate in the atria and thus do have a P wave. Paroxysmal atrial tachycardia (option d) differs with a regular but rapid (150-250 beats per minute), shortened PR interval and normal QRS complex (Smeltzer & Bare, 1992; pp. 565-570).

Nursing Process: Analysis
Client Need: Physiological Integrity

8. **The correct answer is b.** The high concentration of glucose in the dialysate draws excess fluid and metabolic by-products through the peritoneal wall by osmosis (option d). In chronic renal failure (CRF), the kidneys are unable to excrete excess fluid (option a) and electrolytes (option c) leading to

imbalances (Ignatavicius & Bayne, 1991; p. 1909).

Nursing Process: Implementation
Client Need: Physiological Integrity

9. **The correct answer is a.** Malignant hyperthermia is a rare familial disorder that is fatal in over 50% of the cases. It is triggered by certain anesthetic agents and consists of hyperthermia, tachycardia, tetanus, and dysrhythmia. People at risk for this problem include those with an unexplained death of a family member after anesthesia or those with a history of muscle cramps, weakness or a history of severe unexplained fever themselves after anesthesia. Night sweats (option b) are usually associated with infectious processes. Untreated hypertension (option c) and cocaine use (option d), while significant, are not related to malignant hyperthermia (Smeltzer & Bare, 1992; p. 433).

Nursing Process: Analysis
Client Need: Physiological Integrity

10. **The correct answer is b.** Activity intolerance may occur since less oxygen is being carried to the tissues. The client is already complaining of fatigue and exertional dyspnea typical of mild to moderate anemia. These symptoms would be manifestations of lowered oxygen supply and inability to tolerate the usual activity patterns. Sensory-perceptual deficit related to organic brain tissue damage (option a) may result from brain oxygen loss associated with strokes or cardiac arrest. High risk for infection related to decreased resistance to pathogens (option c) might be the result

of neutropenia. Fatigue related to impaired physical mobility (option d) is incorrect. The client would have fatigue related to lack of oxygen or impaired physical mobility related to fatigue (Lewis & Collier, 1992; pp. 668, 685, 695, 1707).

Nursing Process: Analysis
Client Need: Physiological Integrity

11. **The correct answer is a.** Metal pins are inserted into the skull and a halo ring is applied for immobilization purposes. Pin care is performed as ordered to remove exudate and decrease risk of infection. Osteomyelitis is a serious complication of skeletal traction. Halo traction does not involve cast application (option b). Pain under a cast may be indicative of infection, hematoma, or compartment syndrome. Pelvic traction involves application of a belt slightly above and encircling the iliac crests (option c). Circulatory status should be assessed in all neurological clients but specific attention to the lower extremities is not indicated with halo traction (option d) (Black & Matassarin-Jacobs, 1993; pp. 1886-1887; Phipps, Long, Woods & Cassmeyer, 1991; pp. 2022-2029).

Nursing Process: Assessment
Client Need: Physiological Integrity

12. **The correct answer is a.** The rubella virus can cross the placental barrier so immunity of the mother is not adequate protection for the fetus (option b). Option (c) is incorrect because a direct Coomb's test is done on the infant to determine if an infant is sensitized to the Rh antigen. This is not related to the

rubella virus. Option (d) is incorrect because the most susceptible time for the fetus is during the first trimester. The teratogenic effects may manifest themselves in the neonate in the form of congenital heart disease or cataracts. There is no assessment data to indicate that surgery is necessary (Olds, London & Ladewig, 1992; pp. 532-533).

Nursing Process: Planning
Client Need: Safe, Effective Care Environment

13. **The correct answer is a.** The signs presented may be from several causes and further assessment is necessary before any analysis and planning can safely be done. Option (b) is incorrect because sedation may cause more confusion and mask symptoms leading to appropriate diagnosis. Options (c) and (d) are incorrect because they presuppose that two different problems exist - respiratory problems and hypovolemia. Correct assessment is necessary before nursing actions take place (Marlow & Redding, 1988; p. 804).

Nursing Process: Assessment
Client Need: Physiological Integrity

14. **The correct answer is c.** A pulmonary angiography requires the injection of an iodine dye. In clients allergic to dye, diphenhydramine (Benadryl), an H_1 antihistamine, may be administered prior to the procedure to decrease the risk of anaphylaxis. Peripheral oxygen supply (option a) is unrelated to the effects of diphenhydramine (Benadryl). It's effect on blood pressure and cardiac output (option b) is influenced by blocking

histamine's release causing vasodilation and increased capillary permeability. Diphenhydramine (Benadryl) blocks the effects of histamine in the bronchioles by decreasing bronchoconstriction, spasm, edema and hypersecretion of mucous (option d) (Ignatavicius & Bayne, 1991; pp. 654-655; Pagana & Pagana, 1992; pp. 604-605).

Nursing Process: Evaluation
Client Need: Physiological Integrity

15. **The correct answer is c.** The following procedure should be used when taking a central venous pressure (CVP) reading. The client should be lying flat in the bed without a pillow (option b). If the client cannot tolerate a flat position, the bed may be elevated up to 30 degrees but the same elevation should be documented and used for every reading. The zero of the manometer should be at the same level as the right atrium which is located at the midaxilla, fourth intercostal space (option c). After the intravenous fluid is introduced and the stopcock turned toward the client, the fluid should slowly fall until it stops at the level to be read. Fluctuations should occur and directly relate to the respiratory cycle (option d). This means the apparatus is functioning normally. Proper reading is taken during the expiratory phase (option a) of the respiratory cycle (Smith & Duell, 1993; pp. 748-750).

Nursing Process: Evaluation
Client Need: Safe, Effective Care Environment

16. **The correct answer is c.** Clients with diarrhea excrete more sodium and water causing dehydration. This increases the

amount of lithium in the circulation and may result in lithium toxicity. To combat this possibility, the client's intake of sodium and fluids should be increased while the dehydrating condition exists. Dry mouth (option a) is a common side effect of many psychotropic medications and does not generally need to be reported. Relief can be obtained by frequent sips of water and sucking of hard candy. Rash and abdominal distention (option b) are unrelated to lithium therapy but may be adverse effects of antipsychotic drugs. Flu-like symptoms (option d) may occur in clients taking antipsychotic medications related to agranulocytosis and leukopenia (Cook & Fontaine, 1991; pp. 135, 138-139).

Nursing Process: Evaluation
Client Need: Physiological Integrity

17. **The correct answer is a.** Fresh fruits and vegetables harbor bacteria not removed by washing. Flowers and potted plants (option c) carry bacteria. Intravenous sites (option b) should be kept clean and changed every other day to avoid infection. Packed red blood cells (PRBC's) may be needed to correct anemia but will not increase the number of white blood cells (WBC's) and therefore will not reduce infection (Smeltzer & Bare, 1992; p. 360).

Nursing Process: Planning
Client Need: Safe, Effective Care Environment

18. **The correct answer is b.** The American Cancer Society advises all women after the age of 50 to have annual mammograms (option c).

Mammograms are not performed by ultrasound technique but do use x-ray; however, the amount of radiation exposure is minimal (option d). Deodorant can alter a mammogram and mimic calcifications (option a) (Smeltzer & Bare, 1992; pp. 1294-1295).

Nursing Process: Evaluation
Client Need: Health Promotion & Maintenance

19. **The correct answer is a.** In intussusception a portion of the intestine telescopes into another part of the intestine. This causes the walls of the intestine to press against each other leading to inflammation, edema, and hemorrhage. The stool mixes with blood and mucus and looks like currant jelly. Constipation results from the swelling and obstructed flow about the intussusception. Gray stools are seen in abnormalities of bile elimination not intussusception (option b). Fatty, foul smelling stools are seen in children with cystic fibrosis (option c). Black tarry stools are seen in abdominal bleeding, such as ulcers (option d) (Whaley & Wong, 1991; p. 1516).

Nursing Process: Assessment
Client Need: Physiological Integrity

20. **The correct answer is a.** Universal precautions (blood and body precautions) advocates that all blood and body fluids are potentially infectious. Infections such as hepatitis B are transmitted by direct or indirect contact with infectious blood or body fluids. Universal precautions decrease the risk of transmission. Respiratory isolation (option b) is used to prevent

transmission of infectious diseases spread by droplets in the air such as measles, mumps, meningococcal meningitis and pneumonia. Enteric precautions (option c) are used to prevent transmission of hepatitis A. Good handwashing alone (option d) is not sufficient to prevent transmission of contaminated blood and body fluids. The Center For Disease Control (CDC) requires protective barriers (gloves, gowns, aprons, masks and goggles) be worn as indicated during client contact (Phipps, Long, Woods & Cassmeyer, 1991; pp. 614-615).

Nursing Process: Planning
Client Need: Safe, Effective Care Environment

21. **The correct answer is c.** Noisy breathing or snoring occurs when the tongue is obstructing the airway. This is alleviated by the head tilt, jaw thrust. The nurse should not delay by calling the anesthesiologist (option b), but should open the airway first, apply oxygen and continue to monitor. Oxygen therapy will be ineffective at this point since the airway is not patent and raising the head of the bed will cause the head to fall forward, further blocking the airway (options a and b). Inserting a nasal airway will cause an unnecessary rise in intracranial pressure (option d) and should be avoided, if possible (Smeltzer & Bare, 1992; p. 440).

Nursing Process: Implementation
Client Need: Safe, Effective Care Environment

22. **The correct answer is a.** The indirect Coomb's test is done on the maternal blood to determine if Rh positive antibodies are present. The test is negative which indicated she does not have any Rh positive antibodies in her circulation, which could only have come from the fetus. The negative antibody titer indicates there are not any anti-Rh positive antibodies circulating. Rhogam is recommended to be given at 28 weeks and after delivery to decrease possible transplacental bleeding concerns. Option (b) is incorrect as the results indicate the mother is not sensitized. Option (c) is incorrect because hydrops fetalis is an Rh hemolytic disease meaning the mother is sensitized. Symptoms of hydrops fetalis include marked fetal edema, congestive heart failure of the neonate and jaundice. Option (d) is incorrect because erythroblastosis fetalis is the most severe hemolytic disease of Rh sensitization. Test results indicate the mother is NOT sensitized. Treatment of severe erythroblastosis fetalis usually includes a fetal exchange transfusion (Ladewig, Long & Olds, 1990; p. 322).

Nursing Process: Implementation
Client Need: Physiological Intergrity

23. **The correct answer is b.** The Good Samaritan Law allows a nurse to act in an unforseen emergency situation to assist others. The nurse is held to the same standards as would be reasonably expected by any registered nurse under similar conditions. The Good Samaritan Law does not apply to emergencies in health care institutions. Health care

professionals may act in an emergency but are not required to do so by law. In this case, the most action the nurse could take would be to assess the infant and start cardiopulmonary resuscitation (CPR) if the child indeed is not breathing (options a, c and d). That would be the reasonable standard once intervention has started (Gillies, 1989; p. 446).

Nursing Process: Planning
Client Need: Safe, Effective Care Environment

24. **The correct answer is c.** Orthodox Jewish law conforms to kosher dietary rules. One rule states that meat and milk or milk products cannot be served together. Therefore, the only option that does not contain a milk product is vegetable soup. All other options contain a dairy product: cottage cheese (option a), sour cream (option b), and butter (option d) (Ellis & Nowlis, 1989; pp. 709-710).

Nursing Process: Planning
Client Need: Physiological Integrity

25. **The correct answer is a.** The nurse should participate actively in the care of a client in crisis. The object of assisting a client in crisis is to help in productive problem solving. This includes identifying alternatives and discussing consequences of those alternatives so the client can make an informed decision about the problem. Allowing the client to leave the emergency room without assisting the client to make an informed decision may have serious consequences (option b). Allowing the client to walk without the nurse's intervention

(option c) is asking the client to take care of himself. The client may increase his anxiety rather than becoming calmer. Changing the subject (option d) may be counterproductive at this point. The nurse's role is to help the client focus on goals pertaining to the crisis so it may be resolved (Cook & Fontaine, 1991; p. 223).

Nursing Process: Implementation
Client Need: Health Promotion & Maintenance

26. **The correct answer is a.** Men over the age of 40 should be screened for prostate cancer, a leading cause of cancer deaths. Decreased sexual libido (option b) does not normally occur until the 60's or 70's. Testicular self-examination should be done monthly (option c). However, an adult male who contracts mumps may develop orchitis with resulting atrophy. Hearing loss (option d) should occur if the ear infection is severe or prolonged. Screening would occur if disease or age related symptoms were present (Smeltzer & Bare, 1992; pp. 1325, 1332, 1339, 1594).

Nursing Process: Implementation
Client Need: Health Promotion & Maintenance

27. **The correct answer is b.** The most common side effect of epidural anesthesia is hypotension. Many caregivers attempt to ward off hypotension by preloading their pregnant clients with 500-1000 ml of intravenous fluid (usually ringer's lactate) prior to the administration of epidural anesthesia. Option (a) is incorrect because an epidural does not penetrate the dura

mater to cause a change of pressure in the cerebral spinal fluid (CSF) like spinal anesthesia may. Option (c), tachycardia, is not related to epidural anesthesia. Option (d), seizures, are not commonly seen in epidural anesthesia administration (Ladewig, London & Olds, 1990; pp. 458-459).

Nursing Process: Evaluation
Client Need: Physiological Integrity

28. **The correct answer is a.** Drug holidays are recommended at least two times a year for clients on neuroleptic medications to decrease the risk of tardive dyskinesia. Prevention of tardive dyskinesia is a crucial aspect of administering neuroleptic medications. Treatment of neuroleptic malignant syndrome includes immediate discontinuation of the neuroleptic medication (option b). Clients do not develop dependence on neuroleptic drugs (option c) and brief drug holidays will not decrease photosensitivity (option d) which is a side effect of the medication (Johnson, 1993; pp. 284-285).

Nursing Process: Analysis
Client Need: Physiological Integrity

29. **The correct answer is a.** With a metered dose aerosol inhaler, dosage must be delivered as the client inhales so the white mist is taken into the pulmonary capillaries. Holding breath would produce a questionable dosage intake (option b). Option (c), powdered residue, and option (d), tablet, may be true of turbo inhalers which deliver a dose of fine white powder (Baer &

Williams, 1992; p. 652).

Nursing Process: Evaluation
Client Need: Physiological Integrity

30. **The correct answer is b.** Lacrimation or tearing of the eye on the same side as the headache may occur. The prodromal phase of visual and speech disturbances (option a) occurs with migraine headaches. Clients with cluster headaches prefer to pace, walk, or sit during the attack (option c). Cluster headaches usually occur during napping or rapid eye movement (REM) sleep (option d) (Ignatavicius & Bayne, 1991; p. 874).

Nursing Process: Planning
Client Need: Physiological Integrity

PRACTICE SESSION: 10

Instructions:

Allow yourself 30 minutes to complete the following 30 practice questions. Use a timer to notify yourself when 30 minutes are over so that you are not constantly looking at your watch while completing the questions.

1. Ben, a 10 year old, has sustained a 7% partial thickness burn on his right leg. According to the American Burn Association, this is classified as a minor burn and can be treated at home. The nurse understands that Ben's parents need further teaching when they state:
   a. "If we see any drainage from the wound, we will need to report it to the doctor right away."
   b. "Ben can take gym in school just like before."
   c. "Before we change the dressing we'll soak it in warm water so it doesn't stick."
   d. "We'll wrap the new dressing with several layers of gauze to protect the burn."

2. A 35 year old male with extensive metastatic renal carcinoma telephones the nurse with complaints of urinary incontinence and lower back pain with movement. Which of the following instructions should the nurse give him?
   a. "Force fluids to 3000 cc and make an appointment with the physician."
   b. "Apply moist heat to back and look for blood in urine."
   c. "Go to the emergency room for evaluation."
   d. "Stay on bedrest for 24 hours or until pain subsides."

3. A client is diagnosed with disseminated intravascular coagulation (DIC). The physician orders a STAT platelet count. What other laboratory test should the nurse monitor to assess the progression of DIC?
   a. White blood cell with differential count.
   b. Osmolality.
   c. Fibrin split products.
   d. Serum protein electrophoresis.

4. A 28 year old client is admitted with acute exacerbation of asthma. The physician administers an intravenous loading dose of theophylline (Aminophylline). The nurse evaluates that it would be safe to send the client for a chest x-ray:
   a. immediately after the medication is given.
   b. 15 minutes after the intravenous dose.
   c. 30 minutes after the loading dose.
   d. 60 minutes after intravenous administration.

5. Sarah, a four month old, is admitted with dehydration from gastroenteritis. Rehydration therapy has begun. Which of the following signs and symptoms would indicate an improvement in Sarah's status?
   a. Urine specific gravity 1.008.
   b. Hematocrit 49%.
   c. Serum sodium 139 mEq/L.
   d. Serum potassium 4.9 mEq/L.

6. The physician orders a heparin sodium (Heparin) infusion of 25,000 units in 500 ml of 5% dextrose and water at 18 ml per hour. What will be the concentration of heparin sodium (Heparin) per hour?
   a. 750 units per hour.
   b. 800 units per hour.
   c. 900 units per hour.
   d. 1100 units per hour.

7. When conducting an assessment interview with a depressed client, the nurse will most likely see which of the following cognitive impairments?
   a. Flat affect.
   b. Obsessional pessimistic thoughts.
   c. Self-medicating behaviors.
   d. Persecutory beliefs.

8. A 72 year old male client is receiving 5-fluorouracil for the treatment of colon cancer. He is diagnosed with stomatitis as a complication. Instructions are given to the client on the stomatitis by the nurse. Which of the following statements indicates the client has an adequate understanding of this complication?
   a. "Spicy foods help stimulate saliva and actually decrease the irritation."
   b. "Lubrication of the lips with petroleum jelly should be avoided."
   c. "Stomatitis is an inflation of the lower gastrointestinal tract."
   d. "Stomatitis occurs because the cells in my mouth divide rapidly."

Situation:
Mr. Joshua Weinstein, 62 years old, is admitted to the hospital with cough productive for large amounts of yellow sputum, fever of 101°F (38.2°C), pulse 74, and regular. Mr. Weinstein states he was getting over the flu and woke up feeling sick. The client also complains of some chest pain that worsens on inspiration. (The next three questions refer to this situation.)

9. Based on the assessment data, the priority nursing diagnosis is:
   a. ineffective airway clearance.
   b. fluid volume deficit.
   c. knowledge deficit.
   d. activity intolerance.

10. Arterial blood gases show that Mr. Weinstein is hypoxic. Oxygen 5 liters by mask is ordered. The nurse would question this order if which of the following is present?
    a. History of cardiac tamponade.
    b. History of emphysema.
    c. Presence of bloody sputum.
    d. Presence of bradycardia.

11. Mr. Weinstein asks how he can keep from getting sick like this again. The nurse would teach him about:
    a. immune globulin.
    b. tetanus toxoid.
    c. varicella-zoster immune globulin.
    d. influenza vaccine.

12. Emily, a 9 year old, has just had a relapse of acute lymphocytic leukemia (ALL). Her parents have been told that Emily's prognosis is very poor. During Emily's first hospitalization, the nurse remembers how Emily's parents were supportive of Emily and got along with each other. Now they seem to be fighting all of the time and nothing any nurse does for Emily is good enough. The most appropriate reaction by the nurse would be to:
    a. tell Emily's parents that the nurses are doing the best that they can and there is no need to take their anger out on them.
    b. tell them that Emily needs them to be supportive; when they were supportive the first time, Emily got better.
    c. ignore the behavior; anger is a normal phase of the grief process.
    d. set up a time with Emily's parents to discuss how they are feeling and what interventions they think might be helpful in Emily's care.

13. A 72 year old client is admitted for open reduction of a wrist fracture. That night she is found wandering in the hallway near the fire alarm. When the nurse calls the client's name, the client says, "If you come any closer to me I"ll pull this fire alarm. You're a drug addict. I saw you taking drugs out of the cabinet." The best response by the nurse would be,:
    a. "I'm concerned you'll hurt your arm. I'll ask someone to take you back to your room."
    b. "Older adults often become confused when they're in a new place. I'll help you back to your room."
    c. "Please don't pull the fire alarm. You'll wake up everyone else."
    d. "You are in City Hospital. I am not a drug addict. I'll escort you to your room."

14. A client is admitted with a diagnosis of syndrome of inappropriate antidiuretic hormone (SIADH). The nurse would expect to see what laboratory finding?
    a. Serum sodium 125 mEq/L.
    b. Serum potassium 2.7 mEq/L.
    c. Serum glucose 250 mg/dl.
    d. Serum chloride 110 mEq/L.

Situation:

Mr. Tyrone Washington, 25 years old, has been diagnosed with being in the icteric phase of hepatitis A. He returned from a vacation several weeks ago where he ate shellfish which is presumed to be the cause. Assessment data includes the following: fatigue, weight loss, jaundice, hepatomegaly and right upper quadrant pain. (The next two questions pertain to this situation.)

15. Mr. Washington asks the nurse if his liver is permanently damaged. The best reply of the nurse would be:
    a. "The liver cells have necrosed and liver failure may occur."
    b. "Liver function tests may remain abnormal for several years."
    c. "The liver will be fine since you have no renal disease."
    d. "Liver cells will regenerate if complications don't occur."

16. Mr. Washington is placed on a high calorie, low fat diet. The low fat diet is related to the:
    a. tendency to lose weight.
    b. inability to tolerate proteins.
    c. lack of bile in the intestines.
    d. need for B-complex vitamins.

17. A family of four, two adults and two children, are brought to the emergency room with suspected carbon monoxide poisoning. The nurse should prepare to:
    a. stop oxygen when carboxyhemoglobin levels are more than 5%.
    b. administer 100% oxygen at hyperbaric pressure.
    c. draw blood for carbon dioxide levels.
    d. report the incident to the health department.

18. Assessment of an arteriovenous fistula for hemodialysis includes evaluation of:
    a. thrill and bruit of the fistula.
    b. mobility and strength of the arm.
    c. color and temperature of the hand.
    d. rhythm and rate of radial pulse.

19. Danny, a three year old, needs to have a pre-operative intramuscular injection. Which of the following would be the best choice for the administration of the medication?
    a. Place one hand over the greater trochanter, make a V with the index and forefinger and inject into the V using a 1 ½ inch needle.
    b. Have Danny's dad hold his arm still while injecting with a 1 ½ inch needle into the deltoid.
    c. Discuss with the physician the possibility of ordering another route of administration.
    d. Have another nurse hold Danny's greater trochanter and knee and inject into the muscle between with a 1 inch needle.

20. Mr. Charles Petrovich, 62 years old, is admitted to the cardiac care unit with an acute myocardial infarction. The electrocardiogram shows a bundle branch block. The difference between a normal sinus rhythm and a bundle branch block is that:
    a. the bundle branch block is always preceded by a normal P wave.
    b. the bundle branch block has a prolonged QRS complex.
    c. normal sinus rhythm contains a longer PR interval.
    d. normal sinus rhythm usually occurs with an acute myocardial infarction.

21. A client placed on a client controlled analgesic (PCA) pump asks why this machine works so well. The nurse explains that:
   a. the client can deliver an unlimited amount of medication as needed to achieve pain relief.
   b. PCA pumps eliminate the highs and lows of drug concentrations.
   c. the analgesia interrupts pain conduction where the sensory fibers exit from the spinal cord.
   d. the client can manually regulate the power source to vary the amplitude and frequency of the electrical stimulation.

22. A 30 year old woman has just undergone a subtotal thyroidectomy for hyperthyroidism. Four days post-operative, her pulse rate is 120/minute, respirations 28/minute, temperature is 102°F (38.9°C), and she has a slight hand tremor. These signs are an indication that the client may have:
   a. hypercalcemia and tetany related to removal of one or more of the parathyroid glands.
   b. hypokalemia and tetany related to removal of one or more of the parathyroid gland.
   c. malignant hyperthermia related to general anesthesia during the surgery.
   d. hypocalcemia and tetany related to removal of one or more of the parathyroid glands.

23. A 35 year old male client is admitted to the psychiatric unit after threatening to punch a co-worker. On interview, he tells the nurse, "This is all my boss' fault. He is the reason for all of my problems. I have to take matters into my own hands before he ruins my life." The appropriate action by the nurse at this time would be to:
   a. notify the client's boss of potential danger.
   b. call the client's place of employment to check his work history.
   c. ask the client if he has been thinking of harming his boss.
   d. decrease the client's environmental stimuli.

24. A client who has been on a respirator for two days experiences acute respiratory distress accompanied by distended neck veins. The best action of the nurse is to:
   a. hand ventilate the client.
   b. prepare for chest tube insertion.
   c. call the physician immediately.
   d. perform emergency chest decompression.

25. A 42 year old male is seen in the cancer prevention and early detection clinic. He tells the nurse that his father died of colorectal cancer and asks her what the risk factors for this type of cancer are and how to prevent it. Which of the following information given by the nurse is correct?
   a. A history of rectal polyps that have been removed does not increase the risk for colon cancer.
   b. Colorectal cancer is one of the few cancers that is not believed to be familial.
   c. Maintaining a high protein diet could help to lower risk for developing colon cancer.
   d. Flexible sigmoidoscopy is recommended after the age of 50.

26. A client who is gravida 2, para 1 is 32 weeks pregnant. She presents with a family history of diabetes on her obstetrical history. The physician suspects gestational diabetes. She has been continually showing a 2+ glucose on her urine for the past week. Which of the physician's statements would the nurse question?
   a. "She is going to need continued observation on the effect the diabetes is having on the pregnancy so we are going to have non-stress test (NST) done weekly."
   b. "Because we need to keep your sugars under control, I'm going to prescribe tolbutamide (Orinase), an oral hypoglycemic agent, for you to take daily."
   c. "I'm going to have you take a glucose tolerance test (GTT) to get more specific data on your sugars."
   d. "Infants born to mother's with diabetes run a higher risk of neonates having respiratory distress syndrome (RDS) and/or hyperbilirubinemia."

27. Two weeks post-operatively, a 49 year old woman who has had a left nephrectomy develops a deep vein thrombosis (DVT) in her right leg. She is subsequently placed on an intravenous heparin sodium (Heparin) infusion at 1100 units/hr. Which of the following laboratory values indicates that she is therapeutically anticoagulated?

a. Prothrombin time (PT): Client 10.9 seconds. Control 10.0 seconds.
   Partial thromboplastin time (PTT): Client 21.0 seconds. Control 21.0 seconds.

b. PT: Client 9.0 seconds. Control 9.0 seconds.
   PTT: Client 25.0 seconds. Control 20.0 seconds.

c. PT: Client 25.0 seconds. Control 10.0 seconds.
   PTT: Client 20.0 seconds. Control 20.0 seconds.

d. PT: Client 10.0 seconds. Control 10.0 seconds.
   PTT: Client 48.0 seconds. Control 20.0 seconds.

28. A 17 year old female is brought into the emergency department following a motor vehicle accident. She has sustained multiple injuries. She is unconscious, does not appear to be breathing and is bleeding profusely from a crushed left leg and lacerated left arm. She has a patent intravenous line in her right arm. Which of the following actions should be the priority of the nurse?

a. Ask the paramedics if the client sustained any neck injuries.

b. Place pressure over the left arm laceration.

c. Prepare the client for an endotracheal intubation.

d. Connect the client to a cardiac monitor.

29. Jamie, 8 years old, is scheduled for an elective adenoidectomy. On physical examination, she is noted to have a greenish yellow vaginal discharge. Antibiotics are ordered and surgery is canceled. Which of the following interventions is most appropriate at this time?

a. Interview all members of Jamie's household separately.

b. Enroll Jamie's mother in a parenting skills class.

c. Reschedule the adenoidectomy for two days after the last dose of antibiotics.

d. Teach Jamie's parents how and when to give the antibiotics prescribed.

30. A client experiencing panic attacks is taught relaxation techniques. The nurse understands that these techniques are often helpful because:

   a. they distract the client from thinking about underlying issues.

   b. they help the client control symptoms and this allows exploration of unconscious conflicts.

   c. they help the client understand that anxiety is a normal response to stress.

   d. they help the client see that they never have to feel anxious.

STOP You have now completed Practice Session: 10. Now take a few minutes and correct your answers. Calculate your accuracy rate by dividing the number of questions you completed correctly by the total number of questions you completed (30).

Correct answers ÷ total number of questions completed = accuracy rate.

_____ ÷ _____ = _____

PRACTICE SESSION: 10

ANSWERS AND RATIONALES

1. **The correct answer is a.** Drainage from the wound is expected and is not necessarily a sign of infection. Activity levels should not be altered in minor burns (option b). Warm water soaking of the dressing decreases the pain associated with the removal (option c). The burn should be wrapped with several layers of gauze to protect it (option d) (Mott, Sperhac, & James, 1990; p. 1170).

   Nursing Process: Evaluation
   Client Need: Physiological Integrity

2. **The correct answer is c.** Urinary incontinence is a sign that spinal cord compression may be taking place. This is an oncologic emergency and this client should be evaluated immediately. With prompt evaluation and treatment neurological function may be preserved. All other options (options a, b and d) involve waiting and may result in permanent damage (Smeltzer & Bare, 1992; p. 380).

   Nursing Process: Implementation
   Client Need: Safe, Effective Care Environment

3. **The correct answer is c.** Disseminated intravascular coagulation (DIC) is the result of an imbalance between hyper- and hypocoagulability from disease or injury. The altered clotting mechanism results in systemic or localized intravascular formation of fibrin clots. As fibrinogen is depleted in the clotting process, fibrin split products (FSP) or fibrin degradation products (FDP) are formed through fibrinolysis. The FSP's have an anticoagulant effect and inhibit clotting. When FSP's are present in large amounts in the serum, it is indicative of increased fibrinolysis associated with DIC. A DIC screening includes bleeding time, platelet count, partial thromboplastin time (PTT), prothrombin time (PT), fibrinogen, FDP or FSP, red blood smear and euglobulin lysis time. A white blood cell (WBC) with differential count, osmolality and protein electrophoresis (options a, b and d) are not included in a DIC screen (Pagana & Pagana, 1992; pp. 799-800; Phipps, Long, Woods & Cassmeyer, 1991; pp. 275-277, 349).

   Nursing Process: Assessment
   Client Need: Physiological Integrity

4. **The correct answer is d.** After rapid-release tablet or liquid or an intravenous injection, onset of action for theophylline (Aminophylline) is one hour. As the medication begins to work, the client may go to x-ray with less danger of respiratory distress. Options (a), (b) and (c) may be too soon to ensure client safety (Baer & Williams, 1992; pp. 660-661).

   Nursing Process: Evaluation
   Client Need: Safe, Effective Care Environment

5. **The correct answer is a.** In dehydration the urine specific gravity is increased; therefore, an improvement in the child's condition would bring the specific gravity to normal levels (1.002 - 1.030). In dehydration the hematocrit is elevated because of the volume loss (normal range: 35-45%) (option b). The serum sodium levels remain within normal limits (135-145 mEq/L) in dehydration because the loss is an isotonic loss (option c). The serum potassium remains within normal limits (3.5 - 5.0 mEq/L) because of impaired renal function (option d) (Mott, Sperhac, & James, 1990; pp. 1435, 1452; Whaley & Wong, 1991; p. 1280).

Nursing Process: Evaluation
Client Need: Physiological Integrity

6. **The correct answer is c.** To calculate 900 units per hour several calculations must be completed:
1) calculate units per ml using proportions:
500 ml:25,000 u = (X) u:1 ml. This equals 50 u/ml.
2) calculate ml/minute (min):
18 ml:60 min = (X) ml:1 min. This equals 0.3 ml/min (volume per hour).
3) calculate u/min.:
50 u/ml times 0.3 ml/min = 15 u/min times 60 min/hr = 900 u/hr (volume/min x 60 min/hr).
The physician's order would have to be 15 ml/hr to equal 750 u/hr (option a), 16 ml/hr to equal 800 u/hr (option b) and 22 ml/hr to equal 1100 u/hr (option d) (Kee & Marshall, 1992; pp. 168-172).

Nursing Process: Planning
Client Need: Psychosocial Integrity

7. **The correct answer is b.** Cognitive changes that frequently occur in depressed individuals include slowed thoughts, decreased concentration, ruminative thoughts that are pessimistic in nature and often focus on self blame and an attitude of hopelessness. Option (a) is an affective change that occurs usually in schizophrenics. Option (c) is a behavioral change rather than a cognitive change but does often occur in depressed clients. Option (d) usually occurs in clients experiencing paranoia (Haber, Leach-McMahon, Price-Hoskins & Sideleau, 1992; pp. 550-552).

Nursing Process: Assessment
Client Need: Physiological Integrity

8. **The correct answer is d.** The cells in the mouth proliferate rapidly which makes it susceptible to the effects of chemotherapy. Spicy foods (option a) should be avoided as they will cause irritation. Lips should be lubricated (option b) to prevent sores from forming. Stomatitis (option c) refers to an inflammation of the mouth (Smeltzer & Bare, 1992; pp. 354-363).

Nursing Process: Evaluation
Client Need: Physiological Integrity

9. **The correct answer is a.** The client states he is coughing up large amounts of sputum which suggests ineffective airway clearance. There is no evidence for fluid volume deficit (option b), knowledge deficit (option c), or activity intolerance (option d) (Smeltzer & Bare, 1992; p. 565).

Nursing Process: Analysis
Client Need: Physiological Integrity

10. **The correct answer is b.** Higher levels of oxygen are contraindicated in clients who have chronic obstructive pulmonary disease (such as emphysema) because the respiratory drive will be compromised. The other options (options a, c and d) would not prevent oxygen therapy (Smeltzer & Bare, 1992; p. 579).

Nursing Process: Analysis
Client Need: Safe, Effective Care Environment

11. **The correct answer is d.** Pneumonia that follows a viral infection such as flu can often be prevented through immunization with the influenza vaccine. Immune globulin (option a) prevents hepatitis A in exposed individuals. Tetanus toxoid (option b) prevents tetanus from contaminated wounds. Varicella-zoster immune globulin (option c) is used to prevent chickenpox in immunosuppressed children (Smeltzer & Bare, 1992; pp. 586, 989, 1894, 1933).

Nursing Process: Implementation
Client Need: Health Promotion & Maintenance

12. **The correct answer is d.** Parents of a terminally ill child need help dealing with their feelings and complaining about their child's care can restore some sense of control in the uncontrollable situation of a child dying. Telling the parents that the nurses are doing the best that they can is defending, a nontherapeutic response. It also avoids the parents' need for support (option a). Telling them to be supportive of Emily because that is how she got better the first time is false reassurance, a nontherapeutic response. It also avoids the need for the parents to discuss their feelings (option b). Ignoring the behavior will not support the parents through the grieving process. Opportunities to express emotions with the nurse, not at the nurse, will help the parents deal with their feelings allowing more emotional reserve to meet the needs of their child (option c) (Whaley & Wong, 1991; pp. 1057-1059).

Nursing Process: Implementation
Client Need: Physiological Integrity

13. **The correct answer is a.** The client is in a state of delirium with cognitive changes probably related to the new hospital environment. The client should be approached in a matter of fact way. Messages should be given firmly and clearly, especially when the client is confused and upset. This response also provides empathy about the reason for the hospitalization and also suggests she may talk with someone else that she doesn't perceive as threatening. Teaching/explaining should not be done while the client is confused and agitated (option b). The client generally is not capable of reasoning appropriately due to the cognitive changes which accompany delirium but will be able to accept these ideas when more lucid. Asking the client not to do what she has threatened to do (option c) is based on the assumption she can make that judgement. This response also places the nurse in a power struggle where the client feels threatened and will act to decrease that anxiety in any way she can. It is better for the nurse to take charge of the situation until the client becomes calmer. The client does need

to be reoriented to her surroundings (option d). In this case, however, the client may not believe the information since she feels threatened by the nurse. Rather, the client's anxiety may be decreased by relating to someone else with whom she may feel more secure at the time (Stuart & Sundeen, 1991; pp. 584-586).

Nursing Process: Implementation
Client Need: Physiological Integrity

14. **The correct answer is a.** In syndrome of inappropriate antidiuretic hormone (SIADH), there is a decreased serum sodium level due to increased water retention and increased sodium excretion. The normal serum sodium level is 136-145 mEq/L. Potassium, glucose and chloride should remain within or slightly below normal range (options b, c and d). Normal potassium is 3.5 - 5.0 mEq/L. Normal glucose is 70 mg/dl. Normal chloride is 100-106 mEq/L. (Ignatavicius & Bayne, 1991; pp. 241, 380, 1594).

Nursing Process: Assessment
Client Need: Physiological Integrity

15. **The correct answer is d.** Liver cells become damaged during hepatitis but will regenerate and begin to function normally during the convalescent period. Liver cell necrosis and consequent liver failure followed by death occur with fulminant hepatitis (option a). Liver function tests will remain abnormal (option b) if the client contracts chronic persistent hepatitis which is a common complication of viral hepatitis. Clients with chronic renal disease who contract hepatitis B (option c) are prone to

chronic active hepatitis (Lewis & Collier, 1992; p. 1125).

Nursing Process: Implementation
Client Need: Physiological Integrity

16. **The correct answer is c.** Inflammation of the liver may cause an interruption in the flow of bile which results in the symptoms such as light colored stools and dark urine. Therefore, dietary fat is often poorly tolerated. The high calorie diet is related to the tendency to lose weight (option a). Inability to tolerate proteins (option b) is related to the liver's ability to break down the proteins and is dictated by the client's individual needs. There is a need for both B-complex vitamins (option d) and vitamin K and supplements are often used (Lewis & Collier, 1992; p. 1127).

Nursing Process: Analysis
Client Need: Physiological Integrity

17. **The correct answer is b.** Carbon monoxide poisoning is an emergency situation and 100% oxygen must be administered immediately at atmospheric or hyperbaric pressure to hasten carbon monoxide elimination. Carbon monoxide binds to hemoglobin 200 times faster than does oxygen, therefore oxygen will not be transported to vital organs. Signs and symptoms relate to hypoxia: intoxicated appearance, muscle weakness, confusion, headache and dizziness. Carbon monoxide bound to hemoglobin is called carboxyhemoglobin. Carboxyhemoglobin levels, not carbon dioxide (option c), are drawn at intervals. The hyperbaric oxygen is administered until carboxyhemoglobin levels are less than 5% (option a). The

health department should be notified if the poisoning is accidental so that the building may be checked for problems. However, this would not be the immediate priority (option d) (Smeltzer & Bare, 1992; p. 1972).

Nursing Process: Planning
Client Need: Safe, Effective Care Environment

18. **The correct answer is a.** The fistula must be patent to be functional. Adequate circulation through the fistula is determined by palpating the thrill and auscultating the bruit. The mobility and strength of the arm (option b) is not affected by a fistula. It is important to assess the color, temperature, and radial pulse to assure adequate circulation of the hand distal to the fistula (options c and d) (Ignatavicius & Bayne, 1991; p. 1904).

Nursing Process: Assessment
Client Need: Physiological Integrity

19. **The correct answer is d.** This describes the vastus lateralis. It is the site of choice for intramuscular injections in children because it is easily accessible and there are no important nerves or blood vessels in this area. Although the ventrogluteal site (option a) can be used, it is not recommended because of its close proximity to the sciatic nerve. Also a 1 ½ inch needle is too large for children. It increases the possibility of coming into contact with the bone. Parents should not be used to restrain children during invasive procedures (options b). Another route is not necessary (option c) (Mott, Sperhac

& James, 1990; pp. 896-898; Whaley & Wong, 1991; pp. 1228-1231).

Nursing Process: Implementation
Client Need: Physiological Integrity

20. **The correct answer is b.** The bundle branch block is the same as a normal sinus rhythm with the exception of the length of the QRS complex which usually exceeds 0.10 seconds. Both the bundle branch block and the normal sinus rhythm are preceded by a normal P wave initiated by the sinoatrial (SA) node (option a). A prolonged PR interval of 0.20 seconds or longer is usually indicative of a first degree atrioventricular (AV) block (option c). An acute myocardial infarction may produce a normal sinus rhythm, bundle branch block or a heart block (option d) (Phipps, Long, Woods & Cassmeyer, 1991; p. 640).

Nursing Process: Analysis
Client Need: Physiological Integrity

21. **The correct answer is b.** Patient controlled analgesic (PCA) pumps are extremely effective in managing post-traumatic and post-operative pain because they eliminate the highs and lows of drug concentrations associated with intermittent parenteral dosing. Serum drug levels of the analgesic are maintained; therefore, a consistent sensation of pain relief is achieved. The client activates the pump as needed to deliver a predetermined amount of analgesia. The pump is designed to limit the total amount infused over several hours and controls the frequency of administration to prevent an overdose

(option a). The analgesia unit which interrupts pain conduction where the sensory fibers exit the spinal cord (option c) is called intraspinal analgesia. This type of analgesia targets the fibers which connect to the spinal cord. Electrical stimulation to treat pain (option d) relates to the transcutaneous electrical nerve stimulator (TENS) (Ignatavicius & Bayne, 1991; p. 130; Phipps, Long, Woods & Cassmeyer, 1991; pp. 314, 317, 2019).

Nursing Process: Implementation
Client Need: Physiological Integrity

22. **The correct answer is d.** If the parathyroid glands are accidentally removed during the thyroidectomy, the client can develop muscular twitching or spasms and hyperactivity of the nervous system due to hypocalcemia. These symptoms may occur one to seven days post-operatively as a result of decreased calcium levels (options a and b). Malignant hyperthermia (option c) commonly occurs intra-operatively or immediately post-operatively as a result of general anesthesia (Black & Matassarin-Jacobs, 1993; pp. 426, 1822-1824).

Nursing Process: Analysis
Client Need: Physiological Integrity

23. **The correct answer is c.** When homicidal behavior is suspected, the nurse assesses the client's potential for violence. Asking the questions directly role models verbalization, rather than acting out behavior. The nurse does not have enough assessment data regarding the client's homicidal potential to alert his boss (option a). Obtaining the client's work history (option b) and

decreasing environmental stimuli (option d) are not appropriate at this time. There is no evidence that the client is overstimulated (Johnson, 1993; p. 501).

Nursing Process: Implementation
Client Need: Safe, Effective Care Environment

24. **The correct answer is a.** When acute respiratory distress occurs along with neck vein distension, cyanosis and tracheal shift are evident, a tension pneumothorax has probably occurred. The client should be removed from the machine and ventilated by hand. Then the physician should be notified (option c). Equipment for chest tube insertion should be gathered (option b) so it will be ready for immediate use by the physician. Emergency chest decompression (option d) should only be attempted after specific training and if the physician will be delayed (Smith & Duell, 1993; p. 906).

Nursing Process: Implementation
Client Need: Safe, Effective Care Environment

25. **The correct answer is d.** Sigmoidoscopy is recommended every 2 years after two consecutive negative tests (one year apart). Family history, high fat, protein and beef, and history of rectal polyps (options a, b and c) are all considered risk factors for the development of colon cancer (Smeltzer & Bare, 1992; p. 949).

Nursing Process: Implementation
Client Need: Health Promotion & Maintenance

26. **The correct answer is b.** Option (b) should be questioned as oral hypoglycemics are considered teratogenic to the fetus. Option (a) is true as nonstress test (NST) or biophysical profile (BPP), may be done to assist in planning the course of pregnancy and the timing of delivery. Option (c) is correct as the glucose tolerance test (GTT) is diagnostic for gestational diabetes. Option (d) is correct as respiratory distress syndrome (RDS) appears to result from high levels of fetal insulin which inhibit some fetal enzymes necessary for surfactant production. Hyperbilirubinemia results from the immature liver enzymes to breakdown the circulating bilirubin which is causes from fetal polycythemia. The polycythemia results from the maternal glycosolated hemoglobin's inability to release oxygen (Olds, London & Ladewig, 1992; p. 458).

Nursing Process: Analysis
Client Need: Safe, Effective Care Environment

27. **The correct answer is d.** The effect of heparin sodium (Heparin) is determined by measuring the partial thromboplastin time (PTT). The partial thromboplastin (PTT) in a client therapeutically anticoagulated on heparin sodium (Heparin) is one and a half to three times the normal value or control (options a, b and c). The prothrombin time (PT) measures the effect of coumarin derivatives, the most common being warfarin sodium (Coumadin) (Black & Matassarin-Jacobs, 1993; p. 1306;

Fischbach, 1992; pp. 117-122; Hamilton, 1982; pp. 59-61).

Nursing Process: Evaluation
Client Need: Physiological Integrity

28. **The correct answer is c.** Prepare the client for endotracheal intubation. Airway is always the priority over everything else. Asking the paramedics if the client sustained neck injuries is not a reliable way to determine this (option a). All multiple trauma victims should be treated as though they have a cervical injury until proven otherwise. Controlling hemorrhage (option b) and cardiac monitoring (option d) are important interventions after an airway is established (Smeltzer & Bare, 1992; pp. 1964-1965).

Nursing Process: Planning
Client Need: Safe, Effective Care Environment

29. **The correct answer is a.** Jamie demonstrates clinical manifestations of gonorrhea, a sexually transmitted disease. Sexual abuse should be suspected and investigation consisting of separate interviews with all household members is indicated. Parenting skills are taught, if needed, after a thorough investigation (option b). Rescheduling the surgery is not the priority and avoids the immediate problem of suspected sexual abuse (option c). While the nurse would teach when and how to give the antibiotics prescribed, it also avoids the problem of suspected sexual abuse (option d) (Mott, Sperhac & James,

1990; pp. 602-603).

Nursing Process: Implementation
Client Need: Physiological Integrity

30. **The correct answer is b.** Relaxation techniques which involve tensing and relaxing muscles can help the client develop a sense of control over the intensity of their symptoms by recognizing the physical tension that accompanies the feeling of anxiety. Once this occurs, the precipitating factors that are barriers may become more conscious and thus more available for exploration (option a). Although anxiety is a normal response to stress, these clients are experiencing immobilizing and dysfunctional behaviors (option c). Telling clients to ignore or stop feeling anxiety (option d) will not work and are not therapeutic functions of relaxation exercises (Haber, Leach-McMahon, Price-Hoskins & Sideleau, 1992; pp. 404, 419).

Nursing Process: Analysis
Client Need: Psychosocial Integrity

PRACTICE SESSION: 11

Instructions:

Allow yourself 30 minutes to complete the following 30 practice questions. Use a timer to notify yourself when 30 minutes are over so that you are not constantly looking at your watch while completing the questions.

1. A 23 year old client is pregnant for the first time. The nurse should educate the client about which diet plan?
   a. If her diet is adequate, folic acid and iron are the only supplements she will need.
   b. Because of the added burden of the fetus on her system, she will need to consume megadoses of vitamins daily.
   c. She will need to restrict her intake of proteins to prevent pregnancy induced hypertension.
   d. Recommended weight gain is 20 lbs. for pregnancy so she may have to restrict calories.

2. A 34 year old male client with end stage renal disease is found to have a blood pressure of 195/110. The physician orders nifedipine (Procardia) 10 mg. Which of the following should the nurse tell the client about the medication?
   a. "I am going to inject some medicine in your IV to reduce your blood pressure."
   b. "Hold this under your tongue and I'll be able to check your blood pressure again in 30 minutes."
   c. "Calcium channel blockers can cause flushing, headaches and dizziness."
   d. "Nifedipine (Procardia) helps calcium get into your heart and blood vessels and relaxes them."

3. An 84 year old client is hospitalized with severe respiratory problems necessitating a tracheostomy. The client also has a nasogastric tube for feeding purposes. What precautions should the nurse take when giving care?
   a. The tube feedings should be administered while the client is in the supine position.
   b. The tube feedings should be given via a large bore nasogastric tube.
   c. The tracheostomy cuff should be inflated during feeding.
   d. The tracheostomy cuff should be deflated during feeding.

4. A 62 year old client is on long-term theophylline (Aminophylline) therapy. The client's theophylline (Aminophylline) level is 22 mcg/ml. The nurse would:
   a. administer the prescribed dosage of theophylline (Aminophylline) as ordered.
   b. administer the theophylline (Aminophylline) and a respiratory treatment together.
   c. order an immediate repeat theophylline (Aminophylline) level and inform the physician.
   d. hold the next dose of theophylline (Aminophylline) until clarified with the physician.

5. A 7 month old infant has beta thalassemia major or Cooley's anemia. Which of the following signs and symptoms would the nurse expect to see on assessment?
   a. Increased appetite and microcephaly.
   b. Hypertrophied musculature in the calves.
   c. Hematuria and swollen, painful joints.
   d. Palpable spleen and jaundice.

Situation:
Ms. Diane Fryer, 28 years old, comes to the emergency room in active labor. She is admitted to the labor suite accompanied by her husband. During the assessment, the mother admits to "occasional" intake of cocaine. (The next two questions refer to this situation).

6. The nurse would assess for what signs of cocaine dependence in the neonate?
   a. Meconium staining and precipitate delivery.
   b. Shrill cry and decreased moro reflex.
   c. Poor sucking and microcephaly.
   d. Irritability and hypersensitivity.

7. The pediatrician decides to wean the infant off the cocaine gradually. The nurse would expect which drug to be ordered?
   a. Cocaine.
   b. Paregoric.
   c. Glucose.
   d. Methadone.

8. The nurse approaches a client diagnosed with Alzheimer's disease and asks her to change clothes and get ready for bed. The client yells "No, I won't." and continues muttering and stamping her feet. The best approach by the nurse would be to:
   a. say nothing but start unbuttoning the client's blouse.
   b. acknowledge the client's wishes and approach the client again in a few minutes.
   c. firmly state the instructions for a second time.
   d. explain to the client that it is important for her to get adequate rest to maintain her health.

9. The nurse would best position a client with increased intracranial pressure in:
   a. Trendelenburg position.
   b. prone position.
   c. Sims position with right hip flexed.
   d. supine position head of bed elevated.

10. A 42 year old female status post-right mastectomy as a result of breast cancer returns to the clinic for a routine mammogram. The mammogram was negative. On her way out she tells the nurse that she wants to have a child. Because of her history of breast cancer, the client should be referred to which of the following agencies?
    a. Y-Me.
    b. National Hospice Organization (NHO).
    c. Ronald McDonald House.
    d. Ostomy Society.

11. As the community health nurse, which of the following diseases would be considered reportable according to international quarantine regulations?
    a. Cancer.
    b. Rabies.
    c. Influenza.
    d. Smallpox.

12. A 49 year old female client with a diagnosis of septic shock is placed on triple intravenous antibiotic therapy Which of the following would indicate that she is responding well to therapy?
    a. Arterial blood gas: pH 7.30, $PaCo_2$ 50 mm Hg, HCO_3 24 mEq/L.
    b. She has a cardiac output of 3.0 L/min.
    c. She has a urine output of 30 cc/hr.
    d. Her systemic vascular resistance is below normal.

13. A nurse comes upon an accident on a deserted highway. The nurse tries to get help to transport the victims quickly to a trauma center because:
    a. vasoconstriction occurs to increase blood pressure and stroke may occur.
    b. permanent damage to vital organs can occur due to hypoxemia.
    c. shock has occurred and is not reversible.
    d. compensating mechanisms for shock only occur in the early stage.

14. A 42 year old client is admitted to the oncology surgical floor and is scheduled for a right mastectomy with axillary lymphadenectomy. Which of the following should be included in the pre-operative teaching?
    a. Keep the affected arm elevated and immobile for 3 days after drains are removed.
    b. Blood pressures may be performed in the right arm after 6 months.
    c. Refrain from having manicures on the right hand.
    d. Wear tight fitting clothes to protect from cold exposure.

15. A client is ordered to have 1000 cc of 5% dextrose and ¼ normal saline solution with 40 mEq of potassium chloride (KCl) over eight hours times three bags; an antibiotic in 50 cc intravenously every four hours at 8 a.m. and 12 noon. He is presently not permitted anything by mouth. He voids 300 cc at 7 a.m., 100 cc at 10 a.m., receives 2 cc of a medication intramuscularly at 11 a.m., voids 250 cc at 12 noon and 200 cc at 2:30 p.m. He also has coughed up 200 cc of sputum through the shift. How would the nurse record the intake and output for the 7 a.m. to 3:30 p.m. shift?
    a. 1100 cc intake; 850 cc output; record the sputum in the nurse's note.
    b. 1140 cc intake; 850 cc output plus 200 cc of yellow sputum.
    c. 3100 cc intake; 1050 cc output.
    d. 1140 cc intake; 850 cc output.

16. A 55 year old client has had surgery and is in the recovery room. The nurse would evaluate that the pharyngeal airway can be removed when the client:
    a. responds to verbal stimuli.
    b. demonstrates stable vital signs.
    c. can deep breathe and cough adequately.
    d. gags and pushes out the airway.

Situation:
Mrs. Phyllis Demmler, 27 years old, is hospitalized due to an acute episode of Crohn's disease. In order to rest the gastrointestinal system, oral feedings have been suspended and Mrs. Demmler is being fed through total parenteral nutrition (TPN). The TPN is being infused through a large vein in her arm. (The next two questions refer to this situation).

17. The nurse has just hung a new bag of TPN. The team leader should ask which of the following questions?
    a. "What was the glucose level in the urine when you changed the bag?"
    b. "Did the nurse from the intravenous team change the site dressing?"
    c. "Did you ask the client to do the valsalva maneuver when you changed the bag?"
    d. "Did you change the tubing and check for phlebitis when you changed the bag?"

18. Mrs. Demmler's urine registers as 3+ for glucose at the midnight urine check. The best explanation for this finding is that:
    a. there is a higher amount of glucose in the urine than is expected for a TPN solution.
    b. this is an expected finding for TPN infusion but should continue to be monitored.
    c. the finding is abnormally high but giving insulin would result in hypoglycemia during the night.
    d. glycosuria of 3+ is normal for the first few days the TPN is infused.

19. A client sustained a closed head injury. The nurse assesses for which early sign of impending neurological deterioration?
    a. Loss of corneal reflex.
    b. Increased visual acuity.
    c. Bilateral pupil equality and reactivity.
    d. Ipsilateral pupil dilation.

20. A woman who has a history of emphysema is brought to the emergency room hypoventilating. A set of arterial blood gases (ABG's) reveals that she is in respiratory acidosis which is uncompensated. What would the nurse expect to find?
    a. pH below normal, pCO_2 above normal, HCO_3 above normal.
    b. pH above normal, pCO_2 normal, HCO_3 above normal.
    c. pH below normal, pCO_2 normal, HCO_3 below normal.
    d. pH below normal, pCO_2 above normal, HCO_3 normal.

21. A client arrives on the psychiatric unit who is psychotic and threatens to hit nursing staff if they will not let her go home. If the client attempts to hit the nurse, the therapeutic response would be:
    a. "If you hit me you will lose all off ward privileges."
    b. "Do not hit me. We will help you gain control if you cannot do so on your own."
    c. "This behavior is inappropriate and will not be tolerated."
    d. "What is happening that makes you want to hit me?"

22. The nurse caring for a client with a radium implant finds that the implant has fallen out onto the bedsheets. The initial action of the nurse should be to:
    a. notify the physician immediately and prepare the client for reimplantation.
    b. don lead gloves, remove the implant with forceps and place it in the proper container.
    c. cover the implant with a towel and then with a lead apron.
    d. place a lead apron onto the client and over the implant.

23. A 56 year old male hypertensive client is started on propanalol (Inderal). Which of the following statements made to the nurse indicates the need for further teaching?
    a. "Propanalol (Inderal) blocks the sympathetic nervous system."
    b. "The purpose is to decrease my heart rate which causes a drop in blood pressure."
    c. "Normal side effects might be insomnia, weakness and fatigue."
    d. "People with asthma can not take propanalol (Inderal)."

24. A client on antipsychotic medication is experiencing fever, muscular rigidity, diaphoresis, and disorientation. The initial response of the nurse should be to:
    a. increase fluids to decrease fever.
    b. administer an anti-dyskinetic agent as per doctor's order.
    c. call the physician to draw blood work for possible agranulocytosis.
    d. hold the antipsychotic medication and immediately call the physician.

25. A client diagnosed with borderline personality disorder is manipulating staff members against each other. The appropriate intervention for this behavior would be to:
   a. inform the client that this behavior will not be tolerated.
   b. try to determine which staff members are inconsistent in their approach to the client.
   c. insist that the client focus on his own issues.
   d. invite the client to present his complaints at the next staff meeting.

26. A baby girl is placed under phototherapy for a serum bilirubin of 12 mg/dl on day 2 of life. The care plan should include:
   a. keeping the baby under the phototherapy lights for 24 hours straight, keeping eye patches over eyes while under phototherapy, and observing for hyperthermia and hypothermia.
   b. observing for signs of dehydration, assessing eyes once per shift for the presence of conjunctivitis, and keeping eyes and genitals covered while under phototherapy.
   c. keeping the baby in the nursery under "strict" observation.
   d. weighing the baby every 6 hours, starting an intravenous line on the infant, and keeping the infant NPO.

27. Tara Barovich, 3 years old, has been admitted for tube insertion to both ears due to recurrent ear infections. She is the only child of older parents. After Tara goes into operating room, Mrs. Barovich begins to cry, "I must be a terrible mother. She wouldn't need surgery if I didn't let her get all those infections." The best reply of the nurse would be:
   a. "You won't have to worry about this after the surgery."
   b. "How did you cause Tara's ear infections, Mrs. Barovich?"
   c. "You think you somehow caused her to have this surgery, Mrs. Barovich?"
   d. "The doctor will explain ways that you can keep her from getting infections."

28. Erin is spending her sixth birthday in the hospital with plumbism (lead poisoning). She is receiving daily injections of Ca EDTA and her Glasgow coma scale score is 15. Erin's parents bought her a bicycle for her birthday. Erin asks the nurse if she can ride the new bicycle in the halls. The best response is:
   a. "You may as long as you wear a helmet and an adult is with you."
   b. "You are still very sick and you might lose your balance."
   c. "You could hurt yourself in the hospital. You are better off waiting until you get home."
   d. "Bicycle riding is not allowed in hospitals."

29. A 49 year old male with probable leukemia has undergone bone marrow aspiration. The nurse evaluates a problem has occurred when which of the following was documented?

a. The superficial skin was injected with procaine (Novocain) followed by injection of the periosteum.

b. The client complained of tenderness at the site after 24 hours.

c. The client complained of a sharp pain as the plunger is pulled back.

d. The site of the aspiration was the lateral aspect of the 5th lumbar vertebrae.

30. A client admitted with cirrhosis of the liver is placed on lactulose (Cephulac). The nurse evaluates the effectiveness of lactulose (Cephulac) by monitoring which laboratory test?

a. Ammonia.

b. Urine glucose.

c. Creatinine.

d. Arterial blood gases

STOP You have now completed Practice Session: 11. Now take a few minutes and correct your answers. Calculate your accuracy rate by dividing the number of questions you completed correctly by the total number of questions you completed (30).

Correct answers ÷ total number of questions completed = accuracy rate.

_____ ÷ _____ = _____

ANSWERS AND RATIONALES

1. **The correct answer is a.** Assessment of diet should be the first step in the process. A client consuming recommended daily requirements will only need folic acid and iron to prevent maternal anemia and fetal defects. Option (b) is incorrect because megadoses are contraindicated as toxic levels of vitamins may be harmful to the developing fetus. The recommended weight gain for normal weight pregnant clients is 24 to 32 pounds (10 to 14 kg). Protein and calorie restrictions (options c and d) can be dangerous (Olds, London & Ladewig, 1992; pp. 406-407, 412, 423).

   Nursing Process: Implementation
   Client Need: Health Promotion & Maintenance

2. **The correct answer is c.** Nifedipine (Procardia) is a calcium channel blocker. These drugs slow the intake of calcium into the heart (option d) and blood vessels decreasing peripheral vascular resistance. Nifedipine (Procardia) comes in a capsule and may be given orally, but is usually given sublinguilly (option a). Nifedipine (Procardia) is rapidly absorbed and can have a potent hypotensive effect; therefore, blood pressure should be checked every five minutes until it is stable (option b) (Smeltzer & Bare, 1992; p. 764).

   Nursing Process: Implementation
   Client Need: Physiological Integrity

3. **The correct answer is c.** The tracheostomy cuff should be inflated during the tube feeding so that material is not aspirated into the lungs (option d). Tube feedings should be administered with the client in an upright position (option a). This aids the feeding process and prevents aspiration. When a client has a tracheostomy, tube feedings are usually administered through a smaller bore feeding tube or a jejunostomy (option b). The inflated cuff on the tracheostomy may push against the esophagus and cause swallowing difficulties and discomfort if the esophagus is less flexible because of a large tube (Ignatavicius & Bayne, 1991; p. 2022).

   Nursing Process: Implementation
   Client Need: Physiological Integrity

4. **The correct answer is d.** The onset and action of theophylline (Aminophylline) is related to serum concentration. Serum concentration is dependent upon the drug's absorption and excretion rates. Theophylline (Aminophylline) is mainly metabolized in the liver with 10% excreted unchanged in the urine. The rate of metabolism varies greatly among clients. Decreased metabolism may result from liver disease, congestive heart failure, or prolonged fever. Smoking and high protein diets may increase rate of excretion. Drug interactions may also increase the risk of toxicity or enhance subtherapeutic levels. Therefore, dosages of theophylline (Aminophylline) need to be individualized according to serum concentration levels. Normal

serum concentration levels are between 10 to 20 mcg/ml. The nurse should clarify the dosage of theophylline (Aminophylline) prior to administration if the level is not within therapeutic range (option a). Administering the prescribed dose of theophylline (Aminophylline) with the respiratory treatment may be detrimental if the client's level is not therapeutic (option b). Adverse reactions such as nausea, vomiting, diarrhea, irritability, anxiety, palpitations, headache and seizures may occur if toxicity is present. Ordering laboratory tests without a physician's order is outside the scope of nursing practice (option c) (Baer & Williams, 1992; pp. 658-667).

Nursing Process: Implementation
Client Need: Physiological Integrity

5. **The correct answer is d.** In beta thalassemia there is defective hemoglobin production. The bone marrow forms red bloods cells that are fragile and easily destroyed. Jaundice is caused by increased bilirubin. Bilirubin is a product of hemoglobin breakdown. The spleen enlarges with the increase in red cell destruction. Hypertrophied musculature in the calves is seen in muscular dystrophy, not beta thalassemia (option b). Bleeding disorders are usually manifested by swollen joints and hematuria (option c). As the bone marrow becomes hyperplastic in an attempt to replace red blood cells, it expands the marrow cavities causing an enlarged head. Although this is a form of anemia, appetite is not affected (option a) (Mott, Sperhac & James, 1990; pp. 1317, 1884).

Nursing Process: Assessment
Client Need: Physiological Integrity

6. **The correct answer is d.** Withdrawal signs of cocaine include irritability, hypersensitivity, poor feeding, disturbed sleep pattern, increased pulse, increased respirations, and diarrhea. Meconium staining and precipitate delivery (option a) are often seen with maternal use of marijuana. Shrill cry and decreased moro reflex (option b) are seen with heroin use or methadone maintenance. Poor sucking and microcephaly (option c) are seen as part of the fetal alcohol syndrome (Bobak, Jensen & Zalar, 1989; pp. 986-990).

Nursing Process: Assessment
Client Need: Physiological Integrity

7. **The correct answer is b.** Paregoric or phenobarbital may be used to wean the infant. The dosage is gradually decreased until the drug is gone from the system evidenced by no further signs or symptoms. Cocaine (option a) should not be used because of its addictive and agonizing side effects. Glucose (option c) would not be used since no severe hypoglycemia is involved. Methadone (option d) is a narcotic drug which is given to an adult who has been addicted to heroin. Methadone would not be given to assist clients in ridding themselves of the drug but to block the physical craving for the drug. This drug would also produce withdrawal symptoms (Bobak, Jensen & Zalar, 1989; pp. 984-989; Varcarolis, 1990; pp. 660, 664).

Nursing Process: Analysis
Client Need: Physiological Integrity

8. **The correct answer is b.** This response will assist the client to maintain control over her environment and allow time for transition. Usually waiting a few minutes gives time for adjustment and the client will be more able and willing to comply. The waiting period also gives the nurse time to think through the approach used for the request in case the nurse's behavior precipitated the problem. If the nurse continues to act on the request by unbuttoning the client's blouse (option a), the resulting behavior may lead to agitation and further power struggle where the client may become unmanageable without extra assistance. Restating the request firmly (option c) pushes the client toward feeling a loss of control which the client may try to assert in another way, such as behavioral problems. If instructions need to be repeated they should be stated in exactly the same way as originally stated with a calm and supportive manner. "Firm" statements may be misinterpreted as anger which further upsets the client. Reasoning with the client (option d) may be misinterpreted as insistence and again results in power struggle (Stuart & Sundeen, 1991; pp. 587-588).

Nursing Process: Implementation
Client Need: Physiological Integrity

9. **The correct answer is d.** Positioning the body in the supine, neutral position, avoiding flexion at the neck, hips and knees will prevent obstruction of venous return from the brain. Elevating the head 30 degrees will decrease intracranial pressure by gravity drainage from the brain and head. Options (a),

(b) and (c) are contraindicated in treating increased intracranial pressure. All obstruct venous return from the brain causing spikes in intracranial pressure. An increase in intrathoracic, intraabdominal or neck pressure is sensed through the open venous cerebral system. The increased pressure impedes drainage from the brain, thus increasing intracranial pressure (Ignatavicius & Bayne, 1991; p. 931; Phipps, Long, Woods & Cassmeyer, 1991; pp. 476, 1800).

Nursing Process: Implementation
Client Need: Physiological Integrity

10. **The correct answer is a.** Y-Me is the national organization for breast cancer information and support. The national hospice organization (option b) assists by supporting terminally ill clients and their families. Ronald McDonald House (option c) provides a dwelling for clients and families. The ostomy society (option d) provides support for clients with colostomies and ileostomies usually related to cancer of the colon (Smeltzer & Bare, 1992; p. 1300).

Nursing Process: Implementation
Client Need: Health Promotion & Maintenance

11. **The correct answer is d.** Even though smallpox has officially been declared as eradicated, the disease must be monitored in case it reappears. The other diseases of cancer (option a), rabies (option b) and influenza (option c) may be reportable depending on the laws of individual states but are not reported internationally (Spradley, 1990; p. 248).

Nursing Process: Implementation
Client Need: Health Promotion & Maintenance

12. **The correct answer is c.** Clients with septic shock often have renal failure and 30 cc/hr is a normal minimum urine output. The arterial blood gases (ABG's) given are of a client with respiratory acidosis (option a). A normal cardiac output is approximately 5.0 L/min (option b). A low systemic vascular resistance (SVR) is consistent with continuing shock (option c) (Smeltzer & Bare, 1992; p.332).

Nursing Process: Analysis
Client Need: Physiological Integrity

13. **The correct answer is b.** Shock continues to progress towards death if the underlying cause remains untreated and normal compensatory mechanisms are not supported by outside intervention. Death results because vital organs, especially the heart, do not receive sufficient oxygen and functioning decompensates. Vasoconstriction (option a) occurs and increases blood pressure in the early phase of shock to continue providing oxygen to tissues. Shock is reversible (option c) if treated before severe hypoxemia occurs. Shock can be reversed during the early stage, the compensatory stage and the intermediate stage (option d) (Ignatavicius & Bayne, 1991; p. 405).

Nursing Process: Analysis
Client Need: Physiological Integrity

14. **The correct answer is c.** Manicures place the client at risk for cuts or scrapes. Compromise of skin integrity to an extremity where nodal dissection has been performed increases risk for infection to occur. Blood pressures (option b) and constricting clothing (option d) on the affected extremity could compromise circulation and should be avoided indefinitely. Once drains have been removed (option a) passive exercise is vital to prevent joint stiffness (Smeltzer & Bare, 1992; pp. 1309-1310).

Nursing Process: Implementation
Client Need: Physiological Integrity

15. **The correct answer is a.** Intravenous fluid over eight hours equals 1000 cc; two doses of antibiotics (50 cc each) equals 100 cc. Total is 1100 cc intake. The 40 mEq of KCl are part of the intravenous solution and not added separately. The 2 cc injection is not counted as intake. Urine output is 300 cc, 100 cc, 250 cc, and 200 cc which equals 850 cc. The sputum characteristics are described in the nurse's note but not included in output (options b, c and d) (Potter & Perry, 1989; pp. 651-652).

Nursing Process: Evaluation
Client Need: Physiological Integrity

16. **The correct answer is d.** A pharyngeal airway may be removed when the client begins to gag or when the client removes the airway himself by pushing it out with his tongue. Most clients are semiconscious and will respond to verbal stimuli upon entry to the recovery room (option a) but this does not indicate adequate oxygenation. Vital signs should be stabilizing while the client is in the room or the physician should be

267

notified (option b) but stable vital signs (pulse and blood pressure) do not indicate adequate airway. Clients are often instructed to cough and deep breathe (option c) to clear anesthesia and promote proper ventilation but do not ensure adequate ventilation (Lewis & Collier, 1992; p. 281).

Nursing Process: Evaluation
Client Need: Safe, Effective Care Environment

17. **The correct answer is d.** Tubing should be changed every time the new bag is hung. This prevents bacterial growth in the system. Filters should be changed every 24 hours. The peripheral intravenous site should be checked frequently for phlebitis. The site is usually changed every 48 hours. If the intravenous site is a central vein such as the jugular or subclavian veins, the valsalva maneuver is used to minimize air embolus when the new tubing is being attached. Since Mrs. Demmler's site is in her arm, the valsalva maneuver is unnecessary (option c). Dressings are often ordered to be changed every other day to once per week on the central venous line (option b). Glucose and acetone in the urine should be checked every 4 to 6 hours, not just when the bag is changed (option a) (Lewis & Collier, 1992; pp. 1022-1023).

Nursing Process: Evaluation
Client Need: Physiological Integrity

18. **The correct answer is a.** Glycosuria of 3+ is considered to be an abnormally high finding for all clients, including those with TPN. Within the first few days after TPN is started, glycosuria may be 1+ or 2+ but findings of 3+ or 4+ should be considered abnormal (options b and d). Insulin should be administered into the bag or subcutaneously according to a sliding scale as prescribed by the physician. Since TPN infuses around the clock, insulin administration at midnight should not result in hypoglycemia (option c) (Lewis & Collier, 1992; pp. 1022-1023).

Nursing Process: Analysis
Client Need: Physiological Integrity

19. **The correct answer is d.** The oculomotor nerve, cranial nerve III, controls pupillary responses which carry sensory, motor, parasympathetic and sympathetic fibers. The pupilo-constrictor fibers of the oculomotor nerve are the first to be compressed by herniating tissue. Since the source of increasing intracranial pressure (ICP) (edema, hemorrhage, tumor) tends to be compartmental in the early stages, the pupillary dysfunction is ipsilateral to the edema or space-occupying lesion. The nurse should consider lateral or local herniation syndrome if ipsilateral pupil dilation is present. Bilateral pupil equality and reactivity are normal pupillary responses (option c) associated with normal ICP. A loss of corneal reflexes is mediated by the brain stem including oculocephalic and oculovestibular reflexes (option a). Decreased visual acuity (not increased, option b) occurs in the early stages of increasing ICP. Blurred vision and diplopia may also be present. These findings are due to early hemispheric pressure increases on visual pathways (Hickey, 1986; p. 256; Ignatavicius & Bayne, 1991; p. 928; Phipps, Long,

Woods & Cassmeyer, 1991; pp. 1796-1799).

Nursing Process: Assessment
Client Need: Physiological Integrity

20. **The correct answer is d.** The pH below normal indicates an acid state, while the elevated p CO_2 level indicates the client is retaining CO_2, therefore has an increase in H+ ion concentration. The normal HCO_3 level indicates that no metabolic compensation has yet taken place. The other options include partially compensated respiratory acidosis (option a); uncompensated metabolic alkalosis (option b); and uncompensated metabolic acidosis (option c) (Fischbach, 1992; pp. 840-854; Ignatavicius & Bayne, 1991; pp. 327-335; Kenner, Guzzetta & Dossey, 1985; pp. 498-503).

Nursing Process: Analysis
Client Need: Physiological Integrity

21. **The correct answer is b.** Setting limits on a client's inappropriate behavior and letting her know that staff is available to help her control impulsive and aggressive behavior is the most therapeutic. Options (a) and (c) are punitive and confusing to the client. Option (d) expects the client to have a clear understanding of the meaning of her behavior which at this point is highly unlikely (Varcarolis, 1990; p. 516).

Nursing Process: Planning
Client Need: Psychosocial Integrity

22. **The correct answer is b.** When a dislodged radium implant falls out there is an increased risk of exposure to harmful radiation. The implant should be placed in a lead shielded container (option c) as soon as possible using the proper procedure to minimize risk. The physician should then be notified (option a). Lead aprons should be worn by anyone (option d) assisting with procedures involving radioactive materials and exposure should be monitored (Smith & Duell, 1993; pp. 101-102).

Nursing Process: Implementation
Client Need: Safe, Effective Care Environment

23. **The correct answer is b.** The purpose of the propanolol (Inderal) is to decrease blood pressure. Propanolol (Inderal) blocks the beta receptors in the sympathetic nervous system. This causes a drop in heart rate and blood pressure. All of the other statements about propanolol (Inderal) are true (options a, c and d) (Smeltzer & Bare, 1992; p. 761).

Nursing Process: Evaluation
Client Need: Physiological Integrity

24. **The correct answer is d.** Fever, muscular rigidity, diaphoresis and disorientation are all symptoms of neuroleptic malignant syndrome, a potentially lethal side effect of antipsychotic medications. Immediate recognition and action are required to prevent death. Muscular rigidity and disorientation should not occur with agranulocytosis (option c), rather fever, sore throat, malaise or mouth sores would be indicated with this side effect. An anti-dyskinetic agent (option b) would be appropriate for an acute

dystonic reaction or akathesia. Increasing fluids to decrease the fever (option a) would be indicated but option (d) would be the initial response (Haber, Leach-McMahon, Price-Hoskins & Sideleau, 1992; p. 372).

Nursing Process: Implementation
Client Need: Psychosocial Integrity

25. **The correct answer is c.** Clients with borderline personality disorder often encourage division among staff members (splitting) in order to avoid their therapeutic issues. The multidisciplinary treatment team must work together to provide a consistent approach for the client. Options (b) and (d) do not accomplish this and would encourage the client's splitting behavior. All members of the treatment team must help the client focus on his own issues rather than project their feelings to staff. Simply telling the client to stop the behavior (option a) without helping the client to see why the splitting is harmful would not be therapeutic since it provides no understanding or constructive alternative behavior (Haber, Leach-McMahon, Price-Hoskins & Sideleau, 1992; pp. 485-486).

Nursing Process: Implementation
Client Need: Psychosocial Integrity

26. **The correct answer is b.** The nurse will observe for signs of dehydration from the drying effects of the lights. Eyes should be observed for signs of conjunctivitis as a result of wearing eye patches continually except when feeding. The eyes are kept covered as it is not known whether the ultraviolet light is harmful to the retina or if there are long term side effects from the lights. Genitals are kept covered for the same reason. Option (a) is incorrect. It is recommended that eye patches be removed at least one time per shift for assessment and for socialization purposes. Option (c) is incorrect as most facilities have a phototherapy unit which can be transported to the mother's room so the mother, with a few instructions, can provide care and bonding can be promoted. Option (d) is incorrect as only a daily weight is indicated. The serum bilirubin is not high enough at 48 hours that an intravenous is warranted. Fluids should be pushed in order to flush the bilirubin out of the infant's system (Olds, London & Ladewig, 1992; pp. 1044, 1052).

Nursing Process: Implementation
Client Need: Safe, Effective Care Environment

27. **The correct answer is c.** This answer verbalizes the implied message and requests validation of the nurse's understanding of what was communicated. Option (a) is nontherapeutic because it implies that the child will never have any more ear infections which is false reassurance. Option (b) asks for Mrs. Barovich to explain her actions and may be confrontive. Option (d) places teaching responsibility on the physician when the nurse is capable of doing the teaching and this is within the nurse's scope of practice (Cook & Fontaine, 1991; pp. 60-62).

Nursing Process: Implementation
Client Need: Psychosocial Integrity

28. **The correct answer is a.** Helmets are necessary to prevent head injury in the event of an accidental fall. Erin's Glasgow coma scale score indicates that she has no neurological deficits from the lead poisoning (option b). Allowing children to ride bicycles in the halls of hospitals promotes motor coordination development (options c and d) (Mott, Sperhac & James, 1990; pp. 548, 550; Whaley & Wong, 1991; p. 1726).

Nursing Process: Implementation
Client Need: Health Promotion & Maintenance

29. **The correct answer is d.** This indicates that the test was done incorrectly. This is not a site used for aspiration. The usual sites are the sternum or iliac crest. The injection process was correct (option a) for best results. While most clients do not have pain after the procedure they may experience aching for approximately two days (option b). The actual aspiration causes a brief sharp pain (option c) (Smeltzer & Bare, 1992; p.786).

Nursing Process: Analysis
Client Need: Physiological Integrity

30. **The correct answer is a.** Lactulose (Cephulac), an ammonia-detoxicating agent, acts to lower blood ammonia concentration levels in clients with hepatic encephalopathy. Lactulose (Cephulac) causes acidification of the colonic contents; therefore, increasing ammonia content in the gastrointestinal tract. Ammonia levels may be reduced by 25-50%. As ammonia levels are decreased, the client's mental status improves. Lactulose (Cephulac) is a disaccharide sugar consisting of galactose and fructose. However, lactulose (Cephulac) is mainly excreted in the feces with only a small unchanged amount in the urine. Therefore, monitoring urine glucose is not required during administration (option b). A serum creatinine level is used to diagnose impaired renal function (option c). Lactulose (Cephulac) does not have a direct effect on renal function. Arterial blood gases determine acid-base disturbances of the respiratory and metabolic systems. Lactulose (Cephulac) is unrelated to this laboratory test (option d) (Baer & Williams, 1992; pp. 719-720).

Nursing Process: Evaluation
Client Need: Physiological Integrity

PRACTICE SESSION: 12

Instructions:

Allow yourself 30 minutes to complete the following 30 practice questions. Use a timer to notify yourself when 30 minutes are over so that you are not constantly looking at your watch while completing the questions.

1. The physician has admitted a female client with a diagnosis of central abruptio placenta. The nurse would expect to assess:
   a. no overt vaginal bleeding, rigid abdomen, acute abdominal pain, hypotension.
   b. bright red vaginal bleeding, non-rigid abdomen, no pain.
   c. massive vaginal bleeding, rigid abdomen, acute abdominal pain, profound shock.
   d. blood clots passing through the vagina, boggy uterus, widening pulse pressure.

2. The nurse is planning care for a client with chronic renal failure with a fistula in his right arm. Care should include:
   a. elevating the right arm on a pillow.
   b. stabilizing the right arm in a splint.
   c. placing the call light by the left hand.
   d. taking blood pressures on the left arm.

3. A client diagnosed with amyotrophic lateral sclerosis (ALS) is admitted to the medical unit. The client has a four year history of the disease. The nurse's priority assessment area should be:
   a. respiratory status.
   b. potential for injury.
   c. muscle atrophy.
   d. dysphagia.

4. The nurse evaluates that the client understands post-operative lobectomy teaching when the client states the importance of:
   a. wearing his oxygen.
   b. change in smoking habits.
   c. tolerating foods and fluids.
   d. early ambulation.

5. Brian, a 9 year old, was involved in a motor vehicle accident. He is known to have phenylketonuria (PKU). He has been advanced to a full PKU "diet as tolerated". Which of the following meals would be most appropriate for Brian?
   a. Hamburger, french fries, and apple juice.
   b. Hot dog, cottage cheese, and skim milk.
   c. Pizza, carrot sticks, and lemonade.
   d. Spaghetti with tomato sauce, tossed salad, and grape juice.

6. A client with cancer is receiving morphine sulfate (Morphine) for chronic pain. The nurse should instruct the client to:
   a. eat low protein foods.
   b. drink fluids liberally.
   c. avoid taking other medications.
   d. watch for signs of addiction.

7. A 56 year old female is being treated for stage III hodgkins disease. The client was treated for sepsis after her first chemotherapy course. For her next treatment she will begin injections of colony stimulating factors (CSF). The nurse does teaching about it. Which of the following client responses shows adequate knowledge of this treatment?
   a. "CSF gives me temporary passive immunity to cancer cells."
   b. "Injections will all be given in the same place."
   c. "There should be no side effects."
   d. "This should help to increase my white blood cell count."

8. A 70 year old client comes to the clinic complaining of hearing changes. The nurse finds that the ear is filled with earwax. This may be a particular problem for older clients because:
   a. softening earwax clogs the ear canal.
   b. they tend to use ear drops too frequently.
   c. the earwax tends to be drier and harder.
   d. increased earwax is a normal part of aging.

9. A diabetic client is admitted with ulcerations on his foot and toes. After several days the toes turn dark and a surgeon is brought in for removal of part of the foot. The client's wife wants to know how and why this happened. The best explanation would be that it is a result of:
   a. a virus from an opportunistic infection.
   b. escherichia coli, a nosocomial infection.
   c. necrosis related to hypoxia in the foot.
   d. anaplasia resulting in abnormal cell growth.

10. A 24 year old male client is on the neurosurgical unit. He is status post-closed head injury from a motorcycle injury two days ago. He is arousable to loud verbal stimuli and follows some commands. He has an intraventricular monitor system leveled at 15 cm above midbrain that can be turned to drain, monitor or do both simultaneously. Which of the following should be part of his plan of care?
    a. Open the drain for 20 minutes if intracranial pressure (ICP) is greater than 25 mm Hg.
    b. Zero the top of the transducer at 2.5 cm above the ear.
    c. Use clean technique to draw daily cerebrospinal fluid (CSF) studies as ordered.
    d. Report an intracranial pressure (ICP) tracing that fluctuates similar to a central venous pressure (CVP) trace.

11. On a home visit for newborn assessment, the nurse notes that an older adult lives with the family. The older adult refuses to interact with or look at the nurse. The nurse observes signs of dehydration and poor skin hygiene. The infant's mother draws attention away from the older adult. The nurse suspects elder abuse. The best action of the nurse would be to:
    a. walk over to the older adult and perform a complete assessment even though the homeowner requests the nurse to leave.
    b. talk with the infant's mother and the older adult together about the difficulties involved in living together with a new infant.
    c. discuss the signs and symptoms of elder abuse with the infant's mother.
    d. call the police and ask them to talk to the family about the penalty for assault and battery.

12. In approaching a client who is blind, the nurse should:
    a. tell the client when the nurse enters or leaves the room.
    b. not use words that imply vision such as "see".
    c. allow the client to explore the hospital room alone to become oriented.
    d. open the bathroom door partway so the client can find the bathroom.

13. A post-inguinal herniorrhaphy client is scheduled for discharge the morning after surgery. The evening before discharge the nurse notes a moderate amount of sanguinous drainage. The best action of the nurse would be to:
    a. reinforce the dressing and mark the drainage area.
    b. notify the physician of the change in condition.
    c. reposition the drain to decrease the amount of drainage.
    d. teach the client about post-operative wound care.

14. On taking a dietary history for a pregnant primipara, the client states she is eating a lot of freezer frost and dirt. Which statement is true regarding her dietary history?
    a. The client is exhibiting pica and the most common concern would be iron-deficiency anemia.
    b. The client is exhibiting lactose intolerance and the most common concern is calcium insufficiency.
    c. Most pregnant women have these same cravings and there are few consequences to mother or fetus.
    d. The client is a vegetarian and may not receive enough protein to sustain a healthy pregnancy.

15. A client with cancer has developed petechiae and a nose bleed. The clotting profile reveals prolonged prothrombin time and partial thromboplastin time; with decreased fibrinogen and platelet levels. The nurse would anticipate which order?
    a. Blood cultures.
    b. Serum uric acid.
    c. Radiation.
    d. Echocardiogram.

16. A client with frequent urinary tract infections is scheduled for an intravenous pyelogram (IVP). After the procedure the nurse would:
    a. check peripheral pulses every 30 minutes.
    b. encourage oral fluids.
    c. administer a laxative as ordered.
    d. put up the side rails on the bed.

17. A black 23 year old is about to be discharged with her baby boy. The client comments to the nurse that she is worried about the possibility of sudden infant death syndrome (SIDS) because she had a brother who died in infancy. The nurse bases her response on which of the following facts about SIDS?
    a. It is associated with an allergic response to cow's milk.
    b. Suffocation results from extra bed linens in the child's crib.
    c. The incidence of SIDS is higher in North American caucasians.
    d. Risk factors include low birth weight and family occurrence.

18. The physician orders 1000 cc D_5W with 20,000 u of heparin sodium (Heparin) to infuse at 50 ml/hour. Calculate the hourly heparin sodium (Heparin) dosage.
    a. 50 u/hour.
    b. 100 u/hour.
    c. 1000 u/hour.
    d. 1500 u/hour.

19. A client diagnosed with angina is placed on a low triglyceride diet. The nurse evaluates that the client understands the diet when he chooses which lunch meal?
    a. Chicken sandwich, iced tea.
    b. Peanut butter sandwich, whole milk.
    c. Split pea with ham soup, cocoa.
    d. Cheeseburger, diet cola.

20. In working with the client with anorexia nervosa, the nurse is aware that the first behavioral intervention utilized after the client becomes medically stable is:
    a. meal planning and nutritional instruction.
    b. fostering the client's independence.
    c. providing assertiveness training.
    d. educating the client on the seriousness of the disease.

21. A 60 year old female is admitted to the general surgery floor from the recovery room following a subtotal thyroidectomy for Grave's disease. The nurse assesses all of the following information. Which one should be reported?
    a. A serum calcium of 8.5 mg/dl.
    b. Client displays a negative Chvostek's sign.
    c. Client displays a negative Trousseau's sign.
    d. Complaint of feeling of fullness at the incision site.

22. The community health nurse is asked to provide care to a group of Mexican-American migrant farm workers. The best approach by the nurse to gain trust of the group would be to:
   a. offer a class on nutrition and illness prevention.
   b. announce a screening for tuberculosis and other communicable diseases.
   c. post signs with the telephone number of the nearest free clinics.
   d. talk with the women about their views of illness and their needs.

23. A 32 year old male client is admitted to the psychiatric unit with hallucinations, delusions, weight loss and unkempt appearance. He says to the nurse, "I'm Clark Kent, really Superman. You may not be able to stop my destructive powers." The best reply of the nurse would be:
   a. "Even Superman accepted help from others."
   b. "Your name is really Jack and I doubt you have any special powers."
   c. "You're worried we may not be able to help you?"
   d. "You seem concerned about losing your identity."

24. A man with lung cancer is admitted to the hospital and determined to be in respiratory acidosis. If the condition is not corrected, the nurse would also look for what type of changes?
   a. The kidneys will compensate to decrease carbonic acid content.
   b. The kidneys will retain fluid which results in edema.
   c. Vasoconstriction occurs which increases peripheral resistance.
   d. Vasodilation shunts blood to capillaries resulting in increased tissue oxygenation.

25. The nurse admits a 32 year old male fire fighter following rescue from a building blaze. The nurse notices singed nares and smoke on the fire fighter's face. This would be an indication of:
   a. possible excessive mucous plug formation.
   b. pulmonary edema.
   c. early signs of respiratory arrest.
   d. possible tracheal burns.

26. The most important concern of a nurse caring for a child with acute glomerulonephritis is assessment of:
   a. previous streptococcus infections.
   b. periorbital edema.
   c. blood pressure.
   d. caloric intake.

27. The nurse receives a telephone report from the emergency room about a client with a history of Parkinson's disease to be admitted to the unit. The nurse would anticipate the client to display which of the following symptoms?
   a. Paralysis, possible coma.
   b. Muscle spasticity, rambling speech.
   c. Tremors, rigidity.
   d. Seizures, bradykinesia.

28. A client is admitted with upper gastrointestinal bleeding related to overuse of salicylates. The nurse would teach the client that:
   a. the esophageal bleeding is induced by alcohol abuse.
   b. irritation from the medicine resulted in stomach erosion.
   c. self-induced vomiting from bulimia created an esophageal tear.
   d. salicylate use resulted in malignant colonic polyps.

29. The nurse observes a mother interacting with her overweight child at mealtime. The nurse counsels the mother that the best way to promote weight loss in her seven year old child is to say:
   a. "If you eat a big meal, the other children will tease you."
   b. "Just one small helping of everything or you'll gain weight."
   c. "The doctor says to lose weight or you'll get sick."
   d. "You may have an extra helping now or a snack later."

30. A 27 year old female is admitted to the hospital with acute bacterial meningitis following upper respiratory infection. She has a headache and is sleepy but has no neurological deficits. She is started on intravenous antibiotics. Which of the following nursing actions would not apply?
   a. Instruct her visitors to wear a mask.
   b. Report immediately any nuchal rigidity.
   c. Discuss antibiotic therapy with her husband.
   d. Keep the room dimly lit.

STOP You have now completed Practice Session: 12. Now take a few minutes and correct your answers. Calculate your accuracy rate by dividing the number of questions you completed correctly by the total number of questions you completed (30).

Correct answers ÷ total number of questions completed = accuracy rate.

_____ ÷ _____ = _____

PRACTICE SESSION: 12

ANSWERS AND RATIONALES

1. **The correct answer is a.** Because the diagnosis is a central abruptio placenta there is no place for the blood to go that resulted from the separation of the placenta from the uterine wall. As a result of this "trapped" blood, the abdomen becomes rigid causing acute abdominal pain. The blood pressure drops due to the hemorrhage. Option (b) is incorrect; these are symptoms of a placenta previa. Option (c) is incorrect because these symptoms correlate with a complete abruptio placenta. This is where the entire placenta separates from the uterine wall. Hence, profound shock results from massive hemorrhage. Option (d) is incorrect as there is bleeding that is not concealed. These signs are usually noted after delivery and are associated with retained placental fragments (Olds, London & Ladewig, 1992; pp. 757, 767, 769).

   Nursing Process: Assessment
   Client Need: Physiological Integrity

2. **The correct answer is d.** In caring for a chronic renal failure client with a fistula, it is essential the integrity of the fistula be maintained. Taking the blood pressure on the right arm can interrupt blood flow through the fistula causing clot formation, leaving the fistula useless. To reduce swelling post-operatively after fistula formation, the arm may be elevated on a pillow but is not necessary once the fistula is healed (option a). The affected arm does not need to be immobilized (option b) and can function without difficulty (option c) (Ignatavicius & Bayne, 1991; p. 1906).

   Nursing Process: Planning
   Client Need: Safe, Effective Care Environment

3. **The correct answer is a.** Clients with amyotrophic lateral sclerosis (ALS) have a progressive motor disease. Muscle weakness increases until the trapezius and sternocleidomastoid muscles become involved. This results in a compromised respiratory status which is the usual cause of death. Once the client is diagnosed with the disorder, death usually occurs within three to five years. Therefore, primary concern of the nurse for this client would be respiratory since the client has been diagnosed for four years. Potential for injury (option b) may be true for other diseases such as Parkinsonism or multiple sclerosis, but would not be priority here. Muscle atrophy (option c), and dysphagia (option d) are all important but the usual cause of death is respiratory complications (Ignatavicius & Bayne, 1991; p. 922).

   Nursing Process: Assessment
   Client Need: Physiological Integrity

4. **The correct answer is d.** Early ambulation is essential to maintain and improve muscle strength as well as to mobilize secretions. Smoking should be stopped at least 48 hours prior to surgery and not start again. A change in

smoking habits will not have much effect unless the client stops smoking altogether (option b). Oxygen, unless needed, and consuming foods and fluids would not aid in the prevention of post-operative complications (options a and c) (Lewis & Collier, 1992; pp. 546-549).

Nursing Process: Evaluation
Client Need: Safe, Effective Care Environment

5. **The correct answer is d.** Phenyl-ketonuria (PKU) is a disease of protein metabolism characterized by the inability to metabolize phenylalanine. Foods containing low amounts of phenylalanine include vegetables, fruits, juices and some breads and starches. Foods containing high amounts of phenyl-alanine are high protein foods such as hamburger, hot dog, cottage cheese, skim milk, cheese or pizza (options a, b and c) (Whaley & Wong, 1991; pp. 375-376).

Nursing Process: Analysis
Client Need: Health Promotion & Maintenance

6. **The correct answer is b.** Narcotics can cause constipation so measures to promote adequate bowel function are essential. Adequate fluid intake, stool softeners, and a high fiber diet may be included in the care of a client taking narcotics. Oncology clients usually need a high protein (option a), high calorie diet and take multiple prescribed medications (option c). Clients should be reassured that addiction is unlikely (option d) and encouraged to use pain

medications as needed (Ignatavicius & Bayne, 1991; pp. 589-590).

Nursing Process: Implementation
Client Need: Physiological Integrity

7. **The correct answer is d.** Colony Stimulating Factors (CSF) is given to stimulate the body's own production of the cells in the blood including white blood cells. Injection sites are rotated (option b) to prevent tissue damage and side effects may be severe (option c). There is no such thing as passive immunity to cancer (option a) (Lewis & Collier, 1992; p. 204).

Nursing Process: Evaluation
Client Need: Physiological Integrity

8. **The correct answer is c.** As the adult ages, earwax (cerumen) tends to be less moist and is harder to remove from the ear (option a). Drier earwax should first be softened with ear drops (option b) so that removal is less traumatic to the ear. Increased earwax (option d) does not seem to be particular to older adults (Lewis & Collier, 1992; p. 352).

Nursing Process: Analysis
Client Need: Health Promotion & Maintenance

9. **The correct answer is c.** These symptoms are related to gangrene, a type of cell death resulting from hypoxia (not viral or bacterial infection, options a and b). Circulation is often impaired in the diabetic client due to fatty deposits on blood vessel walls. Therefore sufficient oxygen might not reach

peripheral areas of the body such as feet and toes. The lack of oxygen creates cell necrosis. Anaplasia (option d), cell growth of immature cells, usually relates to malignant growths (Lewis & Collier, 1992; pp. 102-103, 1304-1305).

Nursing Process: Analysis
Client Need: Physiological Integrity

10. **The correct answer is b.** The transducer should be zeroed at the midbrain. This corresponds to 2.5 cm above the inner canthus of the ear. Once it is zeroed, the bag is raised 15 cm above that point. The drain should only be opened under physician parameters (option a). Normal intracranial pressure (ICP) is 0-10 mm Hg and the trace on the monitor resembles that of a central venous pressure (CVP) tracing with small fluctuations (option d). Often, daily cerebrospinal fluid samples are ordered. However, any entry into the system must be under aseptic technique (option c) (Smeltzer & Bare, 1992; p. 1651).

Nursing Process: Planning
Client Need: Physiological Integrity

11. **The correct answer is b.** Elder abuse often occurs when there is a strain and problems in the family. The older adult may seem as an added burden or responsibility. The nurse should recognize the signs or potential for elder abuse and work with the family to assess and deal with those problems. The nurse should try to work for the safety of the older adult without becoming antagonistic towards or making enemies of the family which may result in

retaliation (options a and c). If needed, the nurse may recruit assistance (option d) to act for the older adult's safety through investigation and possible removal from the home if necessary but threats are not appropriate (Swanson & Albrecht, 1993; pp. 472-476; 480).

Nursing Process: Implementation
Client Need: Safe, Effective Care Environment

12. **The correct answer is a.** The nurse should always inform the client when the nurse or others enter or leave the client's presence. Nurses should not refrain from any language (option b) used with other clients. The nurse should orient the client to the room (option c) by starting at a focal point object such as the bed and telling the client the position of objects in relation to the focal object. Doors should be either open or shut (option d), never partially open because of the potential danger (Lewis & Collier, 1992; p. 349).

Nursing Process: Implementation
Client Need: Health Promotion & Maintenance

13. **The correct answer is b.** An inguinal herniorrhaphy wound site should have little, if any, drainage. Any post-operative wound drainage should decrease over time. An increased drainage in this type of wound signals a significant change in the client's condition and the physician should be notified of possible complications. Since the amount of drainage is unexpected, the nurse should take immediate action while continuing to monitor the client's condition (option a). This type of

surgery does not include a drain. Also, nurses should not be repositioning drains in a first day post-operative client (option c). The client would need discharge teaching about wound care but the drainage is the immediate priority (option d) (Lewis & Collier, 1992; p. 294).

Nursing Process: Implementation
Client Need: Physiological Integrity

14. **The correct answer is a.** Pica is defined as the ingestion of non-edible and/or non-nutritive substances. The most common concern is iron-deficiency anemia because these substances may interfere with iron absorption. Signs and symptoms of lactose intolerance are abdominal distention, loose stools, diarrhea and cramps hence, option (b) is incorrect. In option (c), many women do exhibit this practice but there are definite unhealthy consequences for mother and baby, such as fecal impaction, excessive weight gain, and possible malformation. Option (d) is incorrect as there is no indication the client is a vegetarian (meaning the client will not eat any food from animal sources). It is also incorrect to state vegetarians can not receive sufficient amounts of protein as dairy products and eggs contain protein. Some unrefined grains, legumes, nuts, and some cooked and fresh fruits and vegetables contain proteins if the client is a "strict" vegetarian (Olds, London & Ladewig, 1992; p. 413).

Nursing Process: Analysis
Client Need: Physiological Integrity

15. **The correct answer is a.** These are signs of disseminated intravascular coagulation (DIC) and is common with gram-negative sepsis. DIC is an abnormal activation of the coagulation and fibrinolysis mechanisms leading to systemic bleeding and thrombosis. Blood cultures would assist in diagnosis and treatment of the sepsis which is the underlying cause of the DIC. Serum uric acid (option b) is related to hyperuricemia. Radiation (option c) would be a treatment for superior vena cava syndrome. Echocardiogram (option d) would be a diagnostic tool in cardiac tamponade. DIC, hyperuricemia, superior vena cava syndrome and cardiac tamponade are complications of cancer and cancer treatment (Ignatavicius & Bayne, 1991; pp. 595-597).

Nursing Process: Analysis
Client Need: Physiological Integrity

16. **The correct answer is b.** A dye is given for an intravenous pyelogram (IVP) so functioning of the kidneys can be seen more clearly. Oral fluids should be encouraged to rid the body of the dye. Peripheral pulses (option a) would need to be checked if a renal arteriogram was performed since the artery would be punctured to introduce the dye but excessive bleeding should not be a concern for venipuncture. Laxatives may be ordered (option c) prior to the test for better visualization of the abdomen but would not be necessary afterward. There is no sedation used with an IVP so bedrest with the side rails raised (option d) would not be

required unless other problems were evident (Lewis & Collier, 1992; p. 1179).

Nursing Process: Implementation
Client Need: Physiological Integrity

17. **The correct answer is d.** Risk factors for sudden infant death syndrome (SIDS) include family occurrence of SIDS, birth weight, mothers younger than 20, maternal narcotic addiction, and race. There is a higher incidence of SIDS among blacks and Native Americans (option c). There is no evidence to support a relationship of milk allergy to SIDS especially since SIDS usually occurs at night, not during feeding times (option a). Infants found with faces free demonstrate the same signs and symptoms as do children with covered faces (option b) (Mott, Sperhac, & James, 1990; pp. 1898-1899).

Nursing Process: Analysis
Client Need: Health Promotion & Maintenance

18. **The correct answer is c.**

20,000 u:1000 ml D$_5$W = (X) u:50 ml
20,000 x 50 = 1,000,000 (X)
1,000,000 1,000 = (X)
1000 = (X)
1000 u/hour

(Weaver & Koehler, 1992; pp. 102-103).

Nursing Process: Implementation
Client Need: Safe, Effective Care Environment

19. **The correct answer is a.** It is the only choice without fat in it. Triglycerides are a type of fat where three fatty acids are linked to a glycerol which is used by the body to manufacture glucose. Peanut butter and whole milk (option b), split pea soup and cocoa (option c), and a cheeseburger (option d) all contain fat (Burtis, Davis & Martin, 1988; pp. 117, 119, 442-444).

Nursing Process: Evaluation
Client Need: Physiological Integrity

20. **The correct answer is d.** The initial focus of behavioral intervention in the client with an eating disorder is education. Education is first focused on teaching the client the serious and life threatening nature of the illness. Meal planning and nutritional instruction (option a) do not begin until the client has achieved the goal weight due to the obsessive preoccupation with food and the need to stay thin. Fostering the client's independence (option b) and assertiveness training (option c) are important interventions. However, they are not the first intervention (Haber, Leach-McMahon, Price-Hoskins & Sideleau, 1992; pp. 664-646).

Nursing Process: Planning
Client Need: Physiological Integrity

21. **The correct answer is d.** One of the most serious risks, although rare, is hemorrhage into the neck that compromises the airway. Feelings of pressure or fullness should be reported and a tracheostomy kit kept at the

bedside. Sometimes during thyroid-ectomy the parathyroid glands are disturbed. These glands regulate the calcium level in the blood. When this level falls below 7 mg/dl (option a), tetany may begin as evidenced by a positive Trousseau (option c) or Chvostek sign (option b) (Smeltzer & Bare, 1992; p. 1091).

Nursing Process: Analysis
Client Need: Physiological Integrity

22. **The correct answer is d.** In Mexican-American families, the women in the family are responsible for health care. When approaching any subcultural group, the nurse should first assess the culture of the group, their understanding of illness and health as well as group needs. Most migrant farm workers are more concerned with the basic needs of food and shelter. Health screening and promotion are not as important as working quickly (options a and b). They tend to turn to healing agents within their own families or groups first and outsiders as a last resort. Therefore, the nurse must take the initiative to understand the culture and forge a bond with the group for positive results (option c) (Swanson & Albrecht, 1993; pp. 646-648).

Nursing Process: Implementation
Client Need: Health Promotion & Maintenance

23. **The correct answer is c.** When a client is stating delusional beliefs, verbalizing the underlying feelings is a way of identifying and validating the client's concerns. In his statement, the client

states his fear of what will happen if he reveals more of his symptoms. Option (a) is incorrect because it gives credence to the client's belief of being Superman. Option (b) is incorrect because it is too harsh in how it presents reality. Option (d) is incorrect because the client has not voiced a problem with losing identity but rather losing control (Cook & Fontaine, 1991; pp. 60-62, 553).

Nursing Process: Implementation
Client Need: Psychosocial Integrity

24. **The correct answer is a.** Respiratory acidosis occurs when poor ventilation results in increased carbon dioxide. The increased carbon dioxide and water combine to form carbonic acid which accumulates in the system. The kidneys act as a compensatory mechanism to decrease the amount of carbonic acid by excreting it. Since fluid is being excreted, edema is less likely to occur (option b). Vasoconstriction results in increased peripheral resistance (option c) which forces blood to capillaries andincreases oxygenation (option d) (Smith & Duell, 1993; pp. 612-613).

Nursing Process: Analysis
Client Need: Physiological Integrity

25. **The correct answer is d.** Singed nares and smoke around the nose and mouth indicate possible burns in the trachea. This can lead to edema with total airway obstruction. These signs and symptoms would not be indicative of mucous plug formation as seen in chronic obstructive pulmonary disease (COPD) (option a). There are no signs/symptoms indicating pulmonary edema or respiratory arrest

(options b and c) (Black & Matassarin-Jacobs, 1993; pp. 1987-1988).

Nursing Process: Analysis
Client Need: Physiological Integrity

26. **The correct answer is c.** Hypertension is a serious side effect of acute glomerulonephritis and can lead to seizure activity. Determining a history of streptococcus infection is important in order to make an accurate diagnosis, however in this case, the diagnosis has already been made (option a). Periorbital edema is a common symptom of the disease but is not as dangerous as hypertension (option b). A child with acute glomerulonephritis has a decreased appetite and, although it is important to provide for nutritional needs, it is not the nurse's primary concern (option d) (Whaley & Wong, 1991; pp. 1343-1346).

Nursing Process: Assessment
Client Need: Physiological Integrity

27. **The correct answer is c.** The classic triad of Parkinson's disease is tremor, rigidity and bradykinesia. The other choices (options a, b and c) are not clinical manifestations of the disease (Lewis & Collier, 1992; pp. 1599-1605).

Nursing Process: Assessment
Client Need: Physiological Integrity

28. **The correct answer is b.** Salicylate or aspirin-containing drug use may cause severe irritation to the stomach lining which can result in bleeding. Salicylate use is unrelated to cancerous polyps of the colon and the colon is a lower gastrointestinal area (option d).

Although esophageal bleeding may be caused by chronic alcohol abuse, there is no evidence to support alcohol abuse (option a). Retching and vomiting may result in esophageal tears and clients with bulimia indulge in self-induced vomiting (option c) but again, there is no evidence to suggest this explanation (Lewis & Collier, 1992; pp. 1010, 1043-1044, 1101-1102).

Nursing Process: Implementation
Client Need: Physiological Integrity

29. **The correct answer is d.** This approach allows for guided decision-making within the parameters of weight control guidelines and further allows the child control over the process. The suggestion also patterns what would occur for positive weight maintenance. Options (a) and (c) deal with punitive actions and emphasize external control rather than internal self-awareness and insight into behavior. Option (b) emphasizes the restrictions rather than positive food choice patterns (Bomar, 1989; pp. 172-173).

Nursing Process: Implementation
Client Need: Health Promotion & Maintenance

30. **The correct answer is b.** This action would not be appropriate because nuchal rigidity is an expected finding of meningitis. Bacterial meningitis is highly contagious and the client should be in respiratory isolation (option a) for 24 hours of antibiotic therapy. The room should be dimly lit (option d) because these clients often have photophobia as well. Persons who have close contact with the client (option c)

should be considered for prophylactic antibiotic therapy (Smeltzer & Bare, 1992; p. 1700).

Nursing Process: Implementation
Client Need: Physiological Integrity

PRACTICE SESSION: 13

Instructions:

Allow yourself 30 minutes to complete the following 30 practice questions. Use a timer to notify yourself when 30 minutes are over so that you are not constantly looking at your watch while completing the questions.

1. A man calls the public health clinic and asks how he can minimize the risk of radon in his home. Besides radon testing, the nurse should also suggest:
   a. installing exhaust fans in the house.
   b. checking basement walls for cracks and seal them.
   c. locating possible uranium mines in the area.
   d. allowing furnaces to run longer in the winter to introduce fresh air.

2. A 54 year old female with a 35 year history of cigarette smoking is admitted to the unit with the medical diagnosis of chronic bronchitis. She is anxious with labored breathing patterns. The nurse should plan to teach the client pursed lip breathing to:
   a. promote carbon dioxide elimination.
   b. decrease the need for oxygen use.
   c. strengthen the diaphragm.
   d. strengthen the intercostal muscles.

3. Alex, a 7 year old, has come to the emergency department with his parents because he has a temperature of 104°F (40°C) and he has been difficult to arouse for the past few hours. Alex was diagnosed with varicella two weeks ago. Reye syndrome is suspected. Alex's parents ask how the doctor will know for sure. The nurse knows that the only definitive diagnostic procedure for Reye syndrome is a(n):
   a. ultrasound of the abdomen.
   b. liver biopsy.
   c. computerized tomography (CT) of the brain.
   d. voiding cystourethrogram (VCUG).

4. A hospitalized client has a diagnosis of high risk for infection related to immunosuppression. What instructions should be given?
   a. "You may clean the cat litter box if you wear gloves."
   b. "Do not drink unpasteurized milk."
   c. "You should wash your hands before touching anyone."
   d. "Limit interaction with others."

5. A 27 year old client has been admitted to the psychiatric unit. She has been diagnosed with bipolar disorder, manic phase. The primary assessment data that should be collected on the client is:
   a. physical status.
   b. thought process.
   c. history of illness.
   d. social interactions.

6. A client with pre-eclampsia is being treated with magnesium sulfate intravenously. The nurse evaluates that the medication is effective when the client:
   a. shows a blood level of 10 mEq/L.
   b. is not exhibiting any uterine contractions.
   c. has hyperreflexia and clonus is present.
   d. is sleepy and there is a drop in her blood pressure.

7. A 29 year old male is admitted to the hospital with fever, chills, and shortness of breath. He is given a diagnosis of pneumocystis carinii pneumonia (PCP). He was diagnosed with autoimmune deficiency syndrome (AIDS) two years ago. Given this information, which of the following actions taken by the nurse is appropriate?
   a. Explain to visitors that while AIDS is not transmitted by casual contact, PCP is.
   b. Assign the client to a private room and place him in respiratory isolation.
   c. Explain to the client that the virus that causes PCP is a threat to a non-compromised host.
   d. Tell the family they do not need to take any new precautions.

8. A client is being prepared for an appendectomy. Before surgery, he complains of pain. To relieve the client's pain the nurse would:
   a. apply heat to the abdomen.
   b. place him in Fowler's position.
   c. administer analgesics.
   d. gently massage the painful area.

9. The nurse is planning discharge teaching for a 49 year old man with Cushing's syndrome. Teaching should emphasize the client's need to be monitored for signs of infection because:
   a. excess glucocorticoids result in hyperkalemia.
   b. excess glucocorticoids result in protein tissue wasting.
   c. excess production of glucocorticoids impair the immune and inflammatory responses.
   d. glucocorticoid deficiencies impair the immune and inflammatory response.

10. A nurse is attending a block party when Joyce, the newest member of the neighborhood, begins to ask questions about her daughter Emily. Emily is 8 years old and, although there are many other children her age at the party, she stays very close to her mother. Joyce is concerned because Emily complains of nausea and a headache every morning before school, but is fine on the weekends and in the evening. This has been occurring since they moved a month ago and now the school is concerned that Emily has missed so much school she may not be able to advance. Joyce states that she just doesn't know what to do. The nurse's best response is:

a. "Why don't you set up a meeting with Emily's teacher? It sounds like Emily may not like her and wants to avoid her."

b. "It's important that Emily attends school; the complaints she has are made up and will go away when she gets to school."

c. "Take Emily to school and have her gradually increase her time there, then pick her up at the end of the day."

d. "This is very normal for children who move into a new neighborhood, it will go away on its own."

11. The nurse evaluates that the client understands the early signs and symptoms of cholinergic crisis when the client states he would report:

a. tachycardia and muscle spasms.

b. restlessness and absent salivation.

c. facial flushing and dry skin.

d. acute muscle weakness and respiratory distress.

12. A client diagnosed with schizophrenia is sitting in the lounge laughing and talking occasionally even though he is alone. The client's primary nurse observes the behavior and plans to intervene. The nurse should:

a. leave the client alone to decrease stimulation.

b. allow the client to temporarily retreat from his pain.

c. gently redirect the client to a here and now focus.

d. present reality by reminding the client that nobody is in the lounge with him.

13. Ms. Louise Manetti R.N. is the charge nurse on the day shift. The staff have their assignments and are assisting clients with morning care. Ms. Manetti notices that Ms. White, a student nurse, has been staying in the nurse's station reading charts and has not attended to her client assignment. The initial response by Ms. Manetti R.N. should be to:

a. request a conference with Ms. White's instructor.

b. tell Ms. White to please attend to her assigned clients.

c. ask the nurse covering her clients to do the morning care until Ms. White is prepared.

d. point out Ms. White's behavior to her and ask if there is a problem.

14. Lisa, 2 weeks old, is brought to the emergency department by her parents. She is jaundiced and has had clay-colored stools for the past two days. She is diagnosed with biliary atresia. A Kasai procedure is performed. This procedure is done to:
   a. prevent reabsorption of bile from the intestines.
   b. prevent progressive liver disease.
   c. substitute a biliary duct from the jejunum.
   d. prepare the child for liver transplantation.

15. A client with a subdural hematoma is brought to the emergency department. The nurse would determine a problem is present if the:
   a. pO_2 is 90 mm Hg and the pCO_2 is 30.
   b. pO_2 is 85 mm Hg and the PCO_2 is 40.
   c. pO_2 is 75 mm Hg and the PCO_2 is 50.
   d. pO_2 is 75 mm Hg and the PCO_2 is 40.

16. A 49 year old female is admitted to the orthopedic unit from the recovery room following debridement of an infected leg wound. On admission to the unit her vital signs are normal. Several hours later her temperature is 103°F (39.4°C) and she is complaining of chills. The physician is notified and suspects septic shock. Which of the following is indicative of the early stages of septic shock?
   a. Increased cardiac output, hypotension, tachycardia.
   b. Decreased cardiac output, hypertension, and bradycardia.
   c. Arterial blood gas: pH of 7.35 and $PaCO_2$ of 35 mm Hg.
   d. Oliguria, hypotension and disseminated intravascular coagulation.

17. The nurse caring for a post-operative client is about to perform a dressing change on an abdominal wound. Universal precautions for this client would include:
   a. placing a linen-saver pad under the client to catch any spills or drainage.
   b. wearing a mask throughout the procedure.
   c. placing soiled dressings and gloves in a plastic trash bag.
   d. establishing a sterile field using sterile techniques.

Situation:

Mrs. Sheri Simmons, 34 years old, has come to the prenatal clinic. She is pregnant with her third child. She has a history of gestational diabetes. Urine test is positive for glucose. After further tests the physician determines she again has gestational diabetes. (The next three questions refer to this situation.)

18. The nurse is doing health teaching. The nurse evaluates that Mrs. Simmons understands common complications of gestational diabetes when she knows to report which of the following symptoms?
    a. Painful urination.
    b. Increased fetal activity.
    c. Lower abdominal pain and vaginal bleeding.
    d. Sudden sharp abdominal pain.

19. Mrs. Simmons' pregnancy progresses uneventfully. At 40 weeks gestation she is admitted to the labor suite in active labor. After ten hours Mrs. Simmons fails to progress in labor and oxytocin (Pitocin) is ordered. Mr. Simmons, who is coaching his wife, reports to the nurse that the last pain won't ease. The nurse would suspect a problem is occurring if the contraction lasted longer than:
    a. 30 seconds.
    b. 50 seconds.
    c. 75 seconds.
    d. 90 seconds.

20. Mrs. Simmons delivers a baby girl. The infant is placed in the neonatal intensive care unit. The nurse would observe the neonate for which complication specific to Mrs. Simmons' diabetic condition?
    a. Apathy, jitteriness, hypotonia.
    b. Apneic episodes, weak grasp, ineffective sucking.
    c. Fatigue, rapid and labored respirations.
    d. Abdominal distention, vomiting, diarrhea.

21. A 36 year old female with long hair is receiving chemotherapy for breast cancer. One morning she tells the nurse that clumps of her hair have started falling out. After the nurse teaches the client about alopecia, she makes all of the following statements. Which of them indicates a need for further teaching?
    a. "My hair may come back thicker."
    b. "I may even lose my eyebrows and eyelashes."
    c. "I will lubricate my scalp with some vitamin D ointment."
    d. "In most cases, hair loss is irreversible."

22. Priority nursing interventions for a client having a paracentesis procedure would include:
    a. applying a clean dressing to the puncture site.
    b. monitoring vital signs every 15 minutes during the procedure.
    c. measuring and recording drainage.
    d. placing the client in supine position.

23. A nurse is working with a client who suffers from migraine headaches. Which of the following menu selections would be most appropriate?
    a. Pepperoni pizza, garden salad, whole milk.
    b. Peanut butter on toast, chocolate milk, banana.
    c. Yogurt, unsalted crackers, orange juice.
    d. Chicken breast, buttered noodles, fruit flavored drink.

24. A 38 year old male client is brought to the intensive care unit after a car accident where blunt trauma to the abdomen is present. The priority nursing goal would be aimed at:
    a. controlling anxiety in the client through teaching.
    b. preparing the family for possible surgery and recovery.
    c. monitoring volume status and checking for signs of peritonitis.
    d. collecting specimens and preparing the client for possible surgery.

25. Jonathan, 14 years old, has just had surgery on an osteosarcoma of his left leg. Which of the following statements by Jonathan would indicate a need for further teaching?
    a. "After the radiation treatments I will be able to go back to school."
    b. "If my hair falls out, it will probably grow back curlier after I stop taking the medicine."
    c. "I guess this means I won't be able to finish the football season this year."
    d. "The doctor told me I would have to wear a fake leg."

26. A newly diagnosed client with Hodgkin's disease asks how the disease is spread. The nurse replies:
    a. "The first step is to rule out an infectious process."
    b. "It spreads through the lymph system."
    c. "The cause is unknown but believed to be viral in origin."
    d. "It spreads through the circulatory system to the spleen."

27. A group of clients on a psychiatric unit complain to the nurse that one of the clients is masturbating in the television room and ask that the nurse "do something about it." The nurse should initially respond to this situation by:
    a. matter-of-factly telling the client the behavior is unacceptable.
    b. explaining to the group of clients that everyone needs to alleviate sexual tension.
    c. asking the client if he would like to discuss his sexual concerns.
    d. providing privacy for the client.

28. Following a strong coughing spell, the abdominal wound of a post-operative client who had a bowel resection begins to eviscerate. Which of the following actions by the nurse is most appropriate?
    a. Reinsert the protruding organ and cover the wound with a sterile dressing.
    b. Cover the protruding organ and wound with a dry, sterile dressing.
    c. Reinsert the protruding organ and apply an abdominal binder.
    d. Cover the protruding organ with a sterile towel moistened with sterile normal saline.

29. A 34 year old male client is admitted to the burn unit. He is unable to use hands or arms to communicate due to burn injuries. His breathing is assisted by a tracheostomy and ventilator. The nurse notices he is alert since he responds to verbal commands. The best way to communicate with the client is to:

    a. use a pencil taped to his hand to write on a magic slate.

    b. ask him to point to items on a picture board.

    c. ask the family to help anticipate his needs.

    d. have the client mouth words as the nurse reads his lips.

30. A client has a nursing diagnosis of fluid volume deficit related to hyperthermia and the nurse has instituted actions to relieve the problem. The nurse knows the treatment has been ineffective when the client:

    a. has a core body temperature of 100°F (37.8°C).

    b. refused oral food and fluids.

    c. wakens with wet pajamas.

    d. has dry mouth and sunken eyes.

STOP You have now completed Practice Session: 13. Now take a few minutes and correct your answers. Calculate your accuracy rate by dividing the number of questions you completed correctly by the total number of questions you completed (30).

Correct answers ÷ total number of questions completed = accuracy rate.

_____ ÷ _____ = _____

PRACTICE SESSION: 13

ANSWERS AND RATIONALES

1. **The correct answer is b.** Radon is a colorless and odorless gas which seeps into the basement through cracks in the walls and floors. Radon levels can be greatly reduced through sealing the cracks and covering dirt floors. Furnaces (option d) and exhaust fans (option a) tend to pull in the radon gas rather than get rid of it. Radon is formed from the breakdown of uranium in the soil but locating uranium mines (option c) will not minimize risk in the home (Spradley, 1990; pp. 580-582).

Nursing Process: Implementation
Client Need: Health Promotion & Maintenance

2. **The correct answer is a.** Pursed lip breathing prolongs exhalation by forcing the air through a smaller opening in the mouth. This helps to open the airway and reduces the amount of air trapped in the alveoli thus reducing the amount of carbon dioxide in the body. This process does not help to strengthen the intercostal muscles (option d) or the diaphragm (option c). Pursed lip breathing does help rid the lungs of carbon dioxide but does not decrease the body's need for oxygen (option b) (Lewis & Collier, 1992; pp. 586-597).

Nursing Process: Planning
Client Need: Health Promotion & Maintenance

3. **The correct answer is b.** A liver biopsy will show a change in the mitochondria of the cells which may be caused by different viruses, drugs, exogenous toxins, and genetic factors. This change is indicative of Reye syndrome. An ultrasound may indicate an enlarged liver, a possible complication of Reye syndrome (option a). A computerized tomography (CT) of the head would identify increased intracranial pressure, another clinical sign of Reye syndrome, but would not definitively diagnose Reye syndrome (option c). A voiding cystourethrogram (VCUG) is used to diagnose urinary reflux and ureter strictures, not to confirm Reye syndrome (option d) (Whaley & Wong, 1991; p. 1758).

Nursing Process: Analysis
Client Need: Physiological Integrity

4. **The correct answer is b.** Unpasteurized milk contains bacteria which may not be handled well by an immunosuppressed system. Cat litter (option a) may carry disease which is transmitted by methods other than physical contact (e.g., airborne) so cat litter should not be changed by the client. The client is not infected so will not transmit disease to others (option c). Limiting interaction with others (option d) may isolate the client. Precautions may need to be taken to prevent disease transmission but the client should be encouraged to maintain

a support system (Lewis & Collier, 1992; p. 155).

Nursing Process: Implementation
Client Need: Physiological Integrity

5. **The correct answer is a.** Although psychosocial issues are important (options b, c and d), the activity level of many manic clients often places them in danger of physical exhaustion. Manic clients often lack awareness of their physical needs such as fatigue, hunger and waste elimination. Physical problems can be life-threatening in a manic client and, therefore, take precedence over other problems (Cook & Fontaine, 1991; pp. 408-410, 419).

Nursing Process: Assessment
Client Need: Psychosocial Integrity

6. **The correct answer is d.** Magnesium sulfate is a cerebral depressant. It also decreases central nervous system (CNS) irritability and causes vasodilation which results in the client feeling relaxed, even sleepy, and decreasing the blood pressure. Option (a) is incorrect as therapeutic blood levels for magnesium sulfate are between 4-7 mEq/L. At about 10 mEq/L the knee jerk begins to disappear, and at any higher level toxicity sets in. Option (b) is incorrect as magnesium sulfate may be used to relax the uterus and stop contractions if the client is in premature labor. However, the client's uterine activity is not a measure of effectiveness if the client is pre-eclamptic. In option (c), if the client is hyperreflexic and clonus is present, the central nervous system (CNS) is still very irritable and either the medication levels are not yet

therapeutic, or the medication is not working on this client (Olds, London & Ladewig, 1992, p. 519).

Nursing Process: Evaluation
Client Need: Physiological Integrity

7. **The correct answer is d.** Pneumocystis carinii pneumonia (PCP) is caused by a virus that is an opportunist. That is, PCP does not affect people with uncompromised immune systems (option c). PCP is not spread by casual contact (option a) and the client does not require a private room or respiratory isolation (option b) (Smeltzer & Bare, 1992; p. 1365).

Nursing Process: Evaluation
Client Need: Safe, Effective Care Environment

8. **The correct answer is b.** Before surgery, reduce the client's pain by placing him in Fowler's position thus reducing the pressure. Never apply heat to the abdomen (option a), give cathartics or enemas, or massage the area (option d). These actions could trigger rupture of the appendix and cause peritonitis and other complications. Avoid giving analgesics which can mask the pain of rupture (option c) (Illustrated Manual of Nursing Practice, 1991; pp. 774-775).

Nursing Process: Implementation
Client Need: Physiological Integrity

9. **The correct answer is c.** The client needs to be aware that glucocorticoids suppress the immune and inflammatory responses such that minor symptoms may indicate a severe infection. Excess

glucocorticoids actually cause hypokalemia (option a). Wasting of protein tissues does occur with excess glucocorticoid production (option b) but this has no correlation to increased susceptibility to infection. Glucocorticoid deficiencies (option d) are associated with chronic primary adrenocortical insufficiency (Addison's Disease) (Black & Matassarin-Jacobs, 1993; p. 1765).

Nursing Process: Analysis
Client Need: Physiological Integrity

10. **The correct answer is c.** Emily is exhibiting signs of school phobia. This is treated by gradually returning the child to school on a full-time basis. School phobia is a type of separation anxiety and, based on the evidence given, Emily is having a difficult time separating from her mother, so having her mother drop her off and pick her up from school will demonstrate that she is not abandoning her. There is no evidence to suggest that Emily is having difficulty with her teacher (option a). Although it is important for Emily to return to school to decrease feeling of worthlessness and inability to cope, Emily's symptoms are real and will not go away when she gets to school; they may get worse (option b). Separation anxiety does occur when children move, however Emily has missed enough school that she may not advance to the next grade. When it has reached this point it will not go away without intervention(option d) (Clunn, 1991; pp. 357-358; Whaley & Wong, 1991; p. 860).

Nursing Process: Implementation
Client Need: Psychosocial Integrity

11. **The correct answer is d.** Cholinergic crisis is caused by overmedication with anticholinesterase drugs. Signs and symptoms include: acute muscle weakness, respiratory distress, nausea, vomiting, pallor, diaphoresis, increased salivation, gastrointestinal hyper-irritability, severe cramps, diarrhea and bradycardia (options a, b and c) (Long, Phipps & Cassmeyer, 1993; pp. 1242-1246).

Nursing Process: Evaluation
Client Need: Physiological Integrity

12. **The correct answer is c.** The nurse helps the client regain contact with reality by introducing conversation with a here and now focus. Leaving the client who is hallucinating alone only enhances the client's fear (option a). The nurse does not encourage retreat from reality (option b) nor does the nurse tell the client that the voices are not real. This will only serve to alienate the client and would lead to an argument or power struggle between the client and the nurse (option d) (Johnson, 1993; p. 478).

Nursing Process: Implementation
Client Need: Psychosocial Integrity

13. **The correct answer is d.** The charge nurse should point out to Ms. White that her client's care is not finished and she has been in the nurse's station. This opens communication without putting Ms. White on the defensive so she may feel free to talk if there is a problem. Asking another nurse to do the work for Ms. White is inappropriate (option c). Ms. White is capable of the work and the other nurse may be unduly burdened.

Telling Ms. White to do her work (option b) may be appropriate if there is no verbalized problem. However, if there is a problem that may compromise the client's care and safety, the charge nurse should become aware of it since the client is her primary concern. Requesting a meeting with Ms. White's instructor (option a) may be necessary but the initial response would be to assess the problem in order to maintain the client's well-being (Tappen, 1989; pp. 460-462).

Nursing Process: Implementation
Client Need: Safe, Effective Care Environment

14. **The correct answer is c.** Biliary atresia is the obstruction or absence of a portion of the bile duct. A Kasai procedure is done to substitute a duct from a segment of the jejunum. However, this is a palliative procedure and progressive liver disease still occurs (option b). Cholestyramine, a bile acid binder, is used to prevent reabsorption of bile from the intestines (option a). A Kasai procedure is not a necessary prerequisite for liver transplantation (option d) (Whaley & Wong, 1991; pp. 504-505).

Nursing Process: Analysis
Client Need: Physiological Integrity

15. **The correct answer is c.** A priority for care of a client with a head injury is maintenance of adequate oxygenation. Injury to the brain stem can result in an altered breathing pattern leading to hypoxia and hypercapnia. Arterial blood gases are monitored to detect oxygen deprivation and brain stem involvement. Normal pO_2 is 95-100 mm Hg and all

four options (options a, b, c and d) are below normal oxygen levels for arterial blood. Normal pCO_2 is 35-45 mm Hg. The only option that shows a higher than normal carbon dioxide level is option (c) (Smeltzer & Bare, 1992; pp. 313, 1735).

Nursing Process: Analysis
Client Need: Physiological Integrity

16. **The correct answer is a.** In septic shock there is a decrease in systemic vascular resistance (SVR) and vasodilatation. This results in an initial increase in cardiac output. Cardiac output is partially determined by the resistance the heart must work against or SVR. Other early symptoms of shock are hypotension, tachycardia, fever, chills and tachypnea (options b and d). As septicemia progresses, late signs may include oliguria and disseminated intravascular coagulation (DIC) (option d). Arterial blood gases (ABG's) usually indicate respiratory alkalosis or metabolic acidosis. Option (c) is a normal blood gas result (Smeltzer & Bare, 1992; pp. 612, 1921).

Nursing Process: Assessment
Client Need: Physiological Integrity

17. **The correct answer is c.** Universal precautions include placing soiled dressings and gloves in a plastic bag and disposing of them properly according to institutional regulations. Wearing a mask would be done for respiratory contagious organisms or if splashing is predicted to occur (option b). A linen-saver pad prevents linen changes and soiling of bedsheets but is not involved in universal precautions (option a). Establishing a sterile field using sterile

technique during wound care reduces the risk of nosocomial infections but again is not part of universal precautions guidelines (option d) (Potter & Perry, 1991; pp. 520-527).

Nursing Process: Planning
Client Need: Safe, Effective Care Environment

18. **The correct answer is a.** Painful urination is a sign of a urinary tract infection. This condition must be treated early since diabetics are prone to pyelonephritis. Other common complications include candidiasis (symptoms include vaginal discharge, itching and burning) and pregnancy-induced hypertension (symptoms include rapid weight gain and rising blood pressure). Decreased, not increased, fetal activity (option b) would be characteristic of a complication of fetal distress. Lower abdominal pain and vaginal bleeding (option c) might indicate an ectopic pregnancy. Sudden sharp abdominal pain (option d) would be a symptom of abruptio placentae. All options would be reportable to the physician but only painful urination indicating a urinary tract infection would be considered a common complication of a client with diabetes (Martin & Reeder, 1991; pp. 597, 601-603, 613, 624).

Nursing Process: Evaluation
Client Need: Physiological Integrity

19. **The correct answer is d.** Contractions of longer than 90 seconds duration may signal uterine tetany which can be dangerous to mother and fetus. Immediate reaction is required when this condition exists. In the onset of first stage labor, normal contractions last from 30-40 seconds long. As the labor continues and 4 cm dilatation is evident, contractions last 25-45 seconds long (option a). At 5-7 cm dilatation, contractions occur from 40-60 seconds in duration (option b). From 8-10 cm dilatation through birth, contractions last 45-90 seconds long (option c) (Martin & Reeder, 1991; pp. 216-219, 665).

Nursing Process: Analysis
Client Need: Physiological Integrity

20. **The correct answer is a.** Infants born to diabetic mothers should be observed for hypoglycemia. An infant with hypoglycemia may either appear asymptomatic or have the following symptoms: apathy, jitteriness, tremors, hypotonia, high-pitched weak cry, cyanosis, eye-rolling, or sweating. Apneic episodes, weak grasp, and ineffective sucking (option b) are signs of a premature infant. Fatigue and rapid, labored respirations (option c) indicate respiratory distress syndrome. Abdominal distention, vomiting and diarrhea (option d) as well as gastrointestinal bleeding may indicate necrotizing enterocolitis. Options (c) and (d) are also more specific complications related to pre-term infants (Martin & Reeder, 1991; pp. 764-765, 769-770).

Nursing Process: Assessment
Client Need: Physiological Integrity

21. **The correct answer is d.** This indicates a need for further teaching since hair loss usually reverses after the chemotherapy is stopped. Lubrication of the scalp helps (option c) to maintain

skin integrity. The color and texture (option a) of the new hair may differ. All hair (option b) may be affected by chemotherapy (Smeltzer & Bare, 1992; p. 364).

Nursing Process: Evaluation
Client Need: Health Promotion & Maintenance

22. **The correct answer is b.** The nurse monitors vital signs every 15 minutes during a paracentesis and observes for impending signs of shock due to fluid shifting during and immediately after the procedure. A drop in blood pressure may occur early in the procedure during initial volume loss. Applying a sterile dressing to the puncture site is done after the procedure to prevent infection (option a). Measuring and recording drainage assists in maintaining an accurate intake and output record but is not the priority intervention during the procedure (option c). The client is to be positioned upright at the side of the bed. This upright position allows the intestine to float posteriorly and helps prevent laceration during catheter insertion (option d) (Ignatavicius & Bayne, 1991; pp. 1487-1489).

Nursing Process: Implementation
Client Need: Physiological Integrity

23. **The correct answer is d.** Certain foods containing tyramine, monosodium glutamate, milk products or nitrites may trigger migraine headaches. Option (d) contains none of these. Option (a) contains milk products and pepperoni, a nitrate. Option (b) contains peanut butter and a banana which are tyramine containing foods and chocolate is a nitrate. Option (c) contains yogurt, a milk product (Smeltzer & Bare, 1992; p. 1694).

Nursing Process: Analysis
Client Need: Physiological Integrity

24. **The correct answer is c.** The priority nursing goal would be to monitor volume status and to check for signs of peritonitis which include tender abdomen, rebound tenderness, abdominal muscle tightness and low or absent bowel sounds. The second priority is to assist the physician to instill tubes to monitor fluid volume, cardiac output and collect specimens for diagnostic tests such as blood gases and electrolytes. Duties may also include preparation of the client for surgery if the condition warrants (low hematocrit and hemoglobin, rigid abdomen) (option d). The third priority is emotional support to the client through explanation of procedures and general routine (option a). The fourth priority, but still very important, is family support by explaining equipment and procedures including expectations of surgery and the recovery period (option b) (Phipps, Long, Woods & Cassmeyer, 1991; pp. 1154-1155).

Nursing Process: Planning
Client Need: Physiological Integrity

25. **The correct answer is a.** Osteosarcoma is a radioresistant tumor. Very high doses of radiation will not control tumor growth and may instead cause considerable damage to normal tissue and functional loss. Chemotherapy, a treatment for osteosarcoma, does cause alopecia (hair loss), although the hair

usually grows back thicker, darker and curlier (option b). Returning to the football season would increase the chance of injury (option c). Body image is a major concern for adolescents (option d) (Mott, Sperhac & James, 1990; p. 1839; Whaley & Wong, 1991; p. 1683).

Nursing Process: Planning
Client Need: Physiological Integrity

26. **The correct answer is b.** Hodgkin's disease is of unknown origin which occurs in the lymph system (option d) and may spread to the spleen. Since lymph node enlargement is usually the first sign, infectious processes are ruled out first (option a) before diagnostic workup for Hodgkin's disease. Non-Hodgkin's lymphomas have been explored for possible viral etiology (option c) (Smeltzer & Bare, 1992; pp. 803-805).

Nursing Process: Implementation
Client Need: Health Promotion & Maintenance

27. **The correct answer is d.** The most appropriate intervention for the client who is publicly masturbating is to provide privacy for the client. Nurses need to show respect and appreciation for the hospitalized client's sexual needs as normal. Option (a) tells the client that his sexual behavior is unacceptable rather than telling him that the behavior is acceptable but it must be performed in private. Option (b) avoids the issues of both the client who is masturbating and the client group who is complaining about it. Option (c) may be an appropriate response but the nurse does

not have enough data to indicate the client in this specific situation has a sexual concern. The first intervention would be to provide privacy and then determine if further intervention is necessary (Johnson, 1993; p. 378).

Nursing Process: Implementation
Client Need: Health Promotion & Maintenance

28. **The correct answer is d.** When wound evisceration occurs, usually between the fifth and tenth day post-operatively, the protruding organ should be covered immediately with a sterile towel moistened with sterile normal saline (option b). The nurse does not reinsert the organ (options a and c) but remains with the client for continual assessment. Another nurse should notify the surgeon, and the operating room should be made aware that the client will be returning (Black & Matassarin-Jacobs, 1993; pp. 439-440; Ignatavicius & Bayne, 1991; p. 478).

Nursing Process: Implementation
Client Need: Safe, Effective Care Environment

29. **The correct answer is d.** Since the client is alert and responds to verbal commands, he is also capable of responding to questions. Using lip reading gives the client a link to communicate with health care providers and other support systems and gives the client some control over as much of his care as is possible (option a). Maintaining eye contact and observing facial expression can be important in ascertaining the client's needs and maintaining a rapport with the client.

Options (a) and (b) are incorrect since the client is unable to use arms and hands due to burn injuries. It is generally important to keep the family involved in client care. In this instance the client is alert and some means of communication is available. Asking the family to constantly guess and interpret needs (option c) places extra burden on the family as well as places the client in more of a dependent position than is necessary (Smeltzer & Bare, 1992; pp. 539-540).

Nursing Process: Implementation
Client Need: Physiological Integrity

30. **The correct answer is d.** The question asks for signs of ineffective treatment for fluid volume deficit or dehydration which includes dry lips, tongue and mouth, poor skin turgor, and sunken eyes. A core body temperature of 100°F (37.8°C) (option a) is desirable if the has hyperthermia since the temperature is in a more normal range. Even though temperature is coming to normal range it doesn't mean the fluid volume has also returned to normal yet. Refusing food and fluids (option b) may cause dehydration but is not a sign of dehydration. Damp or wet clothing (option c) may be related to dehydration but is not a sign of it. It may be the result of other problems besides hyperthermia (Lewis & Collier, 1992; p. 1552).

Nursing Process: Evaluation
Client Need: Physiological Integrity

PRACTICE SESSION: 14

Instructions:

Allow yourself 30 minutes to complete the following 30 practice questions. Use a timer to notify yourself when 30 minutes are over so that you are not constantly looking at your watch while completing the questions.

---

1. The nurse is to obtain a sputum specimen. The proper initial direction to give the client is to:
   a. instruct the client that a specimen is needed of the sputum he coughs up and leave a cup at the bedside.
   b. ask the client to rinse his mouth with water, take some deep breaths, cough and expectorate into the cup.
   c. tell the client to breathe deeply several times and cough up something into the specimen cup.
   d. ask the client to give a sputum specimen when the respiratory therapist gives him his treatment.

2. A newly admitted female client has been diagnosed with obsessive compulsive disorder. She tells the nurse she worries constantly that she has accidently run over someone with her car and has spent the last several days retracing her drive to work to make sure she has not hit anyone. In working with this client, the nurse understands that:
   a. reality orientation to the unlikelihood of this occurring would prove useful.
   b. teaching the client that she can control these thoughts will decrease anxiety.
   c. the client does understand that her fears are unrealistic in nature.
   d. helping the client discover and prove that no one was injured is the only immediate action necessary.

3. The parents of an 18 year old boy with Kaposi's srcoma are seen in the outpatient cancer clinic. They ask the nurse about "alternative" forms of cancer therapy. The nurse should base her response on the knowledge that the National Cancer Institute recognizes which of the following?
   a. Laetrile under careful medical observation.
   b. Interferon in clinical trials.
   c. Macrobiotic diet with protein supplements.
   d. Amygdalin with vitamin B_{17}.

4. A female client is admitted to the labor and delivery suite stating her membranes have just ruptured. The nurse palpates the presenting part and ascertains it is the umbilical cord. The priority action of the nurse would be to:
   a. notify the physician.
   b. keep gloved fingers in vagina and attempt to relieve compression on presenting part.
   c. obtain fetal heart rate and start oxygen on the client at 6-10 liters/minute.
   d. notify the client that birth is imminent and prepare for delivery.

Situation:
Mrs. Millie Wolfe, 72 years old, has been hospitalized for productive cough, weakness and shortness of breath on exertion. She states she has lost some weight because she "doesn't feel like eating." She also complains of waking at night to change her nightgown because it is so wet. (The next three questions refer to this situation.)

5. Mrs. Wolfe is diagnosed with pulmonary tuberculosis. She is placed in a private room. The nurse would instruct Mrs. Wolfe in which of the following precautions?
   a. She should wear a mask at all times.
   b. A tissue should cover nose and mouth when she coughs.
   c. The private room is sufficient precaution.
   d. No precautions are necessary since she is on the appropriate medication.

6. Mrs. Wolfe has been given a nursing diagnosis of potential for injury related to possible spread of infection. Which of the following outcome criteria would be appropriate?
   a. Adequate nutrition to maintain body weight.
   b. Decreased anxiety about diagnosis.
   c. Compliance with medication regimen.
   d. Return to pretreatment activity level.

7. Mrs. Wolfe is to be discharged to her home. Her daughter worries that her mother will forget to take her medication. The best action of the nurse would be to:
   a. suggest that the daughter administer the medication to Mrs. Wolfe.
   b. ask the physician to transfer Mrs. Wolfe to a skilled care facility while she is on the medication.
   c. tell the family to limit the length of visits with Mrs. Wolfe until she is completely well.
   d. refer her to visiting nurses to check on Mrs. Wolfe's medication administration.

8. Ms. Jill Brooks, 18 years old, is admitted to the hospital with abdominal pain. Diagnostic tests show cancer which has metastasized to the liver. During morning care, Ms. Brooks says, "I wish I would just die and get it over with. I know there's no hope." The best reply of the nurse would be:
   a. "Are you saying you feel hopeless?"
   b. "You have a realistic outlook of your prognosis. Let's talk about it."
   c. "It sounds like you believe you are being punished."
   d. "It's hard to find out you have cancer. Let's talk about what that means to you."

9. A baby girl is delivered vaginally without complications. First assessment at delivery reveals a pulse rate of 92 by palpation at the stump of the cord. The infant is lying with elbows and hips flexed with knees positioned up toward torso. The color of the torso and face is pink with pronounced acrocyanosis. There is only a weak grimace accompanied by nasal flaring. The initial action of the nurse would be to:
   a. warm the infant.
   b. prepare for resuscitative measures.
   c. apgar score the infant in 5 minutes.
   d. continue to assess the infant.

10. The nurse caring for a client with chronic renal failure (CRF) would expect the medical regimen to include a(n):
    a. vasoconstrictor.
    b. corticosteroid.
    c. iron supplement.
    d. non-narcotic analgesic.

11. Baby boy Devlin was born with cleft lip and palate. The nurse is assessing the infant's ability to suck. The infant may be unable to suck on a regular nipple or breast because:
    a. the deformity may cause damage to the mother's breast.
    b. sucking may cause further damage to the child's mouth.
    c. sucking may cause infection if used by this infant.
    d. he cannot create a proper vacuum in the mouth.

12. A client with a head injury is admitted to the hospital. He is awake and conversing. His pupils are 4 mm and react briskly to light. Which of the following changes in the client's neurological status would indicate a need for immediate intervention by the nurse?
    a. He becomes lethargic and converses less.
    b. Pupils are 4 mm and react sluggishly to light.
    c. Hand grasps and pedal pulses are weak bilaterally.
    d. He is unable to follow complex commands.

13. The community health nurse is asked to visit a family whose adolescent has been diagnosed with an adjustment disorder. The nurse would approach the family with which goal in mind?
    a. Promoting separation of the young adult from the parents.
    b. Committing to new family members.
    c. Maintaining contact with the custodial parent.
    d. Assisting in redefinition of boundaries to allow for independence.

14. The physician orders 1500 ml of normal saline solution to infuse over 12 hours. The intravenous solution is placed on a microdrip. How many drops per minute will the nurse regulate the intravenous solution?
   a. 21 gtts/min.
   b. 25 gtts/min.
   c. 125 gtts/min.
   d. 150 gtts/min.

15. A new graduate nurse asks the charge nurse on an acute psychiatric inpatient setting how the staff determines when a client needs to be secluded or restrained. The charge nurse responds by stating that restraints or seclusion are used to:
   a. increase the client's sensory input.
   b. encourage client compliance with treatment.
   c. build a system of positive reinforcement.
   d. prevent injury to clients and staff.

16. A client newly diagnosed with Parkinson's disease was admitted to a medical unit. While teaching the client about the therapeutic management for his disease he responds, "I will take my medications to cure my Parkinson's disease." The nurse would include which action in the plan of care?
   a. Ask the physician to explain the disease process to the client.
   b. Praise the client for learning so well and give positive reinforcement.
   c. Continue to educate the client including dietary teaching.
   d. Schedule a specific time for the client and family to discuss Parkinson's disease.

17. A 38 year old female was involved in a vehicle accident five days ago and develops respiratory failure. She is intubated and placed on mechanical ventilation. Her arterial blood gases are as follows: pH 7.32; $PaCO_2$ 30 mm Hg; HCO_3 14 mEq/L; PaO_2 60 mm Hg; SaO_2 89%. This client's acid-base dysfunction is:
   a. respiratory alkalosis.
   b. metabolic acidosis.
   c. respiratory acidosis.
   d. metabolic alkalosis.

18. A female nurse is caring for a 28 year old male client newly diagnosed with insulin dependent diabetes mellitus. While the nurse is attempting to conduct diabetic teaching, the client frequently makes remarks such as, "Sit on my bed with me," and "Why don't you give me your home telephone number and we can discuss this over dinner once I'm discharged." Which of the following would be the most therapeutic response by the nurse?
   a. "I think you are avoiding the issue. This information is very important. Please try to pay attention."
   b. "I notice that every time I try to talk to you about your diabetes, you start to flirt with me."
   c. "This is totally inappropriate. We do not have a social relationship."
   d. "You must be feeling lonely. I can understand that this must be difficult for you."

19. Mr. Fred Selkman is admitted with a diagnosis of hyperparathyroidism. Which of the following nursing interventions would be appropriate in this client's care?
a. Assess for a positive Chvostek's sign.
b. Encourage a calcium rich diet.
c. Force fluids to a minimum of 3000 ml per day.
d. Administer levothyroxine (Synthroid) as ordered each morning.

20. Mr. Michael Kasevich is a nursing assistant on the evening shift. He is standing at the desk when a client rings the call bell for assistance to the bathroom. The charge nurse asks Mr. Kasevich to assist the client. Mr. Kasevich remarks, "Oh, that client just wants some attention. He does this all the time. He can wait." The initial response of the charge nurse would be to:
a. inform the head nurse in writing of Mr. Kasevich's behavior.
b. tell Mr. Kasevich firmly to go do it now.
c. go and assist the client to the bathroom and ask Mr. Kasevich to check on him in a few minutes.
d. ask Mr. Kasevich to go with you to care for the client then speak to Mr. Kasevich about his behavior.

21. A woman calls the coronary care unit about her husband who had coronary artery bypass graft (CABG) surgery and was discharged one week ago. She states that her husband has serous mixed with purulent drainage from his saphenous vein incision site and asks what to put on it. The nurse should advise the woman to:
a. cleanse the wound with hydrogen peroxide.
b. stop taking the anticoagulant.
c. call the physician about the drainage.
d. increase the antibiotic dosage.

22. A post-operative client hospitalized for several weeks starts to become disoriented and confused at times, sleeps a great deal of the day, and has anorexia accompanied by weight loss. The nurse might suggest which of the following to the physician?
a. Referral to psychiatric consultation for depression.
b. Move to a rehabilitation hospital to encourage progress.
c. Fewer visits from family and friends to decrease exhaustion.
d. Medication to promote night time sleeping and daylight naps.

23. A client from another country is admitted to a medical unit. The client does not speak English and there is no interpreter available to assist with translation. The best approach in asking assessment information is to:
    a. raise your voice while pantomiming the action.
    b. use pantomime to finish the assessment process quickly.
    c. set the tone by being friendly and informal.
    d. ask the client's family to help locate an interpreter.

24. A client with ascites is being discharged. Dietary teaching would include which of the following?
    a. Drink one eight ounce glass of water every two hours from 8 a.m. to 8 p.m.
    b. Avoid foods like snack foods and frozen vegetables.
    c. Avoid foods like lemon, vinegar, oregano, and pepper.
    d. Take an over the counter antacid after meals.

25. Mrs. Karen Woods, 40 years old, is admitted through the emergency room and diagnosed with Addison's disease. After recovery she is discharged on glucocorticoids and mineralocorticoids. The nurse would instruct Mrs. Woods to observe for which of the signs and symptoms of insufficient replacement?
    a. Vomiting, weakness, polyuria, weight loss.
    b. Weight gain, edema, hypertension, oliguria.
    c. Tachycardia, abrupt headaches, heat intolerance, anxiety.
    d. Dry skin, hoarse voice, bradycardia, weight gain.

26. A 30 year old female client is admitted with pelvic inflammatory disease (PID). A high priority nursing diagnosis would be:
    a. altered sexuality patterns related to loss of body part.
    b. acute pain related to dysuria.
    c. high risk for infection transmission related to vaginal discharge.
    d. fear related to impending surgery.

27. A nurse caring for a client on mechanical ventilation would reposition the client frequently to:
    a. mobilize secretions.
    b. prevent skin breakdown.
    c. ensure adequate ventilation.
    d. prevent contractures.

28. A nursing student is assigned to a client diagnosed with a conversion disorder. She asks the nurse in charge to explain a symptom characteristic of this disorder termed la belle indifference. The charge nurse bases her response to the student on her understanding that la belle indifference is described as:
    a. conscious deception and communication of false physical symptoms.
    b. a fear that one has a serious disease that cannot be detected.
    c. decreased anxiety over a debilitating symptom and resultant disruption in one's life.
    d. the experience of physical symptoms without organic pathology.

29. A 60 year old male client is admitted to the cardiothoracic floor following a right lung wedge resection for lung cancer. He has a right chest tube attached to a Pleur-Evac drainage system. The Pleur-Evac is placed to 20 cm of suction as is ordered by the surgeon. Which of the following actions taken by the nurse indicates a good understanding of chest tube functioning? The nurse:
   a. reports immediately that the chest tube is bubbling continuously.
   b. explains to the licensed practical nurse (LPN) that the fluid in the Pleur-Evac will rise with expiration and fall with inspiration.
   c. gently loops the excess tubing on top of the bed.
   d. puts client's right arm and shoulder through range of motion exercises every six hours.

30. Baby boy Jake is being treated for hyperbilirubinemia with phototherapy. Which of the following findings would the nurse expect to see?
   a. Loose green stools.
   b. Lights six inches above Jake.
   c. Jake's eyes open and alert.
   d. A lactose rich formula.

STOP You have now completed Practice Session: 14. Now take a few minutes and correct your answers. Calculate your accuracy rate by dividing the number of questions you completed correctly by the total number of questions you completed (30).

Correct answers ÷ total number of questions completed = accuracy rate.

_____ ÷ _____ = _____

ANSWERS AND RATIONALES

1. **The correct answer is b.** First rinse the mouth with water so normal mouth flora does not contaminate the specimen (option c). Then ask the client to take several deep breaths and cough deeply so the sputum comes from the lung. The specimen should be placed in a sterile container and sent to the proper laboratory. Leaving the specimen cup without proper instruction often leads to an inadequate or contaminated specimen (option a). Respiratory therapy (option d) may contaminate the specimen depending on the type of treatment (Smeltzer & Bare, 1992; p. 517).

   Nursing Process: Implementation
   Client Need: Physiological Integrity

2. **The correct answer is c.** The client understands that these involuntary (option b) thoughts are meaningless and unrealistic. Telling the client that her worries are unnecessary is not a helpful intervention (option a). Even though clients may try to ignore these thoughts and resultant behavior, they remain preoccupied with them. The nurse can not disprove (option d) or talk the client out of them (Johnson, 1993; pp. 412-413).

   Nursing Process: Analysis
   Client Need: Psychosocial Integrity

3. **The correct answer is b.** Interferon is used to stimulate the immune system and has both direct and indirect effects on cancer cells. It's use is approved for certain cancers especially Kaposi's Sarcoma. Laetrile (amygdalin and vitamin B_{17}) has been investigated by the National Cancer Institute and found to have no therapeutic benefit and actually has many harmful side effects (options a and d). Persons on macrobiotic diets (option c) tend to develop multiple dietary deficiencies (Smeltzer & Bare, 1992; p. 370).

   Nursing Process: Assessment
   Client Need: Physiological Integrity

4. **The correct answer is b.** This is a life saving measure for the fetus. While the nurse is relieving pressure on the cord, another nurse will obtain the fetal heart rate to evaluate the effectiveness of the intervention. Oxygen should be started on the mother by face mask at 6-10 liters/minute in hopes of "hyper-oxygenating" her so the fetus will be oxygenated through the placenta (option c). The nurse will ask another nurse to notify the physician (option a). The nurse will also notify the client of the emergency at hand and prepare her for delivery (option d) (Olds, London & Ladewig, 1992; pp. 769-771).

   Nursing Process: Implementation
   Client Need: Safe, Effective Care Environment

5. **The correct answer is b.** Tuberculosis is spread through the air. Mrs. Wolfe should cover her nose and mouth when

coughing so that the tuberculosis is not spread. The client does not wear a mask (option a). However, the nurse should wear a mask when caring for the client. The private room (option c) would not prevent spread of an airborne infection. The medications take at least 2-3 weeks (option d) before the client is no longer contagious (Ignatavicius & Bayne, 1991; pp. 2041-2044).

Nursing Process: Implementation
Client Need: Safe, Effective Care Environment

6. **The correct answer is c.** Mrs. Wolfe has a potential for spreading the tuberculosis unless she stays compliant with medication. Clients must take several medications over a nine month to one year period. Compliance may be difficult due to drug side effects and length of treatment. Adequate nutrition to maintain body weight (option a) is an outcome criteria for altered nutrition: less than body requirements. Decreased anxiety related to diagnosis (option b) is an outcome criteria for anxiety. Returning to pretreatment activity level (option d) is related to a nursing diagnosis of fatigue (Ignatavicius & Bayne, 1991; pp. 2043-2045).

Nursing Process: Planning
Client Need: Health Promotion and Maintenance

7. **The correct answer is d.** A visiting nurse would be able to check on Mrs. Wolfe's progress. This would include determining her self-care ability such as taking her own medication. The nurse would also be able to reinforce teaching.

There is not enough evidence to determine that Mrs. Wolfe cannot take her own medication (option a). Someone else giving the client medication places the client in a dependent position and will decrease her self-esteem and may decrease her ability to care for herself. Mrs. Wolfe would not need to be transferred to a skilled care facility (option b) unless she is unable to be cared for any other way. Being in her own environment will also help her to get well more quickly. Restricting visitation (option c) is unnecessary once Mrs. Wolfe is released from the hospital and maintains her medication regimen. Lack of visitation may decrease her self-esteem and cause further problems (Ignatavicius & Bayne, 1991; pp. 215-217).

Nursing Process: Implementation
Client Need: Health Promotion & Maintenance

8. **The correct answer is d.** This statement shows empathy for what the client is going through, then offers to listen to how this diagnosis will affect her. It will allow the client to talk about what she wants and help her deal with the diagnosis and treatment at her own pace. Option (a) states what the client has already said and may show the client that the nurse is not listening very well. Option (b) offers no hope and that may not be accurate. Option (c) is a misinterpretation of the client's statement and is not based on theory (Cook & Fontaine, 1991; pp. 60-64).

Nursing Process: Implementation
Client Need: Psychosocial Integrity

9. **The correct answer is b.** The first apgar score reveals a 6 based on scoring a 1 for heart rate as it is present but below 100. Respiratory effort is scored 1 as there are respirations but with effort as manifested in the form of nasal flaring. Muscle tone is scored as a 2 as the infant presents with a normal newborn positioning of elbows and hips flexed with knees positioned towards the abdomen. Reflex irritability is scored as 1 as only a weak grimace was noted. Skin color is scored as a 1 for the infant is not totally pink but has acrocyanosis which is present in approximately 85% of newborns at 1 minutes after birth. A score of less than 8 indicates that the infant is having problems with adjusting to extrauterine life and sustaining itself. Warming the infant (option a) would not be the only action since cold stress has not been assessed as a causative factor. The nurse would continue to apgar the infant at the five minute mark (option c) and continue to assess (option d) however, intervention may be necessary to save the infant (Ladewig, London, & Olds, 1990; pp. 437-440).

Nursing Process: Implementation
Client Need: Physiological Integrity

10. **The correct answer is c.** In chronic renal failure (CRF) there is a decreased production of erythropoietin by the kidneys causing impaired generation of erythrocytes or red blood cells by the bone marrow. Clients with CRF can be hypertensive so the use of a vasoconstrictor (option a) would not be appropriate. Corticosteroids (option b) and non-narcotic analgesics (option d) are not routinely given but may be administered for individual needs

(Smeltzer & Bare, 1992; p. 1127).

Nursing Process: Planning
Client Need: Physiological Integrity

11. **The correct answer is d.** An infant with a cleft lip and palate may be unable to create an effective vacuum by sucking because the deformity does not allow the mouth to fit snugly enough around the nipple or breast. Therefore, the formula will not be drawn into the mouth. A baby with cleft lip may be able to create a proper seal but a cleft palate usually means that sucking would be ineffective. The inability to suck because of the ineffective vacuum may cause frustration but should not damage the mother's breast (option a). Sucking should not cause further damage to the child (option b). In fact, as soon as the baby is able to suck, he should do so. Sucking is encouraged because it strengthens the muscles needed for proper speech. Sucking by itself will not cause infection (option c). After any feeding the mouth is cleansed with water to prevent infection (Marlow & Redding, 1988; pp. 498-499).

Nursing Process: Assessment
Client Need: Physiological Integrity

12. **The correct answer is a.** A change in the level of consciousness is the most significant variable indicating a deterioration of the neurological status. Pupils that are equal, between 2-6 mm and react briskly are considered normal. When the pupillary reaction becomes sluggish, this can indicate progression to unconsciousness. The nurse should note and chart the abnormality, but sluggish pupils are not an immediate concern

(option b). Motor weakness bilaterally can be the result of decreased muscle tone from cerebellar injury or brain stem involvement, or from difficulty following commands (option c). Disorientation and a decline in verbal response indicates a diminished level of consciousness (option d) (Ignatavicius & Bayne, 1991; p.928).

Nursing Process: Analysis
Client Need: Physiological Integrity

13. **The correct answer is d.** According to Carter & McGoldrick's family stages, families with adolescents have the task of redefining their boundaries so that adolescents can learn increasing levels of independence. Adjustment problems can be the result of rigid boundaries. Promoting full separation of the young adult from the parents (option a) is stage 1 when the young adult is unattached and between families. Commitment to new family members (option b) is the task of a family with young children. Maintaining contact with the custodial parent (option c) is a task of divorced families (Danielson, Hamel-Bissell & Winstead-Fry, 1993; pp. 6-7).

Nursing Process: Planning
Client Need: Health Promotion & Maintenance

14. **Step One:**
Total volume divided by the hours to infuse equals ml/hr.

$$\frac{1500\ ml}{12\ hour} = 125\ ml$$

Step Two:
$$\frac{total\ ml\ \ x\ \ drop\ factor}{minutes} = \frac{drops}{minute}$$

$$\frac{125\ ml\ \ x\ 60}{60\ minute} = 125\ gtts$$

(Weaver & Koehler, 1992; pp. 96-98)

Nursing Process: Implementation
Client Need: Physiological Integrity

15. **The correct answer is d.** The purpose of restraint and seclusion are to contain injurious actions; decrease, not increase (option a) sensory input; and reduce difficult interpersonal relationships. Options (b) and (c) imply that seclusion would be used to coerce or punish the client to behave in a certain way which would not be a therapeutic use of restraint or seclusion (Johnson, 1993; p. 511).

Nursing Process: Implementation
Client Need: Psychosocial Integrity

16. **The correct answer is d.** The client does not understand the medication for Parkinson's disease since there is no cure for the disease. A specific discussion with the client including the family would be beneficial to enhance learning. Therapeutic management is aimed at relieving the symptoms. Pharmacotherapy of Parkinson's disease is aimed at correcting an imbalance of neurotransmitters within the central nervous system characterized by dopamine deficiency and acetylcholine excess in the corpus striatum. Option

(a) is incorrect because the nurse can do the teaching and does not need to ask the physician to do it for her since it is within the nurse's scope of practice. Option (b) is incorrect because the client has misunderstood the teaching. Option (c) implies that the client made a correct statement and just continues the teaching without correcting the misinformation (Lewis & Collier, 1992; pp. 1599-1606).

Nursing Process: Planning
Client Need: Health Promotion & Maintenance

17. **The correct answer is b.** The pH shows acidosis. A low $PaCO_2$ produces alkalosis, so it is not the cause of the acidosis. The low HCO_3 indicates a metabolic acidosis. The hypoxemia is producing a lactic acidosis that causes lactate to bind with the bicarbonate (Black & Matassarin-Jacobs, 1993; pp. 302-310).

Nursing Process: Analysis
Client Need: Physiological Integrity

18. **The correct answer is b.** The nurse shares her observation of the client's behavior with the client to open the issue up for discussion. With this response, the nurse gently encourages the client to explore the meaning of his seductive behavior. Option (d) assumes the nurse already knows what the client is feeling when she has not gathered enough assessment data. Option (a) allows the client to avoid the therapeutic issue, as does option (c). Although it is true that the nurse-client relationship is not a social one, this response (option c) does not allow for exploration of the client's

feelings (Stuart & Sundeen, 1991; pp. 650-651).

Nursing Process: Implementation
Client Need: Health Promotion & Maintenance

19. **The correct answer is c.** Hyperparathyroidism is characterized by excess serum calcium and phosphate levels. This leads to formation of kidney stones therefore it is necessary to force fluids to not only decrease the stone formation but it also keeps the client from dehydrating, another sign of hyperparathyroidism. Chvostek's sign is used to assess spasms of the facial muscles caused by low levels of calcium (option a). A low calcium diet is indicated, not a high one (option b). Levothyroxine (Synthroid) is used for clients who have had a thyroidectomy or hypothyroidism (option d) (Black & Matassarin-Jacobs, 1993; pp. 1827-1835).

Nursing Process: Implementation
Client Need: Physiological Integrity

20. **The correct answer is d.** Accompanying the aide ensures that the client's immediate needs are met and that the aide performed his duties responsibly. Then the charge nurse would privately discuss the aide's behavior with him. Option (a), writing a note to the head nurse, may be necessary if the aide's behavior does not change after the charge nurse has dealt with the situation. Option (b), telling him firmly to go do it now, places you in a power struggle with the aide who may refuse or may take it out on the

client. Option (c), doing the assignment then asking the aide to check, would be inappropriate. This reinforces that the aide could wait to do his job and takes the charge nurse away from other duties (Marquis & Huston, 1992; pp. 220-222).

Nursing Process: Implementation
Client Need: Safe, Effective Care Environment

21. **The correct answer is c.** The drainage is purulent which could possibly mean an infection. Medical attention is needed for proper treatment. Cleansing a wound with hydrogen peroxide could possibly damage the tissues if not irrigated properly (option a). To advise a client to stop taking a prescribed medication (option b), or to increase or decrease a medication dosage (option d), is not within the scope of nursing practice (Ignatavicius & Bayne, 1991; pp. 2157-2163).

Nursing Process: Implementation
Client Need: Physiological Integrity

22. **The correct answer is a.** Disorientation, confusion, increased need for sleep, and anorexia accompanied by weight loss are all signs of depression. The nurse should act as soon as possible to foster proper assessment and treatment. There is no evidence to suggest that a rehabilitation hospital (option b) is indicated for this client since the underlying medical problem has not been identified. Family and friend visits (option c) often wane over time and continued contact helps decrease the incidence of depressive symptoms and encourages healing. Although the client is sleeping during the day there is no evidence to suggest night wakefulness. Clients with depression often sleep a great deal. Sedative medication to promote sleep (option d) would foster further depression (Lewis & Collier, 1992; p. 297).

Nursing Process: Implementation
Client Need: Psychosocial Integrity

23. **The correct answer is d.** Often clients with language barriers have already considered their need for interpreters in a foreign country and may have contacts or have ideas on how to reach an interpreter. Often, family and friends of a foreign client will be able to translate on some level as well. Pantomiming the questions using one descriptive word at a time is often helpful to get the idea across to the client. However, many people interpret raised voices (option a) as a sign of frustration or anger. Also, the assessment process will probably take longer due to the language barrier. Assessment should be done thoroughly with these clients to glean information which the client may not be able to tell the nurse (option b). The nurse should approach clients of another culture by being polite and formal (option c) to show respect (Swanson & Albrecht, 1993; pp. 387-388).

Nursing Process: Planning
Client Need: Physiological Integrity

24. **The correct answer is b.** A low sodium diet is recommended to control water retention associated with ascites. Sodium is the major cation in the extracellular fluid. Sodium is responsible for maintaining extracellular

osmolarity. The concentration of sodium in the extracellular fluid determines how and where water is transferred from body compartments. Sodium concentration influences the total solute concentration. Any alteration in extracellular fluid sodium concentration affects fluid volume and distribution of other electrolytes. Option (a) is a typical schedule of forcing fluids. Fluid restrictions are indicated for clients with ascites. Fluid restrictions are initiated when serum sodium levels decrease. The kidneys retain sodium and dilutional hyponatremia results from excessive fluid volume. Fluids may be restricted to 1500 ml per day or less. Eight ounces every two hours for twelve hours equals 2880 ml per day. Foods like lemon, vinegar, oregano and pepper (option c) are often used by clients to flavor food which should not be salted and are not contraindicated in these clients. Antacids (option d) may be given to treat gastrointestinal problems. Many antacids contain high levels of sodium. Clients should be warned to use low sodium antacids (Ignatavicius & Bayne, 1991; pp. 240, 1487; Phipps, Long, Woods & Cassmeyer, 1991; p. 1182).

Nursing Process: Implementation
Client Need: Health Promotion & Maintenance

25. **The correct answer is a.** Anorexia, nausea, vomiting, weakness, depression, dizziness, polyuria and weight loss should be reported to the physician because medication dosage may be insufficient for the client's lifestyle needs. Rapid weight gain, round face, edema, hypertension and low urine output (option b) may indicate excessive medication and should also be reported to the physician for possible dosage change. Tachycardia, abrupt headaches, heat intolerance and anxiety are signs of pheochromocytoma (option c). Dry skin, hoarse voice, bradycardia and weight gain are signs of hypothyroidism (option d). (Phipps, Long, Woods & Cassmeyer, 1991; pp. 1048, 1082-1083).

Nursing Process: Implementation
Client Need: Health Promotion & Maintenance

26. **The correct answer is c.** Clients with pelvic inflammatory disease (PID) should be taught good aseptic technique such as hand washing, proper disposal of perineal pads and avoidance of sexual contact while infected. Normally there is no surgery (option d) nor loss of body part (option a) related to PID. These may occur with other nursing problems related to a mastectomy or hysterectomy. Dysuria (option b) is often a sign of a sexually transmitted disease such as gonorrhea but not PID (Lewis & Collier, 1992; pp. 1391, 1408, 1433-1434).

Nursing Process: Analysis
Client Need: Physiological Integrity

27. **The correct answer is a.** The primary reason for turning and repositioning clients on mechanical ventilation is to mobilize and drain secretions. Secretions in the base of the lung are difficult to drain unless the client is frequently repositioned. Preventing skin breakdown and contractures are important but do not relate to the question (options b and d).

314

Repositioning does not ensure adequate ventilation (option c) (Lewis and Collier, 1992; pp. 626-647).

Nursing Process: Analysis
Client Need: Physiological Integrity

28. **The correct answer is c.** La belle indifference is characteristic of conversion disorders which usually involve the loss or alteration of a body function without physiological cause. Conversions are usually disruptive alterations such as blindness or paralysis. Individuals who experience conversions usually develop an attitude of a lack of concern for the seriousness of their symptoms (la belle indifference). Option (d) is the definition of somataform disorders. Option (b) is the definition of hypochondriasis. Option (a) is the definition of malingering (Johnson, 1993; p. 649).

Nursing Process: Analysis
Client Need: Psychosocial Integrity

29. **The correct answer is d.** Putting the affected arm and shoulder through range of motion (ROM) exercises several times daily will prevent ankylosis of the shoulder and thus decreases post-operative pain. Constant bubbling is normal when suction is added. This would indicate a leak of air in the system if there was no suction (option a). On expiration, the pressure in the client's chest increases and pushes the water in the drainage system down, while on inspiration the pressure in the chest is less and the water will rise slightly (option b). Kinking or looping of tubing can cause back pressure which defeats the purpose of the chest tube

(option c) (Smeltzer & Bare, 1992; p. 548).

Nursing Process: Implementation
Client Need: Physiological Integrity

30. **The correct answer is a.** Loose green stools are common because phototherapy increases bowel motility. Fluorescent lights should be placed 18 inches above the neonate (option b). The nurse would not see the baby's eyes open because a child receiving phototherapy wears eye patches to prevent damage to the retinas (option c). Phototherapy decreases the activity of the enzyme, lactase, that aids in the digestion of lactose. The build-up of lactic acid leads to a low pH stool and diarrhea that can cause dehydration. A lactose-free formula is indicated (option d) (Mott, Sperhac & James, 1990; pp. 1408, 1887).

Nursing Process: Implementation
Client Need: Physiological Integrity

PRACTICE SESSION: 15

Instructions:

Allow yourself 30 minutes to complete the following 30 practice questions. Use a timer to notify yourself when 30 minutes are over so that you are not constantly looking at your watch while completing the questions.

1. A 54 year old male is admitted to the surgical floor and is scheduled for perineal radical prostatectomy as a result of prostatic cancer. Because of the nursing diagnosis of knowledge deficit, which of the following is appropriate to include in his teaching plan?
   a. Post-operatively, sitting is preferable to standing and lying.
   b. Give information regarding the future penile prostheses.
   c. Urinary dribbling will gradually diminish, but after a month no further improvement should be expected.
   d. Once he has returned home there is no need to avoid alcohol or coffee.

2. A 75 year old female is being discharged from the hospital after four weeks of rehabilitation from a hip fracture. The nurse's assessment prior to discharge teaching would be directed towards:
   a. ability to perform self-care activities.
   b. presence of hazards at home.
   c. toilet facilities.
   d. housekeeping activity abilities.

3. A female client at 10 weeks gestation is admitted for continued nausea and vomiting for the past three days. Medical diagnosis is hyperemesis gravidarum. The nurse would plan which actions for the client's initial care plan?
   a. Force fluids, vital signs every 2 hours.
   b. Monitor intake and output, serve 6 small meals throughout the day.
   c. Suction as needed, provide emotional support.
   d. Assess amount and character of emesis, monitor fetal heart rate.

4. A client who is being seen by a nurse in an outpatient mental health clinic states, "I don't know if I need to be here. Am I going crazy or does everyone get this nervous and anxious?" The nurse bases her response to the client on her understanding of distinguishing normal anxiety from anxiety disorders. In anxiety disorders:
   a. the symptoms can interfere with activities of daily living.
   b. the client experiences severe anxiety most of the time.
   c. symptoms can not be treated successfully without medications.
   d. normal coping is effective in relieving the discomfort.

5. Heather, a seven year old, is admitted to the pediatric unit following an acute asthma attack. Heather's primary nurse is completing a care plan with the diagnosis of impaired gas exchange related to ventilation perfusion imbalance. Which of the following implementations would be most appropriate for this care plan?
   a. Place Heather in a cool mist tent.
   b. Encourage increased fluid intake.
   c. Administer theophylline (Aminophylline) as ordered.
   d. Allow Heather to act out her feelings with a doll.

6. Ms. Mendez R.N. is the charge nurse on the evening shift. She notices that Ms. Caldwell comes back 30 minutes late from dinner the past two days. This evening Ms. Caldwell is again late. Ms. Mendez asks the other nurses accompanying Ms. Caldwell to dinner where she is. They say she is in the bathroom. Ms. Caldwell comes back 30 minutes late again. The initial action of Ms. Mendez should be to:
   a. call the supervisor for assistance in making a written report.
   b. say nothing but report it to the head nurse the next day.
   c. ask staff to watch Ms. Caldwell to see if the pattern continues.
   d. tell your observations to Ms. Caldwell and ask what is happening.

7. A client undergoes surgery with spinal anesthesia and complains of a headache. Which of these actions should the nurse take?
   a. Begin intravenous pressors.
   b. Maintain hydration.
   c. Monitor vital signs.
   d. Administer oxygen.

8. The nurse is taking care of a client who is having a closed (percutaneous) renal biopsy. Following the procedure the nurse would place the client in which position?
   a. Right side with a pillow against the abdomen.
   b. Flat supine with a pressure dressing.
   c. Prone position over a sandbag for support.
   d. Prone position with a pressure dressing and a soft pillow.

9. A 19 year old female client is given a diagnosis of acute myelogenous leukemia. Her care plan should include which of the following?
   a. Tell her she can continue to play basketball but more carefully.
   b. Caution her against straining with stool.
   c. Teach her that a normal white count is between 1,000 - 3,000.
   d. Instruct her to eat foods high in calcium and low in protein.

10. The nurse is caring for a client who has just been diagnosed with lung cancer of the oat cell type. The client jokingly asks the nurse for a "little black bottle to end this". The nurse should document which of the following?
    a. The client is using humor appropriately to deal with the new diagnosis and its prognosis.
    b. The client is in the bargaining stage of grief and is trying to bargain with the nurse.
    c. The client is having difficulty dealing with the new diagnosis and is contemplating suicide.
    d. The client needs some health teaching concerning the diagnosis and various treatment options.

11. David, a three year old, is about to be discharged from the same day surgery unit following a hypospadias repair. The nurse knows that David's father needs further teaching when he states:
    a. "He'll soak in the bathtub at least twice per day."
    b. "I'll buy his favorite juice so he will want to drink more."
    c. "I'll make sure his swimming suit is not too tight."
    d. "He won't be able to ride his tricycle for another week."

Situation:
Mrs. Pamela Douglas, 38 years old, is brought to the emergency room complaining of severe vomiting and diarrhea accompanied by fever. After further assessment the physician believes Mrs. Douglas is infected with salmonella. (The next two questions refer to this situation.)

12. Which of the following assessment data would support the diagnosis?
    a. Greenish stools with blood.
    b. Fever of 104°F (40°C).
    c. Eating egg salad at a picnic that day.
    d. Recent meal with shrimp.

13. The appropriate nursing care would be:
    a. universal precautions during the acute phase.
    b. force oral fluids to 3,000 ml per day.
    c. ambulation as soon as possible.
    d. low residue, bland diet.

14. A 42 year old mother of two has recently been diagnosed with cancer of the breast with widespread metastasis. The recommendation after surgery is chemotherapy. Due to poor venous access a subcutaneous port will be implanted for future intravenous treatments. Which of the following responses from the client shows an understanding of vascular access devices?
    a. "I will check daily for signs of infection."
    b. "I will do heparin sodium (Heparin) flushes weekly as instructed."
    c. "I understand my blood samples can not be drawn from the catheter."
    d. "I will have a permanent mark on my skin to help with location of the port."

15. A client is admitted with a medical diagnoses of bronchiectasis. The nurse recognizes that the client understands his discharge teaching when he verbalizes which significant manifestations to be reported to the health care provider?
    a. Dry cough, rib pain.
    b. Loss of appetite, fatigue.
    c. Increased sputum, fever.
    d. Nausea, dizziness.

16. Lori Fleming, 19 years old, comes to the emergency room alone. She tearfully tells the nurse she has been raped by her boyfriend and is afraid to go home and tell her parents. She says, "I should have listened to my father. He never liked that guy." The nurse analyzes this statement as:
    a. an attempt to find some control over the situation.
    b. a way to blame her father for the rape incident.
    c. an opportunity to be independent from her parents.
    d. a type of secondary victimization.

17. A female neonate is brought to the newborn nursery following an uncomplicated delivery. The neonate is diagnosed as having fetal alcohol syndrome (FAS). Nursing care would include which of the following?
    a. Place the neonate under phototherapy lights.
    b. Assess vital signs every hour for the first 48 hours.
    c. Give phenobarbital 15 mg twice per day as ordered.
    d. Offer the neonate two ounces of formula every hour.

18. The home health nurse has been visiting a 62 year old quadriplegic at home on mechanical ventilation. The client has tube feedings by nasogastric tube at 100 ml per hour. The family states the gastric residuals have been 20 to 50 ml per hour every two hours. The nurse suctions the client's tracheostomy and obtains large amounts of yellow thick creamy secretions. The nurse's initial action would be to:
   a. obtain a sputum sample for culture and sensitivity.
   b. stop the feedings and check nasogastric placement.
   c. continue suctioning secretions and tell the family you will stop more frequently to suction.
   d. call the physician for mechanical ventilation adjustment orders.

19. A primary role of the school health nurse is to assist with:
   a. project Head Start.
   b. nutritional counseling program for women, infants and children (WIC).
   c. enrolling underserved children in Medicaid services.
   d. health related curriculum development.

20. A 47 year old male client in the manic phase of bipolar disorder is verbally abusive to staff and other clients. The nurse decides to intervene during the next incident of verbal abuse. The most therapeutic response to this client's behavior would be:
   a. "Let's sit down and discuss your feelings of hostility."
   b. "If you continue abusing others you will have quiet time in open seclusion for 30 minutes."
   c. "Your behavior is inappropriate and will not be tolerated. Stop it immediately or you will be placed in seclusion."
   d. "I can understand that you are upset, but please try to consider other people's feelings."

21. A 52 year old female client has been diagnosed with multiple myeloma. She was admitted for possible hypercalcemia. Which of the following signs and symptoms are indicative of hypercalcemia?
   a. Excitability and paresthesia.
   b. Bone pain and positive Chvostek's sign.
   c. Constipation and weakness.
   d. Serum calcium 9.8 mg/dl.

22. It is suspected that Jessica, a five year old, has oxyuriasis (pinworms). Which of the following would the nurse teach Jessica's parents to do to confirm diagnosis?
   a. Observe Jessica for rectal itching.
   b. Place a piece of cellophane tape to her perianal region at night.
   c. Launder all the family's clothes and linens in hot, soapy water.
   d. Report any bloody stools to the physician immediately.

23. A client falls off a ladder and fractures several ribs. Pain is severe and the physician performs intercostal nerve blocks. The nurse knows the treatment is effective when:
   a. breath sounds are normal bilaterally.
   b. temperature returns to normal.
   c. heart rate is 80 to 100 beats per minute.
   d. the client takes deep breaths.

24. A 25 year old female client has the following intravenous fluid ordered for her by the physician: 1000 ml D_5 with 20 mEq KCl over six hours times four bags. Drop factor is 15 drops per ml. The correct flow rate for the intravenous fluid would be:
   a. 28 drops per minute.
   b. 21 drops per minute.
   c. 56 drops per minute.
   d. 42 drops per minute.

25. A 16 year old male is admitted to the emergency department following a motorcycle accident with a large sucking chest wound. Which of the following initial actions would be appropriate for the nurse to take?
   a. Prepare the client for insertion of a chest tube.
   b. Block the chest wound with a sterile towel.
   c. Insert a large bore needle into the 6th intercostal space.
   d. Auscultate over both lung fields to determine whether he is exchanging air.

26. A client on intravenous solution at a slow rate has suddenly developed fever, nausea, vomiting and headache. After calling the physician the nurse should prepare to:
   a. stop the intravenous infusion and draw blood cultures.
   b. increase the rate of fluid infusion.
   c. restart the intravenous since it is probably infiltrated.
   d. place the intravenous on an infusion pump.

27. Mrs. Audrey Davis, 68 years old, has been taking diltiazem hydrochloride (Cardizem) for her angina. The nurse would need to use caution in administering which of the following drug orders?
   a. Acetosalicylic acid (Aspirin).
   b. Lanoxin (Digoxin).
   c. Vitamin B complex.
   d. Acetaminophen (Tylenol).

28. The nurse evaluates the effectiveness of mannitol (Osmitrol) therapy in a client by which physiologic response?
   a. Bilateral dilated pupils.
   b. Intracranial pressure 8 mm Hg.
   c. Widened pulse pressure.
   d. Heart rate 58 beats per minute.

29. A 30 year old female client is admitted to the neurosurgical floor following transphenoidal craniotomy for removal of a pituitary tumor. Two hours after her arrival, which of the following findings discovered by the nurse should be reported to the physician immediately?
   a. Complaint of mouth and nose pain.
   b. Urine specific gravity 1.005, serum sodium 150.
   c. Large amount of bloody drainage on nasal drip pad.
   d. Inability to breathe through the nose.

30. A 21 year old male client is admitted to the neurosurgical unit with a subarachnoid hemorrhage from a cerebral aneurysm. At the time of admission he is sleepy but has no real focal deficits. He is placed on bedrest and subarachnoid precautions. When the nurse walks into the room the client is agitated, attempting to get out of bed and states, "I am getting out of bed, I can't go this way". Which of these actions should the nurse take?
   a. Say to the client in a calm manner, "I know this is difficult but let me explain to you why it is so important that you stay in bed."
   b. Administer the 1 mg midazolam hydrochloride (Versed) IV PRN agitation that is ordered.
   c. Help him to stand at the side of the bed to void.
   d. Call the physician and report a change in level of consciousness.

STOP You have now completed Practice Session: 15. Now take a few minutes and correct your answers. Calculate your accuracy rate by dividing the number of questions you completed correctly by the total number of questions you completed (30).

Correct answers ÷ total number of questions completed = accuracy rate.

_____ ÷ _____ = _____

ANSWERS AND RATIONALES

1. **The correct answer is b.** After total prostatectomy, impotence is almost always expected and the client should be encouraged to talk about it. In the post-operative period, sitting is discouraged (option a) since it increases abdominal pressure. Urinary dribbling (option c) will continue to improve for about a year. Coffee, alcohol (option d) and spicy foods may cause discomfort (Smeltzer & Bare, 1992; pp. 1329-1330).

   Nursing Process: Planning
   Client Need: Physiological Integrity

2. **The correct answer is b.** A goal for prevention and management of falls focus on reducing environmental hazards. Increased independence and mobility may be important and valuable factors to decrease the risk of falling but are not the priority (options a, c and d) (Carpenito, 1992; pp.525-549).

   Nursing Process: Assessment
   Client Need: Health Promotion & Maintenance

3. **The correct answer is d.** Continue to assess and quantify all emesis and any other output and intake as hyperemesis may lead to dehydration which leads to fluid and electrolyte imbalance. The client may deteriorate and starvation may set in. This causes severe protein and vitamin deficiencies which may cause metabolic changes to both fetus and mother resulting in irreversible changes and/or death. Vital signs may be taken every 2 hours. However, most clients are allowed nothing by mouth when first admitted (option a). Option (b) is incorrect as the client was just admitted and will be allowed nothing by mouth until her electrolytes are within normal limits. Then, the client will progress to small frequent meals as tolerated. Option (c) is incorrect as suctioning is not pertinent since the client is conscious. Emotional support will be needed (Ladewig, London, and Olds, 1990; p. 302).

   Nursing Process: Planning
   Client Need: Physiological Integrity

4. **The correct answer is a.** The experience of anxiety is a natural part of every human life. However, when the anxiety is so pervasive that it begins to interfere with daily existence, an anxiety disorder is present. Option (b) is incorrect because the degree of anxiety varies from person to person and can be at different levels throughout the day. Medication is not always needed for the treatment of anxiety disorders (option c) and behavior patterns used to cope with anxiety disorders are usually maladaptive (option d) (Johnson, 1993; p. 406).

   Nursing Process: Analysis
   Client Need: Physiological Integrity

5. **The correct answer is c.** Asthma attacks are caused by bronchospasm and narrowed airways. Theophylline (Aminophylline) is a bronchodilator that works by relaxing the smooth muscles of the bronchi and pulmonary blood vessels, thus improving gas exchange. Mist tents loosen secretions by providing a high humidity environment but do not lessen bronchospasm (option a). Increased fluid intake also loosens secretions but does nothing to relax smooth muscles (option b). Very often children with asthma are encouraged to work out their feelings with dolls to decrease their anxiety, although this is not the priority in this situation. The theophylline (Aminophylline) will work much faster to open the airway (option d) (Mott, Sperhac & James, 1990; pp. 1022-1037).

   Nursing Process: Planning
   Client Need: Physiological Integrity

6. **The correct answer is d.** Before any action is taken, a full assessment of the situation must be obtained. Although the nurse may be guessing at reasons for being off the unit for so long, Mrs. Caldwell is the person who knows. Asking questions by making observation and showing concern will assist Mrs. Caldwell to make an informed analysis and dictate action. Options (a) and (b) take action without obtaining the facts and are incorrect. Option (c) is a breach of confidentiality (Tappen, 1989; p. 71).

   Nursing Process: Implementation
   Client Need: Safe, Effective Care Environment

7. **The correct answer is b.** Two major complications of spinal anesthesia are hypotension due to blockage of sympathetic nerves and headache from lower cerebral spinal pressure which is the result of leakage of cerebral spinal fluid into the epidural space. Maintaining hydration will increase production of cerebral spinal fluid raising cerebral spinal pressure. Monitoring vital signs (option c), beginning intravenous pressors (option a), and administering oxygen (option d) are measures taken in the treatment of hypotension (Ignatavicius & Bayne, 1991; p. 465).

   Nursing Process: Implementation
   Client Need: Physiological Integrity

8. **The correct answer is b.** After a percutaneous or closed renal biopsy, pressure is placed on the biopsy site for approximately twenty minutes and a pressure dressing is applied. The client is then placed in a supine position and instructed to stay flat without moving for at least four hours thus placing pressure on the biopsy site and preventing hemorrhage, a potential complication. Bedrest is then ordered for 24 hours. Clients are placed on the right side with a pillow after a liver biopsy (option a). The client is placed in a prone position with a sandbag and soft pillow for support while the biopsy is taking place (options c and d) (Phipps, Long, Woods & Cassmeyer, 1991; pp. 1148-1149, 1401-1402).

   Nursing Process: Implementation
   Client Need: Safe, Effective Care Environment

9. **The correct answer is b.** Straining during a bowel movement causes increased intracranial pressure which increases risk for hemorrhage. A client with acute myelogenous leukemia is at higher risk for infection, bleeding and activity intolerance secondary to neutropenia, thrombocytopenia, and anemia. Contact sports should be avoided because of the risk of hemorrhage (option a). A normal white count is between 5,000-10,000 (option c). Protein intake should be encouraged to foster red blood cell maturation. Increased fluids are encouraged (option d) (Smeltzer & Bare, 1992; pp. 783, 802-803).

Nursing Process: Planning
Client Need: Physiological Integrity

10. **The correct answer is c.** The client has been diagnosed with a potentially lethal condition with a poor prognosis since oat cell cancer has a poor treatment record. The client also states a desire to "end this" which points to hopelessness and asks the nurse for a "little black bottle" with which to do it. These factors lead to a nursing diagnosis of potential for violence: self-directed or suicide. The nurse should then assess the client further and chart that the client has expressed thoughts of suicide. Precautions should be taken such as informing the physician and other nursing staff and instituting an observation schedule to ensure the safety of the client. Health teaching may need to be done (option d) but the client's safety is the priority. Bargaining is a stage of the grief process (option b) but usually involves a request in exchange for something else (e.g., "I'll give all my money to the poor if God lets me be cured."). The client is using some humor to deal with the anxiety of asking the nurse for a way "to end this" which is inappropriate (option a) (Cook & Fontaine, 1991; pp. 218, 610-613).

Nursing Process: Analysis
Client Need: Physiological Integrity

11. **The correct answer is c.** Hypospadias is a condition in which the urethral opening is located on the ventral surface of the penis. While loose fitting clothing is important to prevent trauma, swimming is contraindicated until a follow-up visit to the surgeon. Two baths a day as well as increased fluids are recommended for irrigation and to promote wound healing (options a and b). Straddle toys are avoided to prevent trauma to the area (option d). (Whaley & Wong, 1991; pp. 512-513).

Nursing Process: Evaluation
Client Need: Physiological Integrity

12. **The correct answer is c.** Salmonella is a gram-negative bacteria which is found in contaminated foods. Symptoms such as enteritis, vomiting, diarrhea, dehydration, and fever occur within several hours of eating the food. Greenish stools with varying amounts of blood (option a) is characteristic of a shigella infection. Fever of 104°F (40°C) (option b) may be found in typhoid fever. Salmonellosis produces a low grade fever. Eating shrimp (option d) may produce problems with shigellosis or hepatitis A (Smeltzer & Bare, 1992; pp. 1928-1931).

Nursing Process: Analysis
Client Need: Physiological Integrity

13. **The correct answer is a.** Salmonella is a bacterial infection that is transmitted through contaminated food with the entry port being the mouth. Universal precautions and medical asepsis are necessary to keep others from becoming contaminated. The client should take nothing by mouth until abdominal pain subsides, then have liquids as tolerated (options b and d). The client should remain at rest until symptoms subside (option c) (Smeltzer & Bare, 1992; p. 1930).

Nursing Process: Implementation
Client Need: Physiological Integrity

14. **The correct answer is a.** Since the port is a foreign body that was surgically implanted, the client should be taught to look for signs of infection. Implanted ports require heparin flushes every 21 to 28 days (option b) to prevent occlusion and these are usually performed by a health professional. Flushing is also done after any procedures such as drawing blood (option c) or infusion. Ports are easily palpable (option d) so marking is not necessary (Smeltzer & Bare, 1992; p. 357).

Nursing Process: Evaluation
Client Need: Physiological Integrity

15. **The correct answer is c.** Early detection and treatment of lower respiratory track infections prevent them from developing into complications. Clinical manifestations to be reported include increased sputum production, grossly bloody sputum, increasing dyspnea, fever, chills, and chest pain (options a, b and d) (Lewis & Collier, 1992; pp. 519-521).

Nursing Process: Evaluation
Client Need: Health Promotion & Maintenance

16. **The correct answer is a.** Victims of rape often review their situations to find a way of avoiding rapes in the future. This process assists them to gain a sense of control over their lives through problem-solving rather than feelings of helplessness and injustice. There is no evidence to support that she believes her father is at fault (option b), rather that she can rely on him for input. The client has not expressed a need for independence (option c) but rather a fear of going home because of her father's reaction to the rape since reactions of family members to rape often include blaming the victim. Secondary victimization (option d) occurs when nurses and the client's significant others react with disgust and inability to be supportive which further victimizes the client (Varcarolis, 1990; pp. 276-278).

Nursing Process: Analysis
Client Need: Psychosocial Integrity

17. **The correct answer is c.** Children born with fetal alcohol syndrome (FAS) are frequently irritable and display seizure activity. They are managed by preventing excessive stimulation and providing anticonvulsant therapy. Phototherapy (option a) is used for children who have physiologic jaundice. Assessing vital signs every hour (option b) is unnecessary and only increases agitation in the already irritable infant. Although children with FAS are poor feeders, offering a bottle every hour (option d) will not improve the poor sucking. This will only make them

more tired (Whaley & Wong, 1991; pp. 523-524).

Nursing Process: Implementation
Client Need: Physiological Integrity

18. **The correct answer is b.** The thick creamy secretions are indicative that the client has aspirated the feedings. Initial intervention would be to turn off the feedings and check the naso-gastric tube for possible dislodgement. Obtaining a sputum sample would be beneficial, but not an initial action (option a). Telling the family you would stop more frequently to suction does not aid the situation and is inappropriate (option c). Mechanical ventilation adjustment would possibly be needed after analysis of arterial blood gases (option d) (Lewis & Collier, 1992; pp. 643-645).

Nursing Process: Implementation
Client Need: Safe, Effective Care Environment

19. **The correct answer is d.** The school nurse may provide assistance with choosing and/or developing health related curriculum. The nurse may make referrals to Head Start (educational and medical services to low income families with children ages 3 to 5 years) or women, infants and children (WIC) program (food supplement and nutrition teaching) but does not necessarily carry a primary role in these programs (options a and b). Not all underserved children are eligible for Medicaid (option c) so referral may be inappropriate and discourage the families from taking advantage of assistance to which they are entitled (Swanson & Albrecht, 1993; pp. 219-223).

Nursing Process: Implementation
Client Need: Health Promotion & Maintenance

20. **The correct answer is b.** The nurse must set limits on manipulative and acting out behaviors and explain the consequences if these limits are tested. At this point the client is frightened about losing control and needs the nurse to control and structure the environment for him. The client is not able to respond to options (a) and (d) because of this. Option (d) also implies that his behavior is understandable and may be interpreted by the client as acceptable. Option (c) is a punitive response that also lacks the specifics and detail needed to care for this client (Townsend, 1993; pp. 372-373).

Nursing Process: Implementation
Client Need: Psychosocial Integrity

21. **The correct answer is c.** Hypercalcemia is seen in cancer when the bones release large stores of calcium. Symptoms of it include weakness and constipation. A normal serum calcium is 8.5-10.5 mg/dl (option d). Excitability, paresthesia (option a) and positive Chvostek's sign (option b) are all symptoms of hypocalcemia (Smeltzer & Bare, 1992; p. 380).

Nursing Process: Analysis
Client Need: Physiological Integrity

22. **The correct answer is b.** The tape is examined for the presence of eggs in the morning. Rectal itching is a symptom of pinworms, however, it is not diagnostic of pinworms (option a). Hot water laundering is required after a diagnosis

is made (option c). Bloody stools are not seen in pinworm infestation (option d) (Mott, Sperhac & James, 1990; pp. 781-782).

Nursing Process: Implementation
Client Need: Physiological Integrity

23. **The correct answer is d.** Rib fractures are painful and clients tend to take short shallow breaths to lessen the pain. Lung expansion is necessary to prevent atelectasis and infection. Nerve blocks may be used to decrease the pain so clients will breathe correctly and promote proper lung expansion. Binding ribs and narcotic medications are generally contraindicated in rib fractures since they will also interfere with lung expansion. Breath sounds should remain normal bilaterally in a rib fracture (option a) unless the rib has penetrated a lung. Nerve blocks are unrelated to temperature. A low grade fever may be present due to damage (option b). Heart rate (option c) is unrelated to nerve block. Pulse may return to normal after a nerve block because pain is relieved but this is not the primary reason for the procedure (Lewis & Collier, 1992; p. 543).

Nursing Process: Evaluation
Client Need: Physiological Integrity

24. **The correct answer is d.** The flow rate is calculated as follows:

$$\frac{\text{volume of infusion (ml)}}{\text{time of infusion (minutes)}} \times \frac{\text{drop factor}}{\text{(drops/ml)}} =$$

$$= \text{drops/minutes}$$

$$\frac{1000 \text{ ml}}{360 \text{ min}} \times \frac{15 \text{ drops}}{\text{ml}} = \frac{15000 \text{ ml}}{1360 \text{ min}} =$$

$$= 41.66 \text{ or } \frac{42 \text{ drops}}{\text{min}}$$

(D'Angelo & Welsh, 1988; p. 182)

Nursing Process: Planning
Client Need: Physiological Integrity

25. **The correct answer is b.** Open pneumothorax calls for emergency measures and the first priority is to stop the flow of air into the chest through the hole. In this emergency, anything that can block the flow of air should be used. As air enters there is a shift of the heart, vessels, and other lung leading to circulatory and respiratory collapse. While a chest tube will be inserted, the first priority is to stop the flow of air (option a). A large bore needle is used to convert a tension pneumothorax to a simple pneumothorax (option c). Auscultation is not a top priority because the client will soon arrest if this flow of air is not stopped (option d) (Smeltzer & Bare, 1992; p. 597).

Nursing Process: Implementation
Client Need: Safe, Effective Care Environment

26. **The correct answer is a.** Fever, nausea, vomiting and headache of sudden onset are often signs of sepsis related to the intravenous catheter. Other symptoms include chills, increased pulse, lethargy and backache. When this occurs the infusion should be discontinued and blood cultures requested of the physician. Increasing fluid rate (option b) would not help unless the infected catheter is removed. Signs of infiltration (option c) include redness and swelling at the intravenous catheter insertion site rather than a systemic reaction. An infusion pump (option d) does not address the infectious process (Smith & Duell, 1993; p. 727).

Nursing Process: Implementation
Client Need: Safe, Effective Care Environment

27. **The correct answer is b.** Calcium channel blockers like diltiazem hydrochloride (Cardizem) alter contractility of the heart muscle by blocking the flow of calcium into the cell during depolarization. Lanoxin (Digoxin) promotes calcium movement from extracellular to intracellular cytoplasm. The lanoxin (Digoxin) is stored in body tissues especially myocardium and lean body mass. Serum levels of lanoxin (Digoxin) may increase leading to nausea, vomiting and bradycardia. The other medications do not adversely affect diltiazem hydrochloride (Cardizem) (options a, c and d) (Baer & Williams, 1992; pp. 329-330, 333, 528, 530, 787).

Nursing Process: Planning
Client Need: Physiological Integrity

28. **The correct answer is b.** Mannitol's (Osmitrol) effect as an osmotic diuretic is to pull water from the cells to the extracellular fluid and from red blood cells to plasma. A dilution of extracellular sodium is achieved by increasing plasma volume, extracellular volume and circulation time. Mannitol (Osmitrol) is indicated to treat increased intracranial pressure associated with cerebral edema, brain stem compression or herniation. A reduction in intracranial pressure occurs within 15 minutes of administration. Bilateral dilated pupils (option a) are indicative of tentorial herniation associated with increased intracranial pressure. The oculomotor nerve is compressed by the herniating tissue resulting in pupil dilation. Mannitol's (Osmitrol) effect is to decrease intracranial pressure; therefore, decreasing the incidence of herniation. A widened pulse pressure and bradycardia (options c and d) are characteristic of the Cushing's reflex. Both are indicative of impaired autoregulation associated with increased intracranial pressure. Elevation of systolic blood pressure, widened pulse pressure and bradycardia are compensatory mechanisms triggered by ischemia in the vasomotor center in the brainstem (Ignatavicius & Bayne, 1991; pp. 928, 931; Phipps, Long, Woods & Cassmeyer, 1991; p. 1796).

Nursing Process: Evaluation
Client Need: Physiological Integrity

29. **The correct answer is b.** One complication of removal of parts of the pituitary is diabetes insipidus. This is caused by a deficiency in antidiuretic

hormone (ADH). When this is deficient, large volumes of dilute urine (specific gravity < 1.010) are produced. The client loses free water but not electrolytes so hypernatremia and hyperkalemia result. Complaints of mouth and nose pain are normal with this (option a) approach. Nasal packing (option c) is in place with a small drip pad and it is not unusual for the drip pad to get soaked through with bloody drainage several times. Nasal packing causes inability to breathe through the nose (option d) (Smeltzer & Bare, 1992; p. 1106).

Nursing Process: Analysis
Client Need: Safe, Effective Care Environment

30. **The correct answer is b.** Midazolam hydrochloride (Versed) is a benzodiazepine and will provide rapid reduction in anxiety when given intravenously. The goal for this client is to prevent rupture of the aneurysm. When a client is agitated, he has elevated intracranial pressure, thus all measures must be taken to keep him calm and quiet. While it is necessary to explain to him why bedrest is important (option a) this should have been done earlier, and will take too long to produce results. Subarachnoid precautions include strict, absolute bedrest and avoidance of the valsalva maneuver so he should not be helped out of bed (option c). The physician should be informed after action is taken that the client was agitated and sedated; however, this does not necessarily indicate a change in level of consciousness since the client was not cooperative to begin with (option d)

(Smeltzer, & Bare, 1992; p. 1705).

Nursing Process: Implementation
Client Need: Safe, Effective Care Environment

PRACTICE SESSION: 16

Instructions:

Allow yourself 30 minutes to complete the following 30 practice questions. Use a timer to notify yourself when 30 minutes are over so that you are not constantly looking at your watch while completing the questions.

1. The nurse has given a narcotic intravenously to a post-operative client. What instructions should be given to the nurse aide?
   a. "Keep the head of bed elevated 30 degrees and notify the nurse of depressed respiration and drowsiness."
   b. "Avoid giving fluids orally to prevent aspiration."
   c. "Assist client to the bathroom and monitor urine output."
   d. "Check blood pressure every 15 minutes and notify the nurse of a blood pressure below 100."

2. A 30 year old female client has delivered a baby girl who is small for gestational age. Fourteen hours after birth, the nurse assesses that the infant developed jaundice. The next action of the nurse would be to:
   a. begin phototherapy.
   b. monitor the infant's condition.
   c. prepare to draw a serum bilirubin.
   d. notify the physician.

3. Six days ago a 54 year old client was diagnosed with a tumor of the small intestines and had an ileostomy performed. Presently his ileostomy is draining 1800 ml per day of liquid stool. The nurse would assess for:
   a. metabolic alkalosis.
   b. hypernatremia.
   c. metabolic acidosis.
   d. hyperkalemia.

4. Following a thyroidectomy, the client complains of painful muscle spasms and numbness of the hands. Based on these findings, the nurse should suspect the client has:
   a. hypokalemia.
   b. tetany.
   c. hyperthyroidism.
   d. hypercalcemia.

5. Joey, a 9 year old fourth grader, is sent to the school nurse because he is unable to stay awake during class. Despite two telephone calls to Joey's father by his teacher, Joey continues to come to school without his homework done and no lunch. He is also made fun of by his peers because he sucks his thumb and usually has an unkempt appearance. Which of the following actions should the nurse do first?
   a. Ask Joey if he is able to sleep at night.
   b. File a suspected child abuse and neglect report with the authorities.
   c. Call Joey's parents to complete an accurate history.
   d. Examine Joey for signs of physical abuse.

6. A client with chronic renal failure is ordered a low potassium diet. The nurse evaluates that the teaching was ineffective when the client chooses which meal?
   a. Spaghetti with sauce, apple.
   b. Lamb, green bean, peaches.
   c. Pork chop, beets, apricots.
   d. Turkey, peas, plum.

7. A client has delivered a baby two days ago. The nurse notices the client holding the baby and asking questions regarding care. This behavior indicates that the client:
   a. probably attended prenatal classes.
   b. has not understood the discharge teaching.
   c. should be referred for home care follow-up.
   d. is bonding with the infant.

8. A female client is being seen at an outpatient mental health clinic. Her physician starts her on amitriptyline (Elavil). Two days later the client calls the mental health clinic in tears, "It's no use, the medicine isn't helping, nothing is going to help me." The most appropriate response by the nurse would be:
   a. "Often it takes antidepressants three to four weeks to be fully effective."
   b. "I'll call the physician and report this; he may want to increase your dose."
   c. "It sounds like you are really suicidal; perhaps we should schedule an emergency visit."
   d. "This drug may not be appropriate for you; but let's wait a little longer before deciding."

9. The physician orders tobramycin (Nebcin) 30 mg intravenously T.I.D.. A peak level of tobramycin (Nebcin) needs to be drawn this morning on the client. The nurse would draw the blood specimen:
   a. midway between one dose and the other.
   b. immediately before giving the next dose of medication.
   c. immediately after giving the medication.
   d. thirty minutes after the medication infuses.

10. A 62 year old male is admitted to the hospital with a suspected abdominal aortic aneurysm (AAA). The nurse obtains all of the following data during the assessment. Which data should be reported to the physician?
    a. A systolic blood pressure of 150 mm Hg in the arm and 165 mm Hg in the thigh.
    b. A systolic blood pressure of 150 mm Hg in the arm and 120 mm Hg in the thigh.
    c. Client complaint of low back pain.
    d. Client complaint of abdominal throbbing.

11. A client complaining of anorexia, weight loss, weakness, irritability and polyuria is admitted to the hospital. Bloodwork shows an elevated calcium and a low phosphate. The client is diagnosed with hyperparathyroidism. What other assessment data would be necessary on this client?
    a. Activity intolerance.
    b. Hearing.
    c. Hirsutism.
    d. Urine glucose.

12. Julie, a 17 year old senior in high school, stops in to see the school nurse because she has been losing clumps of hair. The nurse notes a butterfly rash over Julie's nose and cheeks. The nurse suspects systemic lupus erythematous (SLE) and sends her to her family physician for further diagnostic evaluation. Which of the following parts of Julie's history would predispose her to SLE?

   a. Sunbathes for two hours after school each day.

   b. Has a fraternal twin.

   c. Drinks a six-pack of beer when out with friends on the weekend.

   d. Admits to a high fat diet.

13. In caring for a post-operative client in the recovery room, the nurse observes his respirations are shallow and irregular, and his lips cyanotic. The client is receiving 4L O_2 per nasal cannula. The initial action of the nurse should be to:

   a. encourage coughing and deep breathing.

   b. place the client in low semi-Fowler's position.

   c. reposition the head and neck to proper alignment.

   d. suction mucus from mouth and pharynx.

14. A client is admitted with a history of bloody stools for three days. Vital signs are: blood pressure, 100/50 mm Hg; pulse, 112 beats per minute; respirations, 24 per minute. Hemoglobin is 10 gm/dl and hematocrit is 32 gm/dl. Arterial blood gases on room air are: pH, 7.72; $PaCO_2$, 82 mm Hg. The most effective way to increase oxygen delivery to the tissues would be to:

   a. apply 6 liters nasal cannula oxygen.

   b. administer packed red blood cells.

   c. place the client in Trendelenburg position.

   d. sedate the client.

15. A 68 year old male is admitted to the surgical floor following a Whipple procedure for pancreatic cancer. He has a nasogastric tube to low intermittent suction and a T-tube to gravity drainage. Which of the following should be included in his care plan?

   a. Explain to the client that steatorrhea and diarrhea will now be normal.

   b. Explain to the client that since his pancreas has been removed he will need insulin injections.

   c. Apply paste or gel around the T-tube site.

   d. Realize he will need smaller doses of narcotics than most clients.

16. Kelly, a newborn, is brought to the emergency department by her parents because she has projectile vomiting after each feeding. The nurse notes an olive shaped mass in Kelly's epigastrium. It is determined that Kelly will need surgery to correct the problem. The goal for Kelly pre-operatively is to:
a. consume and retain a sufficient amount of formula.
b. restore hydration and electrolyte balance.
c. interview the parents regarding feeding patterns.
d. position her in a high Fowlers position after feeding.

17. A client tells the nurse that he is Jesus Christ and shows her marks on his hands where he has been nailed to the cross. The most therapeutic response to this client would be:
a. "You are not Jesus Christ; that is not possible."
b. "How long have you believed you were Jesus?"
c. "This morning you told me your name was John Hansen."
d. "It is difficult for me to believe that you are Jesus Christ."

18. When assessing a post-operative client's breath sounds, the nurse notes bilateral scattered rhonchi at the bases of the lung fields. This finding may be significant of:
a. impending respiratory arrest.
b. bronchospasm.
c. narrowing of large airways during expiration.
d. obstruction of the upper airway.

19. Holly Rubin, 11 years old, fell from her skateboard. X-rays show a wrist fracture. The nurse evaluates that Holly understands proper cast care when she states she will:
a. remove excess padding if the cast feels tight.
b. cover the cast with plastic while she goes swimming.
c. be careful where she scratches beneath the cast.
d. exercise her fingers and shoulders every day.

20. A client's subclavian central venous pressure (CVP) line reading has ranged from 2 to 5 mm Hg over the last week. His vital signs have been stable. His urine output has been ranging from 40 to 50 cc per hour since admission. He is on oxygen therapy of 4L via nasal cannula. The nurse would anticipate which order from the physician?
a. Pulse oximetry.
b. Removal of central venous pressure (CVP) line.
c. Increased diuretic order.
d. Urine culture and sensitivity.

21. A 68 year old male with a long history of farming is admitted to the hospital. During the physical assessment the nurse notes that the client has an exaggerated posterior curvature of the thoracic spine (humpback). This would be indicative of:
a. kyphosis.
b. pectus carinatum.
c. scoliosis.
d. barrel chest.

22. A 48 year old woman is admitted to the psychiatric unit after an overdose of barbiturates. She tells the nurse, "You know, I'm glad I'm alive but I don't know why. My life is such a mess." The nurse understands that the client's behavior is an example of:
a. ambivalence.
b. regret.
c. denial.
d. reaction formation.

23. A 72 year old male is admitted to the medical unit. While performing the physical assessment the nurse finds clubbing of the fingers. This would indicate:
a. peripheral vascular disease.
b. a benign nervous disorder.
c. cardiopulmonary disease.
d. a long smoking history.

24. A nurse arrives to work the night shift on the medical-surgical unit where she has been employed for three years. She receives a message to call the nursing supervisor, who informs the nurse that the pediatrics unit is very busy. The supervisor then informs the nurse of her decision to place her on the pediatrics unit for the upcoming shift. The correct response of the nurse in this situation would be:
a. "I've not been oriented to that unit and my pediatrics background is extremely limited."
b. "If I'm not needed on my unit tonight, I will go home."
c. "I refuse to float to the pediatrics unit and I would like to document my objections."
d. "My duty is to care for clients in this hospital to the best of my abilities."

25. A client 36 weeks pregnant is admitted with a diagnosis of placenta previa. All of the following nursing measures will be instituted in her care except:
a. bedrest with bathroom privileges if no sign of active bleeding is present.
b. monitoring of fetal heart tones via external monitor.
c. monitoring of blood loss, pain and uterine contractility.
d. rectal or vaginal exams.

26. The nurse believes that a client in labor on oxytocin (Pitocin) has uterine tetany. The initial action of the nurse should be to:
a. call the physician.
b. turn off the oxytocin (Pitocin) drip.
c. administer oxygen 6L by mask.
d. prepare the client for immediate cesarian section.

27. A 32 year old male with Hodgkins disease is receiving chemotherapy to prepare him for a bone marrow transplant. In the safe preparation and disposal of chemotherapeutic agents, which of the following actions should the nurse recognize as incorrect in accordance with Occupational Safety and Health Administration (OSHA) standards?
a. Use latex gloves when handling body secretions.
b. Wear a long-sleeved gown when administering the chemotherapy.
c. Double bag the intravenous bag and tubing following administration.
d. Use Leur-Lok fittings on all intravenous connections.

28. During an interaction with the nurse, a female client tearfully reports that she was sexually abused as a child. The nurse knows that one of the most common complaints reported by clients who are adult survivors of sexual child abuse is:
    a. sexual dysfunction.
    b. gender dysphoria.
    c. voyeurism.
    d. change in sexual orientation.

29. The nurse realizes a client with multiple myeloma understands the importance of fluid intake when the client states:
    a. "Fluids improve my circulation."
    b. "Fluids prevent kidney stones."
    c. "Fluids keep my lips moist."
    d. "Fluids help me to cough up phlegm."

30. The physician orders penicillin 400,000 units now. After reconstitution with 6 ml of sterile water, a 5,000,000 unit vial contains 300,000 units/ml. How many ml should the nurse administer?
    a. 0.5 ml.
    b. 0.8 ml.
    c. 1.3 ml.
    d. 1.5 ml.

STOP You have now completed Practice Session: 16. Now take a few minutes and correct your answers. Calculate your accuracy rate by dividing the number of questions you completed correctly by the total number of questions you completed (30).

Correct answers ÷ total number of questions completed = accuracy rate.

_____ ÷ _____ = _____

PRACTICE SESSION: 16

ANSWERS AND RATIONALES

1. **The correct answer is d.** Narcotics given intravenously are likely to cause central nervous system depression leading to hypotension and apnea. Monitoring vital signs and blood pressure can be done by an aide under supervision. Specific instructions and parameters avoid misinterpretation of directions. Phrases such as "depressed respirations" (option a), and "monitor" (option c), can hold different meanings to the sender and receiver of the message. Elevating the head of the bed to facilitate respirations and assisting the client to the bathroom may be included in the client's care. Oral fluids (option b) may be given to clients if they are alert since the fluids assist the body to rid itself adequately of the narcotic (Ignatavicius & Bayne, 1991; p. 135).

Nursing Process: Implementation
Client Need: Physiological Integrity

2. **The correct answer is d.** The physician should be notified if any jaundice occurs so that proper diagnosis and treatment can be ordered. The physician will probably order bilirubin levels to be determined but this is not within the scope of practice of the nurse (option c). Phototherapy may also be ordered but also requires a physician's order (option a). The infant's condition should be reassessed every four hours but prompt treatment will prevent comp-

lications such as damage to the nervous system (option b) (May & Mahlmeister, 1994; pp. 891-894).

Nursing Process: Implementation
Client Need: Physiological Integrity

3. **The correct answer is c.** Metabolic acidosis occurs due to a reduction in plasma bicarbonate (HCO_3) when alkali is lost in large amounts of stool output (option a). Loss of extracellular fluid through the ileostomy causes a sodium deficit (option b). Lower gastrointestinal output is also potassium rich and high output results in potassium deficit (option d). Excessive output will also lead to a volume deficit (Long, Phipps & Cassmeyer, 1993; pp. 951-957).

Nursing Process: Analysis
Client Need: Physiological Integrity

4. **The correct answer is b.** Tetany is a sign of severe calcium deficiency. Hypocalcemia, not hypercalcemia, (option d) may occur if the parathyroid glands were inadvertently removed with thyroid tissue or suppressed due to edema. Parathyroid hormone is responsible for maintaining serum calcium levels. When calcium is deficient, nerve, smooth, skeletal and cardiac muscle dysfunctions occur. Hypokalemia is manifested by weakness, flaccid paralysis, lethargy, diminished deep tendon reflexes, gastrointestinal disturbances and cardiac arrhythmias (option a). Hypothyroidism, not

hyperthyroidism, would be the result of a thyroidectomy (option c) (Phipps, Long, Woods & Cassmeyer, 1991; pp. 555-557).

Nursing Process: Analysis
Client Need: Physiological Integrity

5. **The correct answer is b.** The nurse is a mandated reporter; therefore, as soon as child abuse or neglect is suspected, it must be reported to local authorities. Joey demonstrates several signs of neglect: no lunch, undone homework despite calls to Joey's father, unkempt appearance, self-stimulatory acts (sucking thumb), and excessive sleepiness. It is also important to assess for physical abuse, although it does not always accompany neglect (option d). While further history-taking from Joey and his parents is helpful in building a case, the nurse must first report the situation to the authorities (options a and c) (Whaley & Wong, 1991; pp. 736-738, 742).

Nursing Process: Implementation
Client Need: Health Promotion & Maintenance

6. **The correct answer is c.** If teaching is ineffective, the client does not understand the teaching and will choose a high potassium meal. In option (c), beets and apricots have high levels of potassium. Options (a), (b) and (d) contain low levels of potassium (Burtis, Davis & Martin, 1988; pp. 774-779).

Nursing Process: Evaluation
Client Need: Physiological Integrity

7. **The correct answer is d.** Holding the infant and asking questions regarding care is positive bonding behavior. In effective teaching, questions are normal and show the client has listened to the teaching and is thinking about it (option b). There is no evidence to suggest whether or not home care referral is especially needed for this client. Definite follow-up should occur if negative behaviors are observed (option c). There is also nothing to suggest the person has or has not attended prenatal classes (option a) (Ladewig, London & Olds, 1990; pp. 769-771).

Nursing Process: Analysis
Client Need: Health Promotion & Maintenance

8. **The correct answer is a.** Therapeutic levels are reached within 10 to 14 days but may take three to four weeks to get a good response. Clients need to be educated so they do not have unrealistic expectations about how quickly they will feel better. Continued suicidal assessment would be important in the nursing care of this client; however, telling the client instead of asking is not appropriate (option c). Calling the physician at this point is premature (option b). Telling the client the medication may be wrong for her is outside the scope of nursing practice (option d) (Haber, Leach-McMahon, Price-Hoskins & Sideleau, 1992; p. 574).

Nursing Process: Implementation
Client Need: Physiological Integrity

9. **The correct answer is d.** A peak level is drawn a half hour after a dose infuses when the medication is administered intravenously (IV). Tobramycin (Nebcin) is always given IV or intramuscularly (IM). When a medication is administered, the drug concentration in the plasma increases from zero level and continues to rise until the elimination rate of drug is equivalent to its rate of absorption. This point is known as the peak plasma level. A peak level is done to insure therapeutic levels of the medication are in the blood (Reiss & Evans, 1990; pp. 20-21).

Nursing Process: Planning
Client Need: Physiological Integrity

10. **The correct answer is c.** Low back pain is caused by pressure on the lumbar nerves and usually indicates rapid expansion of the aneurysm that occurs prior to rupture. In most people, the systolic blood pressure is approximately 15 mm Hg higher in the thigh (option a). In clients with AAA, the blood pressure in the thigh is often lower (option b). These clients also complain frequently of a pulsating abdominal mass (option d). While options (b) and (d) are both characteristic of AAA, they do not imply impending rupture (Smeltzer & Bare, 1992; p. 755).

Nursing Process: Analysis
Client Need: Physiological Integrity

11. **The correct answer is a.** Clients with hyperparathyroidism are prone to joint problems and bone pain due to weakness and decreased bone mass. Fractures and arthralgias may occur which decrease tolerance for activity. Problems with hearing (option b) should not occur with these clients. Hirsutism (option c) and glycosuria (option d) would be true for Cushing's disease but not hyperparathyroidism (Lewis & Collier, 1992; pp. 1340, 1344).

Nursing Process: Assessment
Client Need: Physiological Integrity

12. **The correct answer is a.** Systemic lupus erythematosis (SLE) is an immune complex disorder that results in tissue damage with cell lysis. It is thought to be influenced by genetic and environmental factors. These include exposure to ultraviolet light, drugs, stress and pregnancy. Being a twin, drinking alcohol and eating a high fat diet are unrelated to SLE (options b, c and d) (Mott, Sperhac & James, 1990; p. 1277).

Nursing Process: Assessment
Client Need: Physiological Integrity

13. **The correct answer is c.** The first step the nurse takes is to reposition the head and neck. General anesthesia causes relaxation of the muscles of the tongue and pharynx obstructing the airway. After assuring airway patency, it may be necessary to aspirate mucus or vomitus (option d) that is causing an obstruction. In the recovery room it is essential to stimulate all clients to cough and deep breathe (option a) to clear the airway and expand the alveoli. The head of the bed should remain flat (option b) until the client is awake enough to follow commands (Ignatavicius & Bayne, 1991;

p. 440; Smeltzer & Bare, 1992; p. 439).

Nursing Process: Implementation
Client Need: Physiological Integrity

14. **The correct answer is b.** The major determinant of oxygen delivery is hemoglobin. Infusing packed red blood cells would increase the client's oxygen content. Applying nasal cannula oxygen (option a) would help but the need is hemoglobin to carry the oxygen. Placing the client in Trendelenburg position (option c) is inappropriate and would not insure oxygen delivery to the tissues. Sedating the client (option d) has no clinical significance and possibly would lower the blood pressure (Lewis & Collier, 1992; pp. 664-666).

Nursing Process: Implementation
Client Need: Safe, Effective Care Environment

15. **The correct answer is c.** T-tube drainage or bile is very caustic to the skin and all measures to protect it should be taken. Steatorrhea and diarrhea episodes will be counteracted (option a) as the client takes pancreatic enzymes. In a Whipple procedure, the head of the pancreas is removed (option b) and the client may or may not require insulin. Pancreatic cancer is painful and the need for narcotics may be higher (option d) since a tolerance may have been built up pre-operatively (Smeltzer & Bare, 1992; pp. 1116-1119).

Nursing Process: Planning
Client Need: Physiological Integrity

16. **The correct answer is b.** The classic signs and symptoms of pyloric stenosis have been exhibited. The classic signs and symptoms are projectile vomiting after feeding and an olive shaped mass in the epigastrium. This frequent vomiting leads to electrolyte imbalance and dehydration. These must be restored before surgery to correct the stenosis, a pyloromyotomy, can be performed safely. Consuming and restoring formula is a post-operative goal. The child will continue to have projectile vomiting until the surgery is successfully completed (option a). Feeding patterns do not cause pyloric stenosis and is therefore an unnecessary pre-operative goal (option c). Positioning the child after feedings is a post-operative intervention not a pre-operative goal (option d) (Whaley & Wong, 1991; pp. 1513-1515).

Nursing Process: Planning
Client Need: Physiological Integrity

17. **The correct answer is d.** The use of reasonable doubt allows the client to see that you do not share his delusional belief without being argumentative. Options (a) and (c) attempt to use logic and reasoning which are not effective in decreasing a delusional belief system. Option (b) encourages the delusion and allows the client to imagine that you also believe he is Jesus (Haber, Leach-McMahon, Price-Hoskins & Sideleau, 1992; pp. 541-544).

Nursing Process: Implementation
Client Need: Psychosocial Integrity

18. **The correct answer is c.** Rhonchi are more prominent on expiration. The coarse, musical, rattling sounds are caused by fluid, secretions or obstruction

340

of the large airway. Impending respiratory arrest (option a) would include greatly diminished breath sounds. Bronchospasm (option b) indicates wheezes, musical sounds associated with air rushing through narrowed small airways. Upper airway obstruction (option d) indicates pleural friction rubs which are rough, grating scratching sounds caused by inflamed surfaces of the pleura rubbing together (Ignatavicius & Bayne, 1991; pp. 476, 1944; Lewis & Collier, 1992; p. 828; Smeltzer & Bare, 1992; pp. 599-600).

Nursing Process: Assessment
Client Need: Physiological Integrity

19. **The correct answer is d.** Fingers should be flexed often to reduce edema Exercising the shoulder is necessary to prevent complications such as muscle contracture. If the cast feels tight (option a) the client should report this to the physician since it may be a sign of impaired circulation. The client should not remove any padding. The client should not get the cast wet nor cover the cast with plastic (option b). The client should not place foreign objects inside the cast to scratch (option c) since unseen injury may occur (Smeltzer & Bare, 1992; pp. 1790-1793).

Nursing Process: Evaluation
Client Need: Physiological Integrity

20. **The correct answer is b.** The nurse would anticipate the removal of the central venous pressure (CVP) line. Central lines should not be in longer than one week to prevent infection. The client's physiological signs and symptoms are all within normal limits.

The client is not showing signs of respiratory distress so there is no need for pulse oximetry (option a). Urine output of greater than 30 cc per hour is considered adequate (option c). Sending a urine for a culture and sensitivity is inappropriate since there are no signs of urinary tract infection (option d) (Lewis & Collier, 1992; pp. 735-736).

Nursing Process: Analysis
Client Need: Safe, Effective Care Environment

21. **The correct answer is a.** The physical assessment data correlates with kyphosis. This occurs as bone mass decreases with age and collapse of the vertebrae happens. Pectus carinatum is the forward protrusion of the sternum with ribs sloping back at either side and vertical depressions along costochondral junctions (pigeon breast) (option b). A lateral "S" shaped curvature of the thoracic and lumbar spine relates to scoliosis (option c). When a client has a barrel chest his anteroposterior equals the transverse diameter. Ribs are horizontal instead of the normal downward slope (option d) (Jarvis, 1992; pp. 514-515).

Nursing Process: Analysis
Client Need: Physiological Integrity

22. **The correct answer is a.** Almost all suicidal clients are ambivalent about actually committing suicide. The client's comments of feeling happy to be alive but upset that her life is a mess demonstrates that ambivalence. Regret (option b) is incorrect since the client stated she was glad to be alive. Denial (option c) would be a refusal to believe

something exists such as, "My life isn't a mess, it's wonderful." or "I didn't really try to kill myself, it was a mistake." Reaction formation (option d) is manifested as actions in opposition to what the person actually believes (Cook & Fontaine, 1991; pp. 90, 617).

Nursing Process: Analysis
Client Need: Psychological Integrity

23. **The correct answer is c.** Arterial hypoxemia, whether due to cardiac or pulmonary disease, produces widening and thickening of the fingers and toes as well as convex nails. Peripheral vascular disease (option a) would be related to arterial and venous systems, not arterial only. Nervous disorders (option b) do not produce clubbing but may show numbness, tingling or pain in the extremities. A history of smoking (option d) on the fingers may be indicated by nicotine stains (Lewis & Collier, 1992; pp. 578-600).

Nursing Process: Analysis
Client Need: Physiological Integrity

24. **The correct answer is a.** The nurse, using her professional judgement, has the duty to state her abilities to the nursing supervisor. Once she accepts the responsibility to care for the clients on the pediatrics unit, she can be held legally accountable for her actions. The nurse's action of going home (option b) could be considered abandonment of duty. Refusal (option c) is insubordination. The nurse stating that she is prepared to care for the clients on the pediatrics unit (option d) assumes that she would provide the same care as a nurse previously oriented and

experienced in the care of infants and children (Taylor, Lillis & LeMone, 1989; p. 91).

Nursing Process: Implementation
Client Need: Safe, Effective Care Environment

25. **The correct answer is d.** Rectal or vaginal exams are contraindicated so as not to encourage bleeding. Typically, the first bleed is scanty, and may spontaneously subside if no further vaginal or rectal exams are done. However, each subsequent hemorrhage is greater with a more substantive risk to mother and baby. The client would be allowed to use the bathroom (option a) but she must otherwise remain on bedrest to decrease stimuli to the uterus to prevent any further bleeding. The fetal heart rate usually remains stable unless profuse hemorrhage or shock occurs to the mother (option b). Monitoring for blood loss, pain and uterine contraction (option c) will be done by observation (Ladewig, London & Olds, 1990; p. 510).

Nursing Process: Planning
Client Need: Physiological Integrity

26. **The correct answer is b.** Uterine tetany is an emergency situation because it causes fetal hypoxia. One of the main causes of uterine tetany is oxytocin (Pitocin) infusion. (The other cause is abruptio placentae.) The best and fastest method of reversing the condition is to stop the oxytocin (Pitocin) infusion. This prevents further harm to the fetus. After the oxytocin (Pitocin) is stopped, the nurse should: 1) turn the mother on her left side, 2) increase the regular

intravenous infusion rate, 3) notify the physician (option a), 4) administer oxygen (option c), and 5) have a tocolytic drug available to reverse the oxytocin. If the uterine tetany remains unrelieved, the client should be prepared for a cesarian section (option d) for the safety of the fetus (Martin & Reeder, 1991; p. 665).

Nursing Process: Implementation
Client Need: Physiological Integrity

27. **The correct answer is c.** This is the incorrect action. The intravenous bag and tubing should be placed in a leak proof, puncture proof container to protect other workers from exposure. All of the other measures (options a, b and d) are Occupational Safety and Health Administration (OSHA) standards and should be observed (Smeltzer & Bare, 1992; p. 368).

Nursing Process: Implementation
Client Need: Safe, Effective Care Environment

28. **The correct answer is a.** Many adults who were sexually abused as children report residuals such as sexual dysfunction, difficulty trusting others, depression, panic attacks and poor body image. Although adult survivors of sexual child abuse often report a multitude of problems, there is no evidence to suggest the development of voyeurism (option c), gender dysphoria (option b) or change in sexual orientation (option d) (Poorman, 1988;

pp. 231-232; Stuart & Sundeen, 1991; p. 917).

Nursing Process: Analysis
Client Need: Health Promotion & Maintenance

29. **The correct answer is b.** Clients with multiple myeloma are predisposed to hypercalcemia related to bone breakdown from osteolytic lesions. Clients need 3 to 4 liters of fluids to prevent kidney stone formation. The other statements (options a, c and d) are true but not directly related to multiple myeloma (Ignatavicius & Bayne, 1991; pp. 669, 670).

Nursing Process: Evaluation
Client Need: Health Promotion & Maintenance

30. **The correct answer is c.**

desired dose x volume =
on hand dose

= dose to be administered

$$\frac{400,000 \text{ u}}{300,000 \text{ u}} \times 1 \text{ ml} = 1.3 \text{ ml}$$

(Weaver & Koehler, 1992; p. 65).

PRACTICE SESSION: 17

Instructions:

Allow yourself 30 minutes to complete the following 30 practice questions. Use a timer to notify yourself when 30 minutes are over so that you are not constantly looking at your watch while completing the questions.

1. The nurse's assignment for the day includes three clients scheduled to leave the unit as follows: a 32 year old female for abdominal surgery; a 60 year old male for a colonoscopy; and a 72 year old male for pulmonary function testing. The initial nursing action would be to:
   a. facilitate early morning activities of daily living.
   b. encourage the clients to void early.
   c. inform ancillary personnel of clients' dietary status.
   d. implement routine nursing care until an official notification of test/surgery times.

2. A client hospitalized for a week has been confined to bed with traction. He becomes highly anxious. The nurse checks the client's nursing assessment in the chart. Which of the following data is probably contributing the most to the client's present anxiety?
   a. Several hospitalizations for various surgeries as a child.
   b. A history of fears related to closed spaces.
   c. Loss of his job.
   d. Recent marital problems.

3. Mr. Bill Saunders is scheduled to have a coronary angiography to confirm his diagnosis of Prinzmetal's angina. Prior to the test, he will be given an intracoronary injection of ergonovine maleate (Ergotrate). Mr Saunders asks the nurse why he needs this medication. The nurse's best response is:
   a. "It will help the physician monitor the ST segment changes during the procedure."
   b. "It will provoke a spasm of the coronary arteries."
   c. "It will relieve any chest pain associated with the procedure."
   d. "It will help you relax by sedating you before the procedure."

4. A nineteen year old is admitted after a diving accident. He has sustained a spinal cord injury at the C_8 level. The family asks if the client will ever be the same as he was before the accident. The best response by the nurse is:
   a. "He may have paralysis of all four extremities."
   b. "He won't be exactly the same but he will be able to drive a car with help."
   c. "He will be paralyzed and need a ventilator to help him breathe for the rest of his life."
   d. "He will probably make a full recovery after rehabilitation."

5. Kelly, a 7 year old, is being discharged following a five day admission for acute glomerulonephritis. Which of the following comments by Kelly's parents would indicate a need for further teaching?
   a. "I should weigh Kelly every day and report any major changes."
   b. "I will make sure Kelly stays in bed for another week."
   c. "I will bring Kelly back to the clinic so she can have her urine checked."
   d. "I will make sure Kelly doesn't get any extra salt in her diet."

6. A client is admitted to the labor suite in active labor. The physician orders continuous external fetal monitoring. The nurse would remain alert because the major disadvantage of external fetal monitoring is that it does not accurately record:
   a. frequency of uterine contractions.
   b. the intensity of uterine contractions.
   c. the duration of uterine contractions.
   d. baseline fetal heart rate.

7. A 65 year old client is admitted with the diagnosis of acute exacerbation of chronic obstructive pulmonary disease (COPD). He is dyspneic and slightly cyanotic. The nurse instructs the client in purse-lip breathing. This breathing technique:
   a. decreases the need for high flow oxygen concentration.
   b. facilitates coughing and removal of excessive secretions.
   c. diminishes bronchospasms.
   d. improves gas distribution.

8. A client with hepatitis A has shown signs of jaundice for about 24 hours. What type of isolation precautions would be necessary?
   a. Enteric.
   b. Blood.
   c. Blood and body fluids.
   d. No isolation procedures are necessary.

9. The nurse enters a client's room to find him pacing the floor. The client refuses a PRN medication and asks the nurse to leave him alone. A student nurse who observes this interaction asks the nurse how she plans to intervene. The nurse responds that she will:
   a. honor the client's request but closely monitor his behavior.
   b. ask another nurse to offer him the PRN medication.
   c. insist the client take the PRN medication or be placed in seclusion.
   d. call the physician to report the client's escalating behavior.

10. A 24 year old client comes to the emergency room with a dog bite. The best way to screen for rabies would be to:
    a. ask the client if he knows the dog's owner.
    b. perform a baseline neurologic and musculoskeletal assessment.
    c. administer tetanus and rabies vaccine prophylactically.
    d. observe the client for early signs of rabies.

11. A 38 year old male is admitted to the hospital with a diagnosis of Addison's disease. Considering this diagnosis, the client is most likely to have which of the following symptoms?
    a. Buffalo hump with moon face.
    b. Hyponatremia, hyperkalemia and dark skin pigments.
    c. Hypernatremia, hypokalemia and purple striae.
    d. Ecchymosis and increased body hair.

12. An 8 month old is admitted for repair of a tetralogy of fallot (TOF) defect. While drawing blood for pre-operative tests, the baby becomes hypercyanotic. Which of the following actions should the nurse do first?
    a. Administer 4 liters of oxygen via nasal cannula.
    b. Call the physician.
    c. Begin cardiac compressions.
    d. Place the baby in a knee-chest position.

13. When caring for a client with Crohn's disease, the nurse would include what nutritional information?
    a. Increase diet in minerals and vitamins.
    b. 2,000-2,300 calorie intake daily.
    c. A diet low in protein.
    d. High residue diet.

14. A nurse is working with a client diagnosed with passive-aggressive personality disorder. The nurse would expect to see which of the following behaviors?
    a. Indecisiveness, inefficiency and procrastination.
    b. Frustration, impulsivity and chemical abuse.
    c. Aloofness, lethargy and social withdrawal.
    d. Hostility, jealousy and emotional coldness.

15. A 68 year old female is admitted to the surgical intensive care unit because of complications following total abdominal hysterectomy. She is orally intubated and on a volume ventilator. Her ventilator settings are: intermittent mandatory ventilation (IMV) rate of 12, tidal volume 750 ml, 50% Fio2 and 5cm of PEEP. Which of the following would be included in the plan of care?
   a. Check endotracheal cuff pressure every day to prevent tracheal damage.
   b. Check that the tidal volume is approximately 25 ml/kilogram of body weight.
   c. Recognize that on intermittent mandatory ventilation (IMV) the client can not take more than the set number of breaths.
   d. If agitation occurs, remove her from the ventilator and bag with 100% oxygen.

16. Mark, an eight month old, has been diagnosed with acquired immune deficiency syndrome (AIDS). His parents are preparing to care for him at home. Which of the following statements by Mark's parents indicates a need for further teaching?
   a. We will take his rectal temperature every morning.
   b. Gloves will be worn to give him a bath.
   c. His clothes and bedding will be washed separately in hot soapy water with household bleach.
   d. We will make sure he gets a high calorie formula.

17. A nurse is making rounds on her clients and walks into Mrs. Becker's room to find the bedside table and nightstand filled with flowers, magazines, food, tissues and her water pitcher. Mrs. Becker has been hospitalized for the past month. The nurse's initial action would be to:
   a. delegate the cleaning of the area to the unit's housekeeping staff.
   b. continue making rounds; a collection of these items is inevitable when a client is admitted for a month.
   c. discuss with administration the possibility of installing additional shelves for client rooms.
   d. discuss with Mrs. Becker the need to reduce the clutter and assist her in eliminating nonessential items.

18. The nurses on the oncology unit have decided to examine the quality of their discharge documentation. Evaluation should be based on:
   a. what the committee believes is correct at the time of the audit.
   b. standard criteria from a neighboring institution in the same city.
   c. criteria previously established by the oncology unit nurses.
   d. the standards of nursing practice set by the American Nurses' Association.

19. An HIV seropositive client has just delivered a baby girl. The mother states, " I want to breastfeed my baby, is it OK?" The nurse's best response would be:
a. "Yes. Breast milk is the best nourishment for infants."
b. "No, because breast milk has been implicated as a source for perinatal HIV transmission."
c. "The infant will only receive intravenous solutions because she is HIV positive."
d. "You may want to alternate between nursing and bottlefeeding so neither of you will tire so easily."

20. A client is diagnosed with herpes simplex virus keratitis. The nurse should further assess the client for:
a. an accompanying bacterial infection.
b. signs of chickenpox.
c. clear vesicles along the nerve root.
d. probable immunosuppression.

21. An elderly woman is having a total hip replacement. The nurse is explaining the option of an autologous blood transfusion. The nurse would use which of the following explanations?
a. The blood donor is someone from the client's immediate family.
b. The client will donate her own blood.
c. The blood is typed and cross-matched in the laboratory.
d. The blood is donated directly from one person to another.

22. A client comes to the clinic and states, "I think I'm pregnant." What presumptive changes is she most likely experiencing?
a. Nausea and vomiting, breast tenderness and quickening.
b. Chloasma, Goodell's sign, and enlargement of the abdomen.
c. Fetal heartbeat and fetal movement.
d. Abdominal striae, uterine enlargement, and Braxton Hicks contractions.

23. The physician orders a gastrostomy tube feeding of 250 ml of 65% osmolite solution to infuse at 50 cc/hr. How much osmolite solution and water should be mixed to equal 250 ml?
a. 155 ml of osmolite and 95 ml of water.
b. 163 ml of osmolite and 87 ml of water.
c. 175 ml of osmolite and 75 ml of water.
d. 200 ml of osmolite and 50 ml of water.

24. Mr. Raymond Foster, 33 years old, has a central venous pressure (CVP) line inserted into the subclavian vein through to the right atrium. The nurse is taking a reading and knows to record the reading noted when:
a. the client is sitting upright with the heart across from the top of the manometer.
b. the fluid level stabilizes in the manometer.
c. the highest level is reached in the manometer.
d. the stopcock is turned so that the manometer fills with intravenous solution.

25. Which of these assessments of a client receiving hydrocortisone (Cortef) would indicate a drug related problem which needs to be reported to the physician?
   a. Increased urinary output.
   b. Rapid weight gain.
   c. Blurred vision.
   d. Swollen joints.

26. The home care nurse is evaluating the couple's progress one year after the husband had a myocardial infarction Further counseling would be needed if
   a. the client's wife steps in whenever the client tries to perform activities he usually did prior to the illness.
   b. the couple is not restricting their pre-illness sexual practices.
   c. the couple resumed their pre-illness roles and usual duties.
   d. the client has decided to pursue his engineering degree.

27. A 39 year old female client is admitted to the psychiatric unit in a full manic episode. As the nurse assigned to care for this client, which behavior would be the primary concern?
   a. Rapid speech and labile mood.
   b. Irritability and pressured speech.
   c. Poor judgement and flight of ideas.
   d. Constant physical activity and lack of sleep.

28. A 15 year old client says to the nurse, "My parents just don't understand me anymore. They treat me like I'm eight years old. I wish they'd realize I've grown up now and need more room. What should I do?" The best nursing diagnosis for this client would be:
   a. altered growth and development.
   b. defensive coping.
   c. altered family processes.
   d. health-seeking behavior.

29. The physician orders phenytoin (Dilantin) 100 mg intravenously every 8 hours. The graduate nurse indicates the drug was given at a rate exceeding 50 mg/minute. The registered nurse would immediately assess for:
   a. polyuria.
   b. bradycardia.
   c. hypertension.
   d. hypoglycemia.

30. A 45 year old male is a client in the intensive care unit following coronary artery bypass graft. He is on a volume ventilator with settings: intermittent mandatory ventilation (IMV) rate of 10, 50% Fio2, 5 cm of PEEP and tidal volume of 850 mls. Which of the following findings indicate that the nurse should take immediate action?
   a. The client takes a breath and a tidal volume of 350 mls is recorded.
   b. The high pressure alarm sounds when the client coughs.
   c. The actual respiratory rate of the client is 20.
   d. The client's minute volume is less than 8 liters.

STOP You have now completed Practice Session: 17. Now take a few minutes and correct your answers. Calculate your accuracy rate by dividing the number of questions you completed correctly by the total number of questions you completed (30).

Correct answers ÷ total number of questions completed = accuracy rate.

_____ ÷ _____ = _____

ANSWERS AND RATIONALES

1. **The correct answer is c.** Ancillary staff should be advised early of dietary status especially clients who are allowed nothing by mouth to prevent surgery cancellations and/or test delays. Client activities of daily living would then be prioritized and carried out accordingly (option a). Clients may void early if desired but should void immediately prior to surgeries and tests (option b). Clients for surgery or specific tests are prepared according to physician orders. Preparation begins as ordered and is not delayed for official notification of test/surgery times (option c) (Wywialowski, 1993; pp. 171-187).

   Nursing Process: Implementation
   Client Need: Physiological Integrity

2. **The correct answer is b.** Fear related to closed spaces is called claustrophobia. When feeling "closed in" a client will become highly anxious, or panicked, with feelings of impending doom and feelings that he must get out quickly to avoid disaster. The client has been confined to bed with traction and cannot get out which may lead to the same anxiety as feeling claustrophobic. Hospitalizations for surgeries as a child (option a) should not be relevant unless other data of problems related to hospitalizations was evident. Loss of job (option c) would be more likely to manifest itself as depression. Recent marital problems (option d) would be unrelated to hospitalization (Stuart & Sundeen, 1991; pp. 326, 331-333).

   Nursing Process: Analysis
   Client Need: Physiological Integrity

3. **The correct answer is b.** Prinzmetal's angina is caused by a spasm of a major coronary artery. By providing this spasm with ergonovine maleate (Ergotrate), a true diagnosis of Prinzmetal's angina can be made. ST segment changes occur in Prinzmetal's angina but that is not why the medication is given (option a). Nitroglycerin is given to relieve the chest pain (option c). Ergonovine maleate (Ergotrate) is a smooth muscle stimulant, not a sedative (option d) (Lewis & Collier, 1992; pp. 791-793).

   Nursing Process: Implementation
   Client Need: Physiological Integrity

4. **The correct answer is b.** Even though the injury is at the C_8 level, the client should still be able to use shoulders and arms. Hands will be weak but usable. The client will have to use a wheelchair (option d) but should be able to drive a car with special adaptive devices. Paralysis of all four extremities (option a) and ventilator use (option c) would be true for a C_4 spinal cord injury (Danielson, Hamel-Bissell & Winstead-Fry, 1993; p. 278).

   Nursing Process: Implementation
   Client Need: Health Promotion & Maintenance

5. **The correct answer is b.** Bedrest is not indicated. Ambulation does not have an adverse effect on the course of the disease following the acute period of hospitalization. Monitoring of generalized edema is done through daily weights (option a). Follow-up urinalysis is necessary to monitor blood urea nitrogen (BUN), creatinine and hematuria (option c). A complication of glomerulonephritis is hypertension, therefore sodium is restricted in the form of a "no added salt" diet (option d) (Whaley & Wong, 1991; p. 1345).

Nursing Process: Evaluation
Client Need: Physiological Integrity

6. **The correct answer is b.** The external fetal monitor (tocodynamometer) responds to pressure changes in the abdomen, hence it displays frequency (option a) and duration (option d) utilizing a non-invasive technique. It can not record accurate magnitude or intensity of the uterine contractions. The only ways to ascertain intensity of uterine contractions is by palpation of the uterus or by use of an internal uterine pressure gauge. Option (d) is not considered a major disadvantage as most often external fetal monitoring will record baseline fetal heart rate. The baseline fetal heart rate is difficult to obtain via external fetal monitoring if the mother is obese or if hydramnios is present (Ladewig, London & Olds, 1990; p. 398).

Nursing Process: Planning
Client Need: Safe, Effective Care Environment

7. **The correct answer is d.** Purse-lip breathing extends the expiratory phase of breathing. It is thought to improve gas distribution. The client's dyspnea is eased and respiratory rate decreases. Purse-lip breathing would not decrease the need for oxygen, just its distribution (option a). This breathing does not facilitate coughing and removal of secretions; postural drainage is usually administered to do this (option b). Bronchospasms are not diminished with this breathing; medication is usually used to relieve bronchospasm (option d) (Lewis & Collier, 1992; pp. 586-597).

Nursing Process: Analysis
Client Need: Physiological Integrity

8. **The correct answer is a.** Enteric precautions are necessary because feces may be infected for approximately one week after jaundice appears. After that the client may be discharged (option d). Blood and body fluid precautions (options b and c) are necessary for clients infected with hepatitis B (Lewis & Collier, 1992; p. 1129).

Nursing Process: Planning
Client Need: Safe, Effective Care Environment

9. **The correct answer is a.** The client has the right to refuse medication unless his behavior can be defined as a psychiatric emergency. The client's behavior at present does not represent a clear or immediate danger to himself or others. Therefore, it is very doubtful that any physician would perceive this situation as a psychiatric emergency. Asking another nurse to offer him the medication (option b) disregards the client's rights. Insisting the client take medication or be placed in seclusion (option c) may be perceived as a threat

which is both nontherapeutic and illegal. There is no baseline data to indicate that the client's behavior is escalating (option d) (McFarland & Thomas, 1991; p. 936).

Nursing Process: Planning
Client Need: Psychosocial Integrity

10. **The correct answer is a.** The dog's owner should be located so the dog can be isolated and observed for signs of rabies. If rabies is not present, the client will not require further treatment. If the dog has rabies, the animal is destroyed because there is no cure and the rabies virus is contagious. The client will also need to undergo a series of rabies injections to hopefully prevent the disease. A baseline neurologic and musculoskeletal assessment is performed (option b) when initial treatment is done to enable consequent assessment for rabies symptoms. Antibiotics and tetanus are usually given on initial treatment. Rabies vaccine (option c) is not administered unless the disease is found in the animal or if the animal cannot be found. Hopefully the vaccine would be started before (option d) signs of rabies are evident (Black & Matassarin-Jacobs, 1993; p. 2248).

Nursing Process: Planning
Client Need: Physiological Integrity

11. **The correct answer is b.** Addison's disease is caused by a deficiency of adrenal cortical hormones. These hormones include glucocorticoids which help maintain the blood sugar, sex hormones and mineralocorticoids which help the body retain sodium and water. When sodium is lost in the body, potassium is retained. Therefore,

symptoms of Addison's disease include hyponatremia and hyperkalemia. All other symptoms (options a, c and d) are consistent with an abundance of these cortical hormones as in Cushing's disease (Smeltzer & Bare, 1992; pp. 1097-1100).

Nursing Process: Assessment
Client Need: Physiological Integrity

12. **The correct answer is d.** Placing the child in a knee-chest position will reduce the desaturated venous return from the lower extremities and increase systemic vascular resistance which diverts blood flow into the pulmonary artery. Hypercyanotic infants should receive 100% oxygen via face mask, not nasal cannula (option a). Calling the physician may be necessary if cyanosis continues, but is not the priority (option b). There is no evidence to suggest that the child does not have a pulse, therefore cardiac compressions are not warranted (option c) (Whaley & Wong, 1991; pp. 1553-1554).

Nursing Process: Implementation
Client Need: Physiological Integrity

13. **The correct answer is a.** Extra vitamins are needed for healing. These include thiamin, riboflavin, niacin, and ascorbic acid. Minerals such as zinc are needed for tissue synthesis. High protein diet is needed in inflammatory bowel disease because there are large losses of protein from the intestinal mucosal tissue by exudation and bleeding (option c). Daily calorie intake of 2500-3000 is needed to restore nutritional deficit from daily losses in the stool (option b). A low residue diet will help avoid irritation of the mucosal

lining until healing is well established (option d) (Williams, 1989; p. 449).

Nursing Process: Implementation
Client Need: Health Promotion & Maintenance

14. **The correct answer is a.** Passive-aggressive personality traits include delaying tactics, fault finding, procrastination, errors of omission, inefficiency and indecisiveness from an ambivalent affect. Option (b) shows characteristics of an antisocial personality disorder. Option (c) shows characteristics of a schizoid personality disorder. Option (d) shows characteristics of a paranoid personality disorder (Johnson, 1993; pp. 424-427).

Nursing Process: Assessment
Client Need: Psychosocial Integrity

15. **The correct answer is d.** In case of bucking, confusion or agitation, the client should be removed from the ventilator and bagged with 100% oxygen until the cause of the problem can be found and corrected. Endotracheal cuff pressure should be checked every eight hours and kept below 25 cm H_2O (option a). The tidal volume should be approximately 10 to 15 ml/kg (option b). On an intermittent mandatory ventilation (IMV) setting, the machine delivers a set number of breaths at a set volume. The client is free to take breaths at any time for any volume in addition to this (option c) (Smeltzer & Bare, 1992; pp. 556-558).

Nursing Process: Planning
Client Need: Physiological Integrity

16. **The correct answer is a.** Rectal temperatures are an invasive procedure that increases the risk of acquiring an infection in an already immuno-compromised client. Wearing gloves prevents possible contamination from incontinence during the bath (option b). Contaminated cloth diapers and other garments should be washed separately in hot, soapy water with household bleach to prevent spread of infection to other family members (option c). High calorie diets are necessary for all children with AIDS (option d) (Mott, Sperhac & James, 1990; pp. 1253-1262).

Nursing Process: Evaluation
Client Need: Physiological Integrity

17. **The correct answer is d.** Clutter is an environmental safety hazard to both the client and nurse and needs to be dealt with immediately (option a). Ignoring the problem and doing nothing (option b) could possibly lead to a future accident, thus being negligent. Suggestions regarding additional shelves may be useful but would not be the initial action (option c) (Potter & Perry, 1989; p. 1159).

Nursing Process: Implementation
Client Need: Safe, Effective Care Environment

18. **The correct answer is c.** Since universal standards for oncology units have not been established, each institution's oncology unit should set reasonable professional standards with measurement criteria to guide practice. Criteria should be determined before the standard is measured and not established

at the time of the audit (option a). Although criteria from other hospitals can be used as referents (option b), measurement criteria as well as standards will vary and should be specific to the institution. The American Nurse's Association has written general standards that should be followed (option d) but again, standards and measurement criteria should be specific to the institution (Marquis & Huston, 1992; pp. 343-345).

Nursing Process: Evaluation
Client Need: Safe, Effective Care Environment

19. **The correct answer is b.** Because breast milk has been implicated as a source for perinatal transmission, the Center for Disease Control does not recommend breast feeding for HIV seropositive mothers. This response acknowledges the HIV presence without being judgemental of the mother while delivering facts regarding transmission. Option (a) does not acknowledge that there is a disease process in place. Option (c) sounds very judgmental to the mother since there is no proof that the infant is infected. Option (d) is incorrect as breastfeeding could provide for transmission of the virus from mother to infant (Mandeirville & Troiano, 1992; p. 242).

Nursing Process: Implementation
Client Need: Health Promotion & Maintenance

20. **The correct answer is d.** Herpes simplex virus keratitis is a common but severe eye infection. Clear fluid-filled vesicles appear on the conjunctiva and cornea accompanied by pain and light sensitivity. The condition is often found in immunosuppressed clients. It is a viral infection and not known to necessarily occur with bacterial infections (option a). Chickenpox (option b) and vesicles along nerve roots (option c) are related to the herpes zoster virus (Lewis & Collier, 1992; p. 333).

Nursing Process: Assessment
Client Need: Physiological Integrity

21. **The correct answer is b.** Autologous blood is from oneself and used to decrease the incidence of a reaction. Blood transfusions can cause reactions ranging from mild to severe. To prevent severe hemolytic transfusion reactions caused by blood type or Rh incompatibility, the donor's blood and recipient's blood are tested for compatibility. Blood from immediate family members (option a) or directly from one person to another (option d) may not be 100% compatible and may place the client at risk. Blood that is typed and crossmatched in the laboratory (option c), whether to a familiar or unfamiliar donor, is the usual safe method of preparation for blood transfusion (Ignatavicius & Bayne, 1991; p. 465).

Nursing Process: Implementation
Client Need: Physiological Integrity

22. **The correct answer is a.** Presumptive changes are those subjective changes the client may voice. These symptoms may be due to causes other than pregnancy. Nausea and vomiting may stem from gastrointestinal disorders, breast tenderness may stem from elevated estrogen levels and quickening may be attributed to flatus or increased peristalsis. Options (b) and (d) are

incorrect as these are objective signs the examiner may perceive. These changes may also be attributed to causes other than pregnancy. Option (c) is incorrect as these are the only diagnostic changes for pregnancy and therefore conclusive for pregnancy (Olds, London & Ladewig, 1992; pp. 298-301).

Nursing Process: Assessment
Client Need: Health Promotion & Maintenance

23. **The correct answer is b.**
STEP 1:
Desired dose x Volume =
On-hand dose

Total amount of osmolite

$\frac{65\%}{100\%}$ x 250 = 162.5 ml osmolite
(round up to 163 ml)

STEP 2: (Water to be added)
Total amount
- amount osmolite
amount of water

250 ml
- 163 ml
87 ml of water

STEP 3:
163 ml osmolite
+ 87 ml water
250 ml total solution

(Weaver & Koehler, 1992; p. 87).

Nursing Process: Planning
Client Need: Physiological Integrity

24. **The correct answer is b.** The procedure for reading central venous pressure (CVP) measurement is as follows: position the client so that the base of the manometer is level with the right atrium (option a); open the stopcock to the manometer which fills with intravenous solution (option d); turn the stopcock so that the fluid in the manometer may flow to the client; the fluid level falls then becomes stable and the reading is taken at that point (option c); the stopcock is turned so that the intravenous solution again flows to the client (Lewis & Collier, 1992; p. 735).

Nursing Process: Implementation
Client Need: Physiological Integrity

25. **The correct answer is b.** Rapid weight gain along with a round face and fluid retention are signs of Cushing's Syndrome. Cushing Syndrome can be the result of excessive drug therapy and indicates the need for dosage adjustment. The other signs and symptoms (options a, c and d) are unrelated to hydrocortisone (Cortef) therapy (Ignatavicius & Bayne, 1991; p. 1548).

Nursing Process: Evaluation
Client Need: Physiological Integrity

26. **The correct answer is a.** One problem during post-recovery period is that family members are fearful of what might happen if the client resumes normal activities. Family members become comfortable with the altered routines brought on by the illness and are reluctant to change these routines. Sometimes encouragement and support by the nurse is needed to assist family members to the more healthy and usually less burdensome pre-illness routine (option c). Once recovery is complete clients can usually engage in their pre-

illness sexual practices (option b) with little or no variation. There would be no reason for the client not to pursue further education (option d). Often a serious episode of illness makes a person evaluate life goals and pursue new areas in life (Danielson, Hamel-Bissell & Winstead-Fry, 1993; p. 32).

Nursing Process: Evaluation
Client Need: Health Promotion & Maintenance

27. **The correct answer is d.** It would be common to see all of the identified behaviors (options a, b and c) in the manic client but option d causes greatest concern for the nurse because it can lead to physical exhaustion (Varcarolis, 1990; p. 471).

Nursing Process: Analysis
Client Need: Psychosocial Integrity

28. **The correct answer is d.** The client is 15 years old and working on personal identity issues which includes independence. This is a normal statement for the client's growth and therefore options (a) and (b) would be incorrect. The client is seeking advice on how to handle the situation so health seeking behaviors is the proper nursing diagnosis. Altered growth and development (option a) would be used for clients who would show evidence of retarded progress in physical, mental or emotional milestones. Defensive coping (option c) would be true if the client was trying to make excuses for inappropriate behavior such as substance abuse or criminal activities. Altered family processes (option d) may be true if the parents are unable to deal with the teenager's growth or if conflict develops

which harms the family's growth. This diagnosis is also incorrect since the one person is the nurse's client at this time, not the entire family (Snyder, 1992; pp. 15-16).

Nursing Process: Analysis
Client Need: Health Promotion & Maintenance

29. **The correct answer is b.** If the rate of phenytoin (Dilantin) administration exceeds 50 mg per minute, cardiotoxicity develops immediately. Phenytoin (Dilantin) decreases the force of myocardial contractions resulting in depressed atrial and ventricular conduction. In toxic states, cardiac arrest may occur. Acute renal failure is a potential adverse reaction. Polyuria (option a) may be an initial sign of acute real failure; however, is not an immediate reaction following phenytoin (Dilantin) administration. Hypotension not hypertension (option c) is associated with cardiotoxicity. Cardiovascular collapse with vasodilation and cardiac arrhythmias develop when phenytoin (Dilantin) exceeds the recommended rate of administration. Hyperglycemia not hypoglycemia may develop due to phenytoin's (Dilantin's) membrane stabilizing effect on the pancreas inhibiting insulin release (option d) (Baer & Williams, 1992; pp. 298-303).

Nursing Process: Assessment
Client Need: Physiological Integrity

30. **The correct answer is d.** Minute volume is tidal volume multiplied with respiratory rate. On these settings the minute volume should be a minimum of 850 ml x 10, or 8.5 liters. The other findings are normal and require no

action. High pressure alarm will sound briefly when the client coughs (option b). On intermittent mandatory ventilation (IMV), the client receives a set number of breaths at a set volume but may breathe on his own at any additional rate and volume (options a and c) (Smeltzer & Bare, 1992; pp. 536-538).

Nursing Process: Analysis
Client Need: Physiological Integrity

PRACTICE SESSION: 18

Instructions:

Allow yourself 30 minutes to complete the following 30 practice questions. Use a timer to notify yourself when 30 minutes are over so that you are not constantly looking at your watch while completing the questions.

---

1. A nurse takes a client's temperature and finds it to be below normal (97.3° F or 36.2° C). The next action of the nurse would be to:
   a. record the temperature.
   b. ask the client if he drank something cold.
   c. take a rectal temperature as validation.
   d. retake the temperature in an hour.

2. A client is admitted who is very dirty. The nurse asks the nursing assistant to help with the bath and assessment. The nursing assistant states, "I don't want to touch him. Who knows what you can catch from this guy." The best action by the nurse would be to:
   a. write a report on his behavior.
   b. ask him how he feels about the client.
   c. confront his judgmental attitude.
   d. suggest he wear gloves when assisting.

3. A 55 year old female has been admitted for a rhytidectomy. Discharge instructions should include:
   a. laying flat for one week post-procedure.
   b. washing the suture line with soap and water.
   c. washing the hair is allowed after one day.
   d. eating a soft diet to rest the face.

4. A 27 year old female is admitted to the burn unit after a car accident. Her husband asks to visit her. The nurse replies that the husband must first:
   a. ask permission of the physician.
   b. be tested for infection.
   c. put on cap, gown, mask and gloves.
   d. wash his hands.

5. A client has come to the clinic for cryotherapy of a skin lesion. The client should be instructed that:
   a. he should call the physician if blisters appear.
   b. a warm washcloth may ease the discomfort.
   c. the procedure will not be painful.
   d. a local anesthetic will be given beforehand.

6. The nurse is reinforcing teaching about how to walk with a cane. The best way to walk with a cane is to:
   a. use it on the opposite side of the problem leg.
   b. use it on the same side as the problem leg.
   c. move the unaffected leg at the same time as the cane.
   d. slide the cane along the floor to prevent tripping.

7. A nurse is assessing muscle strength of an elderly client. The best way to assess hip muscles would be to:
   a. ask the client to resist while the nurse tries to straighten the client's bent knee.
   b. ask the client to keep his knee straight while the nurse tries to flex it.
   c. ask the client to resist while the nurse tries to push against the foot and ankle.
   d. ask the client to try and lift his leg from the table while the nurse pushes down on it.

8. A 44 year old client with acromegaly is admitted for removal of the pituitary gland. Post-operatively the client should be warned against:
   a. deep breathing.
   b. talking.
   c. coughing.
   d. swallowing ice.

9. A 68 year old female is brought to the emergency room after fainting in the grocery store. The clerk called the emergency number and told paramedics the client complained of back pain. An aneurysm of the ascending aorta is diagnosed. The priority area of concern post-surgery is:
   a. medication administration.
   b. signs of infection.
   c. wound care.
   d. tissue perfusion.

10. A client is prepared for a colonoscopy for histology examination. After the colonoscopy the client should be observed for:
    a. intestinal obstruction.
    b. hypothermia.
    c. bowel perforation.
    d. electrolyte imbalance.

11. A client should be observed for adverse effects of furosemide (Lasix) therapy which include:
    a. fatigue, bounding pulses, hyperactive bowel sounds.
    b. weakness, irritability, nausea and vomiting.
    c. nausea and vomiting, oliguria, tachycardia.
    d. dyspnea, bounding pulses, constipation.

12. The nurse is conducting a group on daily living activities. Which of the following would be signs that the group cohesiveness needs more support?
    a. Group members sit together for lunch even though the group meeting is later that afternoon.
    b. Group members allow a member to stay silent.
    c. Older members don't take the advice of newer members.
    d. Older members state their group is better than other support groups.

13. A 35 year old female is using basal body temperature (BBT) to predict ovulation. She should be instructed to:
    a. record temperature in a diary.
    b. take temperature immediately after voiding.
    c. record for three to four months for accuracy.
    d. avoid intercourse for one week after temperature rise.

14. A 22 year old client has asked the nurse about contraceptive methods. She states she doesn't know which one to choose and asks for the nurse's help. The best response of the nurse would be:
    a. "Most women choose one method and tend to use it for the rest of their lives."
    b. "Any method can be used if you plan to have children later."
    c. "Each method is equally effective in preventing conception."
    d. "Your lifestyle and personal biases play a large part in guiding your choice."

15. A 50 year old client has been diagnosed with chronic laryngitis of unknown etiology. Which of the following measures would be included in the care plan?
    a. Increased fluids to two liters per day.
    b. A humidified living area.
    c. Observation for peritonsillar abscess.
    d. Bedrest.

16. A newly diagnosed diabetic client states she will be attending a wedding and wants to know if she can have alcoholic beverages. The best response by the nurse would be:
    a. "No, alcohol causes acute hyperglycemic episodes."
    b. "With caution, if you are taking an oral hypoglycemic."
    c. "Yes, if you use it as a bread exchange."
    d. "Yes, if consumed between the larger meals."

17. A 22 year old male client on a psychiatric unit is taking trifluoperazine (Stelazine) 10 mg four times per day. He comes to the nurses' station complaining of an inability to sit still and constantly moves his arm while talking to you. The initial action of the nurse would be to:
    a. notify the physician immediately.
    b. administer the PRN antiparkinson drug.
    c. chart that the client has tardive dyskinesia.
    d. take a lying and standing blood pressure.

18. A client is admitted with liver dysfunction. Which of the following nursing orders should be included in the plan of care?
    a. Observe for signs of hyper-albuminemia.
    b. Check for clot formation in extremities.
    c. Drug dosages will typically be lower.
    d. Give lower amounts of fat soluble vitamins.

19. A client is admitted with diarrhea consistent with an infection of the small bowel or ileum. The nurse would expect to assess:
    a. greasy stools.
    b. watery stools.
    c. presence of pus.
    d. presence of oil.

20. A 52 year old male client is admitted for functional neck dissection due to cancer. The client asks what this means. The nurse replies that it is removal of:
    a. lymph nodes.
    b. sternocleidomastoid muscle.
    c. jugular vein.
    d. spinal accessory nerve.

21. A client with a right leg amputation above the knee is learning to transfer from the bed to the wheelchair. The nurse should instruct the client to:
    a. bear all of his body weight on his arms.
    b. stand and pivot until facing the wheelchair.
    c. bear his body weight on his uninjured leg.
    d. stand and pivot until his back is towards the wheelchair.

22. A client is learning how to dress himself in the rehabilitation unit following a cerebral vascular accident. The nurse's approach should be to:
    a. start with gross motor movements practice.
    b. push the client past frustration and fatigue.
    c. allow the client to choose how best to dress.
    d. start by insisting the client self-dress in morning care.

23. An early sign of infection in an older adult would be:
    a. fever.
    b. confusion.
    c. pain.
    d. bradycardia.

24. A 40 year old female client is having a physical examination. What would the nurse expect to be a normal developmental question for this client?
    a. "How do I want to change my life?"
    b. "How do I balance career and family?"
    c. "How can I communicate better with older and younger generations?"
    d. "How do I balance between self and societal needs?"

Situation:
Donna Fuller, 12 years old, is admitted to the pediatric unit because of an asthma attack. She is on oxygen and has an intravenous line with a theophylline (Aminophylline) drip. Donna also has Down's syndrome. (The next two questions refer to this situation.)

25. Donna's condition is stable at present. The physician asks the nurse to teach Donna to use an inhaler. The first part of this process is to:
    a. ask for a return demonstration.
    b. break the procedure into steps.
    c. give Donna a complete overview of the procedure.
    d. reward Donna for each new behavior.

26. That evening the nurse hears a disturbance in Donna's room. She enters the room to find the water pitcher on the floor and blood coming from the arm where the intravenous had been pulled out. Donna is crying and pointing to the bathroom door. The most reasonable explanation is that:
    a. Donna became upset at being alone and couldn't remember how to find the nurse.
    b. Donna is confused due to hypoxia and should be restrained so she cannot injure herself.
    c. Donna is seeking attention for herself through the only way she has probably been rewarded by her parents.
    d. Donna needed to use the bathroom and could not figure out how to get there while attached to the intravenous line.

27. The nurse is performing an assessment in a wellness center. The client is a truck driver who is on the road and away from the family for long periods of time. This data would be documented under which of the following categories?
    a. Maladaptive responses.
    b. Stress consequences.
    c. Coping behavior.
    d. Risk appraisal.

28. A 57 year old client is due to have surgery for resection of a cancerous tumor of the large intestine. The surgery is scheduled for 2 weeks. The client should be instructed on which type of diet?
    a. Clear liquid diet.
    b. General diet as tolerated.
    c. High calorie, low residue diet.
    d. Bland, high protein diet.

29. A six year old girl is recovering from surgery to correct an atrial septal defect. The nurse would suggest which activity at home?
    a. Knitting.
    b. Jumping rope.
    c. Hand puppets.
    d. Pull toy.

30. A nurse notices that other staff members are ordering second meal trays for clients so the nurses don't have to buy lunch. She comments about it to the other nurses who tell her it's common practice and not really stealing. She approaches the head nurse about it but the head nurse has to go to a meeting and says it's probably an isolated incident. The best action of the nurse would be to:

a. go to see the supervisor about the incidents.
b. ask to be transferred to another unit.
c. make an appointment to see the head nurse.
d. ignore the incidents since the head nurse is aware.

STOP You have now completed Practice Session: 18. Now take a few minutes and correct your answers. Calculate your accuracy rate by dividing the number of questions you completed correctly by the total number of questions you completed (30).

Correct answers ÷ total number of questions completed = accuracy rate.

_____ ÷ _____ = _____

ANSWERS AND RATIONALES

1. **The correct answer is b.** If the client's temperature is below normal, the cause should be found if possible. Temperature can fall due to environmental factors, anesthesia or cold food intake. An abnormal temperature finding should result in some action (option a). If the client had something cold, the temperature can be repeated in thirty minutes (option d). Otherwise, it should be repeated immediately. If the same temperature is found, then a different thermometer should be used. If the temperature remains abnormal, then it should be validated by another means (option c) (Perry & Potter, 1986; p. 241).

   Nursing Process: Implementation
   Client Need: Physiological Integrity

2. **The correct answer is d.** The nursing assistant's concern is that he can "catch" something from the client. Centers of Disease Control (CDC) state protective clothing should be used if there is concern of contamination with blood or body fluids which could be true in this case. Writing a report on the nursing assistant (option a) may be needed if he continues to refuse to assist with the client's care. He has already expressed his feelings about the client (option b). Confrontation (option c) will cause defensiveness which may result in further refusal to assist. The nurse should discuss the incident with him once the client is made comfortable (Perry & Potter, 1986; p. 136).

   Nursing Process: Implementation
   Client Need: Safe, Effective Care Environment

3. **The correct answer is d.** The face should be rested to avoid pulling on the suture lines. This includes little talking or chewing. A soft diet is recommended. The client should elevate the head of the bed (option a) when laying down for one week after the surgery. The suture line should not be touched by soap, water (option b) or makeup until fully healed. Hair washing should be avoided for at least 48 hours (option c) after surgery (Black & Matassarin-Jacobs, 1993; p. 2024).

   Nursing Process: Implementation
   Client Need: Physiological Integrity

4. **The correct answer is c.** The husband must put on protective clothing so the client's burns do not become infected by him. Visitors should wash their hands (option d) but that is not enough for protection. Express permission by the physician (option a) is usually unnecessary although the number of visitors is often limited. Visitors are not tested for infection (option b) but will be excluded if they have respiratory or other infections and this plus the rationale should be explained to potential

visitors (Black & Matassarin-Jacobs, 1993; p. 2002).

Nursing Process: Implementation
Client Need: Safe, Effective Care Environment

5. **The correct answer is b.** With cryotherapy, liquid nitrogen is placed on the lesion. No anesthetic is given (option d) but the client should be warned to expect some discomfort (option c). After the nitrogen is applied, blisters will appear (option a). Discomfort can be minimized by applying a warm, wet washcloth to the site at intervals (Black & Matassarin-Jacobs, 1993; pp. 1977-1978).

Nursing Process: Implementation
Client Need: Physiological Integrity

6. **The correct answer is a.** The cane should be placed on the side opposite to the problem leg (option b). The problem leg and the cane should move together (option c) while the unaffected leg bears the weight. This way, when the unaffected leg is off the floor, the problem leg is assisted by the cane to bear weight. The cane should be picked up from the floor and moved (option d) so any obstacles are avoided (Black & Matassarin-Jacobs, 1993; p. 1898).

Nursing Process: Implementation
Client Need: Physiological Integrity

7. **The correct answer is d.** The best way to assess hip muscle strength is to ask the client to use those muscles by pushing against the nurse's hand. Option (a) tests hamstring muscles.

Option (b) tests quadricep muscles. Option (c) tests foot and ankle muscles (Black & Matassarin-Jacobs, 1993; p. 1876).

Nursing Process: Analysis
Client Need: Physiological Integrity

8. **The correct answer is c.** The client should be taught to deep breathe (option a) to expand lungs and prevent pneumonia. However, the client should not cough, sneeze, or blow the nose because these actions can cause misplacement of the graft which protects the brain. Misplacement can cause a leak in cerebrospinal fluid or can allow an entryway for bacteria. Talking (option b) and swallowing ice (option d) are not contraindicated in this type of surgery (Black & Matassarin-Jacobs, 1993; pp. 1855-1856).

Nursing Process: Implementation
Client Need: Safe, Effective Care Environment

9. **The correct answer is d.** Maintaining tissue perfusion is important to keep adequate oxygenation of tissues so tissue death does not occur. Medication administration (option a) and wound care (option c) are also important but will not be necessary if adequate tissue perfusion is not maintained. Signs of infection (option b) should be monitored but would happen later and would not be an early consideration (Smeltzer & Bare, 1992; p. 710).

Nursing Process: Analysis
Client Need: Physiological Integrity

10. **The correct answer is c.** The tissue walls are sensitive and easily torn. A tube has been introduced into the colon and, although the tube is flexible, perforation could occur. Signs of bowel perforation include bleeding from the rectum, pain and fever. Intestinal obstruction (option a) is not known to be a complication of colonoscopy. Hypothermia (option b) and electrolyte imbalance (option d) can be complications of the preparation for colonoscopy since the bowel must be emptied of any contents through enemas and laxatives (Smeltzer & Bare, 1992; p. 837).

Nursing Process: Analysis
Client Need: Physiological Integrity

11. **The correct answer is b.** Furosemide (Lasix) is a diuretic (option c) that does not conserve potassium. Long term use of furosemide (Lasix) can cause hypokalemia. Signs and symptoms of hypokalemia are the result of systemic muscular weakness. Respiratory muscular weakness leads to shallow ineffective breathing and decreased breath sounds. Cardiovascular changes include a rapid thready pulse (options a and d), postural hypotension and electrocardiograph (EKG) changes. Neuromuscular changes to expect are lethargy, irritability, confusion, coma, hyporeflexia and flaccid paralysis. Gastrointestinal effects are nausea, vomiting, abdominal distention, constipation (option a) and paralytic ileus (Ignatavicius & Bayne, 1991; pp. 269-270).

Nursing Process: Evaluation
Client Need: Physiological Integrity

12. **The correct answer is b.** When a group member is silent and the group is upset about it, a cohesive group will confront the behavior of the silent member. Feedback to keep the group steadily working towards its goal is usually taken on by group members. Meeting for lunch outside of group times (option a) shows connectedness and support within the group. Newer members will be accepted but comments will not be taken as seriously (option c) by the older members. Newer members must first show their willingness to learn about the group before being totally accepted as an equal partner in the work. Stating their group is better than others (option d) shows loyalty to the group (Haber, Leach-McMahon, Price-Hoskins & Sideleau, 1992; p. 339).

Nursing Process: Evaluation
Client Need: Safe, Effective Care Environment

13. **The correct answer is c.** The temperature is recorded every day on a graph (option a) so it is easier to visualize and is more accurately predictable. Temperature should be taken immediately upon awakening (option b) before any other activity (smoking, voiding) which could cause a difference in temperature. Intercourse (option d) should be avoided the day immediately before and day of the temperature rise as well as three days afterward (Olds, London & Ladewig, 1992; p. 176).

Nursing Process: Implementation
Client Need: Health Promotion & Maintenance

14. **The correct answer is d.** Lifestyle, personal attitudes, religious beliefs and future plans are all factors in a woman's choice for contraception. The nurse should first assess these areas before doing any teaching. Most women change their method of contraceptive (option a) based on preferences, lifestyle and future childbearing plans. Future plans are important because some contraceptive methods could cause problems that may interfere with childbearing later such as an intrauterine device (IUD) which may cause pelvic inflammatory disease or a tubal ligation which is usually irreversible (option b). Every method is not equally effective in preventing conception (option c). For example, spermicidal creams and foams have limited effectiveness (Olds, London & Ladewig, 1992; pp. 182-184).

Nursing Process: Implementation
Client Need: Health Promotion & Maintenance

15. **The correct answer is b.** The client's environment should be humidified with cool air to decrease any swelling and to keep the throat moistened. Fluids should be encouraged up to three liters per day (option a) so secretions can be more easily expectorated. Peritonsillar abscess (option c) is not necessarily present with chronic laryngitis. Bedrest (option d) may be true for acute laryngitis but unnecessary for chronic laryngitis (Smeltzer & Bare, 1992; p. 486).

Nursing Process: Planning
Client Need: Physiological Integrity

16. **The correct answer is b.** Oral hypoglycemics may react with alcohol to produce nausea, vomiting, headache, hot flush, sweating and thirst. The client should be cautioned about this reaction. Alcohol can cause hypoglycemia (option a) especially if it is consumed on an empty stomach (option d). Clients should be cautioned that it is even more important to eat the prescribed diet and not eliminate breads (option c) so that hypoglycemia does not occur (Smeltzer & Bare, 1992; p. 1029).

Nursing Process: Implementation
Client Need: Physiological Integrity

17. **The correct answer is b.** The client is demonstrating symptoms of akathesia which is a side effect of antipsychotic medications. Trifluoperazine (Stelazine) has a high incidence of extrapyramidal symptoms such as akathesia and dystonia. The common treatment is to administer an antiparkinsonian drug such as benzotropine mesylate (Cogentin) or a muscle relaxant such as diazepam (Valium). The physician should be notified (option a) but it is not an emergency and can be charted and the physician informed when he next makes rounds. Tardive dyskinesia (option c) is a side effect evident after long term use of antipsychotic medication. Symptoms may include chewing motions and lip smacking. Lying and standing blood pressures (option d) should be done routinely since postural hypotension is a side effect of most antipsychotic medications. Symptoms would include dizziness and unsteadiness (Varcarolis, 1990; pp. 510-511).

Nursing Process: Implementation
Client Need: Psychosocial Integrity

18. **The correct answer is c.** Liver dysfunction would include a problem with metabolizing drugs in the liver and the drugs will accumulate in the system. Therefore, a lowered dose of drugs is necessary to avoid overdosing the client. The client will have hypoalbuminemia (option a) due to decreased ability of the liver to produce albumin. Clotting factors are reduced in the system due to dysfunction of liver so evidence of bleeding, not clots (option b), would be necessary. Fat soluble vitamins (option d) are not absorbed as well since bile salts are not released (Smeltzer & Bare, 1992; p. 985).

Nursing Process: Planning
Client Need: Physiological Integrity

19. **The correct answer is b.** Watery stools indicate small bowel disease since fluid is not absorbed. Greasy stools (option a) indicate intestinal malabsorption. Pus (option c) indicates an inflammatory response seen in enteritis or colitis. Oil (option d) indicates pancreatic problems (Smeltzer & Bare, 1992; p. 922).

Nursing Process: Assessment
Client Need: Physiological Integrity

20. **The correct answer is a.** A functional or modified dissection includes the lymph nodes only. Removal of sternocleidomastoid muscle (option b), jugular vein (option c) and spinal accessory nerve (option d) as well as lymph nodes would occur in a radical neck dissection (Smeltzer & Bare, 1992; p. 855).

Nursing Process: Implementation
Client Need: Physiological Integrity

21. **The correct answer is d.** The client should stand on his uninjured leg and help balance himself with his arms (options a and c). The client should then pivot so the back side is toward the wheelchair (option b) and then sit down. If the client's front side faces the wheelchair, the client will still need to turn around again before sitting. This approach leaves more room for imbalance and requires more time and energy (Smeltzer & Bare, 1992; p. 231).

Nursing Process: Planning
Client Need: Physiological Integrity

22. **The correct answer is a.** Start with gross motor movements like putting arms through armholes. The next move would be to progress to finer motor movements such as buttons. The client should be monitored for signs of frustration and fatigue. He should be encouraged and supported but not pushed (option b). The client should have input into how best to dress but the approach likely to foster success (option c) is to allow the client to practice the movements of getting dressed with help and slowly progress toward independent function (option d) (Smeltzer & Bare, 1992; p. 220).

Nursing Process: Planning
Client Need: Health Promotion & Maintenance

23. **The correct answer is b.** Usual signs of infection such as fever (option a) are not seen or appear later in the infectious process. Other signs of infection would include tachycardia (option d), increased respirations and difference in skin color and facial expression. Pain response (option c) is often delayed and may

show itself first through other symptoms (Smeltzer & Bare, 1992; p. 192).

Nursing Process: Analysis
Client Need: Physiological Integrity

24. **The correct answer is a.** Midlife transition occurs between 35-45 years. During this time a major task is examining present lifestyle, its meaning and if changes are needed. Balancing career and family (option b) usually occurs as part of the transition into the adult world, ages 22 to 28 years. Communicating better with older and younger generations (option c) generally is a task of middle adulthood, ages 45-50 years. Balancing between personal desires and societal needs usually occurs around retirement during late adulthood transition, ages 60 to 65 years (Smeltzer & Bare, 1992; pp. 156-162).

Nursing Process: Analysis
Client Need: Health Promotion & Maintenance

25. **The correct answer is b.** Clients who are mentally retarded can learn to be independent in self-care activities. The first step is to break the procedure to be taught into small segments which can be taught and reinforced easily. A complete overview of the procedure (option c) could be hard to comprehend and prove overwhelming to the client. Breaking it into segments makes the task more manageable. For each new behavior taught, a return demonstration (option a) should be asked to check the client's understanding and recall of the teaching. Then a positive reward

(option d) such as praise or hugging should be given to reinforce progress (Marlow & Redding, 1988; pp. 978-979).

Nursing Process: Planning
Client Need: Physiological Integrity

26. **The correct answer is d.** Donna is in a new place and has an intravenous line which inhibits movement. Hospitalizations are problematic for most people and problem solving skills may be impaired and regressive behavior patterns may emerge. This client was trying to get to the bathroom but couldn't figure out how to do it while attached to the intravenous and could not summon help. There is no evidence to suggest she feels alone (option a) or is seeking attention (option c). There is also no evidence of hypoxia and further restraint will cause anxiety and may result in injury (option b) (Marlow & Redding, 1988; p. 976).

Nursing Process: Analysis
Client Need: Physiological Integrity

27. **The correct answer is d.** Health risk appraisal assesses those areas which may potentially cause problems. Work and driving habits are lifestyle factors which can be a source of problems depending on the individual. Maladaptive responses (option a), stress consequences (option b) and coping behaviors (option c) would occur as a result of the driving and work circumstances. These might include hypertension, arthritis, depression, anxiety, migraines, drug addiction, gastrointestinal symptoms,

etc. (Smeltzer & Bare, 1992; pp. 122-125).

Nursing Process: Analysis
Client Need: Health Promotion & Maintenance

28. **The correct answer is c.** Prior to colon surgery a client is placed on a high calorie, low residue diet to provide high energy reserves with little bulk in the colon. Clear liquid diet (option a) would deprive the body of needed calories. General diet as tolerated (option b) is promoted post-operatively as soon as possible. A high protein diet (option d) would promote wound healing post-operatively. A bland diet may be used for upper gastrointestinal disorders such as peptic or duodenal ulcers (Smeltzer & Bare, 1992; pp. 780-781, 835-836).

Nursing Process: Planning
Client Need: Physiological Integrity

29. **The correct answer is c.** This is a quiet activity which matches the ability of a six year old child. It is a diversional activity that can be started or stopped without much effort and results in a project which builds self-esteem. Option (a) would be appropriate for an older age child. Option (b) is too active for a child recovering from this type of surgery. It increases the oxygen needs and therefore increases the cardiac workload. Option (d) would be appropriate for an eighteen month old child (Marlow & Redding, 1988; pp. 476, 727, 1007, 1131).

Nursing Process: Implementation
Client Need: Physiological Integrity

30. **The correct answer is c.** The nurse approached the head nurse when she was busy and had to attend a meeting. The nurse should make an appointment to see the head nurse when there will be time to discuss the incident properly and neither party is rushed. Going to the supervisor (option a) might be necessary if the nurse is not satisfied with the meeting with the head nurse. Transferring to another unit (option b) and ignoring the situation (option d) do nothing to remedy the situation (Joiner & Corkrean, 1986; pp. 92-93).

Nursing Process: Implementation
Client Need: Safe, Effective Care Environment

PRACTICE SESSION: 19

Instructions:

Allow yourself 30 minutes to complete the following 30 practice questions. Use a timer to notify yourself when 30 minutes are over so that you are not constantly looking at your watch while completing the questions.

1. A nurse is in a movie theater when an adult male starts choking. His wife starts yelling for help. The nurse should:
   a. make a fist and push it into the client's midsection.
   b. stand behind the man and place fist into the area above the navel.
   c. find the xiphoid process and place the heel of the hand against it forcefully.
   d. lay the victim on the floor and begin with ventilation and chest compression.

2. A client returns to the unit after having a cystoscopy under local anesthesia. The client calls the nurse and asks if he can go to the bathroom. The best reply would be:
   a. "Yes, but remember to measure the urine output."
   b. "Yes, but report any burning or pink-tinged urine."
   c. "No, because you may be weak or dizzy."
   d. "No, you must stay on bedrest."

3. A local community is considering water fluoridation. The nurse testifies that water fluoridation:
   a. may cause overdose in preschool children.
   b. acts as a barrier to bacteria.
   c. guards against acid from sugar breakdown.
   d. is not needed for most adults.

4. A 79 year old female is admitted for possible pacemaker insertion due to sinus bradycardia. The nurse explains that sinus bradycardia in older adults is often related to:
   a. increased lipid accumulation.
   b. atherosclerosis.
   c. fewer pacemaker cells.
   d. decreased arterial wall flexibility.

5. A 27 year old client is about to undergo a bone marrow aspiration. The client asks the nurse if the test will be painful. The best response of the nurse would be:
   a. "No, a local anesthetic is given before the procedure."
   b. "No, you should only feel pressure."
   c. "Yes, but only during the aspiration."
   d. "Yes just a pinprick when the needle is inserted."

6. A client is admitted to the psychiatric unit in a manic episode. She talks loudly and rapidly to anyone who will listen to her. She blasts the radio and starts jogging down the hallway threatening to "mow down anyone who gets in my way." In planning care for this client, the nurse recognizes that:
   a. she must set firm limits on the client's use of the radio.
   b. a quiet area is needed to decrease stimulation.
   c. ignoring this behavior will allow the client to become distracted.
   d. involvement in a group exercise program will utilize her excess energy.

7. A client is admitted to the hospital. At the bath the next morning a rash is found in skin folds. The physician diagnoses scabies. What precautions on the unit should be taken?
   a. All clients and unit staff should be treated.
   b. All people having physical contact with the client should be treated.
   c. Only sexual partners should be treated.
   d. Anyone touching the client's personal items should be treated.

8. A client has just been placed on humidified oxygen by nasal cannula. The best way to check effectiveness of the oxygen therapy is to check for:
   a. decreased consciousness level.
   b. decreased respiratory rate.
   c. increased pulse.
   d. increased color.

9. The nurse is delivering a community inservice on how to prevent Lyme disease. She tells the group to:
   a. limit high purine foods in the diet.
   b. keep wood piles close to the house.
   c. keep pets off the furniture.
   d. use energy conservation techniques.

10. A female client calls the clinic and states she is upset over finding nipple discharge during her breast self exam. Which of the following nipple discharges might be related to breast cancer?
    a. green.
    b. milky-watery.
    c. yellow.
    d. pink-serous.

11. A client has just delivered an infant girl by spontaneous vaginal delivery and is admitted to the post-partum unit. She states she needs to urinate and is assisted to the bathroom. She complains that she passed several large clots and questions if this is normal. The nurse suspects a postpartal hemorrhage. The nurse would also assess for:
    a. high blood pressure, low grade temperature.
    b. backache, low grade temperature.
    c. excessive bright red bleeding, high blood pressure.
    d. high temperature, boggy fundus.

12. The initial goal of diabetic education for a client newly diagnosed with insulin dependent diabetes mellitus is:
    a. the client will demonstrate how to administer insulin.
    b. the client will demonstrate how to do daily foot care.
    c. the client will state the importance of exercise in managing diabetes.
    d. the client will plan a daily menu to prevent complications of the disease.

13. The nurse is caring for a client who had a cerebrovascular accident (CVA). The nurse would document self-awareness under which neurological assessment category?
    a. Consciousness.
    b. Mentation.
    c. Movement.
    d. Sensation.

14. A client is to undergo laser surgery to remove the gall bladder. The client asks the nurse how the gall bladder is removed. The nurse responds that the gall bladder is removed by:
    a. using the laser to cut the organ into pieces that are absorbed into the system and discarded.
    b. severing it from the body with the laser and removing it by forceps through small incisions.
    c. pulling it through an incision made over the position of the gall bladder.
    d. freezing the severed organ and pulling it out in pieces.

15. A client comes to the emergency room after slitting his wrists, stating he has changed his mind. One wrist is superficially cut but the second wrist is bleeding profusely. The nurse applies a pressure dressing. The nurse should also:
    a. bandage the other wrist.
    b. monitor vital signs every 30 minutes.
    c. replace the dressing if seepage occurs.
    d. elevate the arm with the pressure dressing.

16. The physician notes that a client is highly anxious and has decided to place him on medication. Which of the following medications would the nurse expect to be ordered?
    a. Alprazolam (Xanax).
    b. Clomipramine (Anafranil).
    c. Doxepin (Sinequan).
    d. Propanolol (Inderal).

17. An 82 year old woman is admitted to the hospital after contracting peritonitis from a ruptured appendix. Her son asks why she waited so long to get help. The nurse responds that:
    a. older adults may not feel pain due to compromised pain receptors.
    b. the client may have been afraid she would die in the hospital.
    c. it must be difficult when observing a loved one go through a serious illness.
    d. she probably misinterpreted the pain due to organic brain changes.

18. A client is admitted with acute upper gastrointestinal hemorrhage. The nurse might clarify which of the following orders with the physician?
    a. Urinary catheter to straight drain.
    b. Prepare for angiography.
    c. Complete blood count.
    d. Barium contrast x-ray.

19. A nurse is performing a physical assessment on a client with suspected lymph system problems. The correct way to assess for lymph node enlargement would be:
    a. softly rolling the skin with the index and third fingers.
    b. firm palpation of superficial lymph node areas.
    c. application of pressure to axillary and inguinal areas.
    d. usually palpated if the client complains of tenderness.

20. The nurse recognizes that the teaching about myasthenia gravis has been effective when the client states,
    a. "I'll stay on a full liquid diet."
    b. "I'll enjoy playing basketball."
    c. "I'll program rest periods at work."
    d. "I'll increase medication during stressful periods."

21. A nursing assistant asks you why a client with organic mental disorder strikes out when he is asked if he's ready to bathe or change clothes. The best response would be:
    a. "He feels exposed and vulnerable without his clothes."
    b. "He's unaware of the need to bathe."
    c. "He probably never bathed this often."
    d. "He reacts this way to unexpected demands on him by strangers."

22. Betsy, 5 years old, is in the burn unit. She becomes confused and pulls on the tubes. The physician orders oxygen and Betsy is placed in soft wrist restraints while she is confused. Her father comes to visit and questions the use of restraints on his daughter. The best reply of the nurse would be:
    a. "Betsy was pulling out her tubes. We don't want to have to replace them."
    b. "Betsy is a little confused right now. When she falls asleep the restraints can be removed."
    c. "Betsy was having some problems that caused a little confusion and she was pulling on her tubes. The treatment will correct it quickly and we'll remove the restraints."
    d. "Betsy was trying to remove her tubes. Now that you're here, you can watch her for me and the restraints can come off."

23. A client suffered a fractured mandible in a car accident and has his jaws wired until the mandible heals. Wire cutters are placed at the bedside along with a picture of the wires to be cut. The nurse plans to cut the wires:
   a. if the client has a respiratory infection.
   b. only on orders of the physician.
   c. only if respiratory arrest occurs.
   d. after seven weeks of healing.

24. A client is being discharged after an induced abortion. Which of the following discharge instructions should be given by the nurse?
   a. Thoughts of depression are abnormal and should be reported to the physician.
   b. Douching is permitted after one week.
   c. The client should return for a checkup in two weeks.
   d. A post-abortion pregnancy test should be negative.

25. Pam Kline is a 22 year old woman who has developed iatrogenic Cushing's syndrome secondary to her long term therapy on prednisone (Deltasone). The prednisone (Deltasone) is used as an additional immunosuppressant for her liver transplant of four years ago. Which of the following observations by the nurse warrants immediate attention?
   a. Blood pressure 132/82.
   b. Oral temperature 38.9°C (102°F).
   c. Labile affect.
   d. Complaint of severe stomach pain that dissipates when she eats.

26. The nurse is checking an electrocardiogram tracing of a newly admitted client. An electrolyte imbalance would probably be observed in:
   a. the QT interval.
   b. the PR interval.
   c. the QRS complex.
   d. the PQRS interval.

27. In assessing a male client for secondary erectile dysfunction the nurse would ask:
   a. if he has ever been able to have a satisfactory erection.
   b. what medications he is presently taking.
   c. his knowledge of how to do a testicular self-examination.
   d. if he knows any qualified sex therapists.

28. A Native American client is visiting from another city. She goes into labor and is brought to the nearest hospital. This client would probably feel more comfortable if:
   a. her husband assists her through the delivery.
   b. she wears a long sleeved robe and a surgical cap.
   c. only females are in attendance at the birth.
   d. she drinks warm fluids during labor.

29. A client had surgery and the nurse is preparing to irrigate the wound and change the dressing as ordered by the physician. Before irrigating with the antiseptic solution, the nurse should:
   a. remove the dressing and discard it in a small paper bag.
   b. give the client the prescribed analgesic 15 minutes before removing the dressing.
   c. go to the chart and check the client's allergy sheet.
   d. wash hands, don gloves, remove old dressing and proceed with wound irrigation.

30. A nurse being interviewed for a job asks to see the mission and philosophy of the hospital because:
   a. these define the aims and values of the hospital.
   b. they operationalize the hospital's functions.
   c. these statements comprise the hospital's plan.
   d. they state specific actions to be taken.

STOP You have now completed Practice Session: 19. Now take a few minutes and correct your answers. Calculate your accuracy rate by dividing the number of questions you completed correctly by the total number of questions you completed (30).

Correct answers ÷ total number of questions completed = accuracy rate.

_____ ÷ _____ = _____

ANSWERS AND RATIONALES

1. **The correct answer is b.** If the client is unable to dislodge the object, the nurse should perform the Heimlich maneuver. The nurse should stand behind the victim (option a), place her hands around the victim, place the fist (thumb-side towards the victim) into the middle of the area above the navel and below the bottom of the xiphoid process, and make several thrusts up and in until the foreign body is expelled (option c). Ventilation (option d) will be ineffective while the foreign body is present (Lewis & Collier, 1992; pp. 875-877).

   Nursing Process: Implementation
   Client Need: Safe, Effective Care Environment

2. **The correct answer is c.** The client may experience episodes of orthostatic hypotension after the cystoscopy. Therefore, the client should have assistance until effects of all anesthesia have elapsed (options a and d). The client should not be up without assistance (option b). Burning on urination and pink-tinged urine are expected after surgery and should be documented (Lewis & Collier, 1992; p. 1180).

   Nursing Process: Implementation
   Client Need: Physiological Integrity

3. **The correct answer is c.** Fluoride acts by helping the tooth enamel be less likely to be affected by acid produced from the interaction between sugar and bacteria (option b), thus reducing the chance of decay and infection. The usual dose of one part fluoride per million in the community's drinking water will not cause overdose in children (option a) but will help protect adults (option d) as well (Lewis & Collier, 1992; p. 981).

   Nursing Process: Implementation
   Client Need: Health Promotion & Maintenance

4. **The correct answer is c.** Age-related changes that may cause bradycardia include a decrease in pacemaker cells, fibrosis and some calcification of the conduction system. Increased lipid accumulation (option a), atherosclerosis (option b) and decreased arterial wall flexibility (option d) due to decreased elastin are all age-related changes but do not cause sinus bradycardia (Lewis & Collier, 1992; pp. 721-722).

   Nursing Process: Analysis
   Client Need: Physiological Integrity

5. **The correct answer is c.** The area at the iliac crest is anesthetized where the needle is inserted so discomfort there is minimized (options a and d). The needle is inserted into the marrow and a syringe is attached. The marrow is then

aspirated. During aspiration, the client usually feels a pulling type of intense pain which lasts a few seconds (option b). The needle is removed and pressure is applied to stop bleeding (Lewis & Collier, 1992; p. 662).

Nursing Process: Implementation
Client Need: Physiological Integrity

6. **The correct answer is b.** The nurse needs to help control the client's environment. Manic clients are easily overstimulated by lighting, noise level and other people. This client needs to be removed from the stimulating environment to prevent threatening and aggressive behavior. Manic clients can not often tolerate activity that is highly structured or competitive (option d). Setting limits is appropriate for this client; however, controlling only one aspect of the environment (the radio) will not decrease stimulation enough for compliance (option a). Ignoring the client's behavior (option c) will only create increased stimulation and possibly exhaustion (Haber, Leach-McMahon, Price-Hoskins & Sideleau, 1992; pp. 590-594; Stuart & Sundeen, 1991; p. 447).

Nursing Process: Planning
Client Need: Psychosocial Integrity

7. **The correct answer is b.** Scabies is transmitted by direct personal contact and seldom by contact with the client's personal items (option d). Since all clients or unit staff did not have direct personal contact (option a), they do not all need treatment. Sexual partners (option c) should be treated but are not the only people to be treated (Lewis &

Collier, 1992; p. 391).

Nursing Process: Implementation
Client Need: Safe, Effective Care Environment

8. **The correct answer is b.** When oxygen therapy is effective, then signs of hypoxia are decreased. Decreased hypoxia includes decreased respirations because the body doesn't have to breathe as fast to try and bring in extra oxygen. Other signs include lowered anxiety level, increased level of consciousness (option a), decreased pulse since the heart doesn't have to beat as fast to distribute the little oxygen in the system (option c), normal blood pressure and improved color (option d). Increased color could also mean increased blue which is a sign of hypoxia (Perry & Potter, 1986; p.391).

Nursing Process: Evaluation
Client Need: Physiological Integrity

9. **The correct answer is c.** Pets should wear flea and tick collars and be kept off furniture to decrease transmission of the tick that causes Lyme disease. High purine foods are limited (option a) in treatment of gouty arthritis. Energy conservation measures (option d) are used in nursing care of clients with systemic lupus erythematosis. Wood piles (option b) should be away from the house so the ticks don't become transmitted into the house (Lewis & Collier, 1992; pp. 1738, 1746).

Nursing Process: Implementation
Client Need: Health Promotion & Maintenance

10. **The correct answer is d.** Serous or any bloody discharge may be related to breast cancer although there are also benign disorders which cause bloody discharge such as intraductal papilloma. Yellow (option c), watery-milky (option b) and green (option a) discharge may be related to fibrocystic disease (Lewis & Collier, 1992; pp. 1382-1383).

Nursing Process: Analysis
Client Need: Physiological Integrity

11. **The correct answer is d.** Blood pressure changes may not be an early indicator of hemorrhage; however, if it did not change, it would be decreased due to lack of blood (options a and c). First the temperature raises rapidly with hemorrhage (options a and b). The fundus would also be boggy from inability to involute. Backaches would be caused from a large infant which puts the uterus at risk not to involute totally or may contribute to uterine atony (Ladewig, London & Olds, 1990; pp. 797, 799).

Nursing Process: Assessment
Client Need: Physiological Integrity

12. **The correct answer is a.** The American Diabetes Association recommends a three level approach to diabetic education. The first level includes those measures to ensure the daily survival of the client such as insulin administration. The second level deals with home management after some experience is gained in living with the disease (option d). Level three consists of life style changes (options b and c) (Lewis & Collier, 1992; pp. 1313-1314).

Nursing Process: Planning
Client Need: Physiological Integrity

13. **The correct answer is a.** Self-awareness and arousal would be documented under consciousness. Mentation (option b) would include areas such as thinking, language and problem-solving. Speaking and walking would belong in the movement category (option c). Smelling, touching and hearing would be areas related to sensation (option d) (Lewis & Collier, 1992; p. 1491).

Nursing Process: Implementation
Client Need: Physiological Integrity

14. **The correct answer is b.** Small incisions are made at several places in the abdomen for instruments such as a laproscope with camera, forceps and laser. The camera guides the surgery. The laser severs the gall bladder and cuts it into pieces. It is then pulled through the small incisions with forceps (option a). Option (c) describes traditional gall bladder surgery. Freezing (option d) occurs in cryosurgery (Lewis & Collier, 1992; p. 1160).

Nursing Process: Implementation
Client Need: Physiological Integrity

15. **The correct answer is d.** Once the pressure dressing is applied, elevate the affected extremity to decrease the blood supply going to the extremity, thus slowing the flow of blood. The other wrist would need to be bandaged (option a) but the priority is to stop the bleeding of the more serious wound. Vital signs (option b) should be

monitored every 15 minutes for this type of injury. Once the pressure dressing is applied, it should not be removed to replace it (option c) but may be reinforced (Perry & Potter, 1986; pp. 1069-1070).

Nursing Process: Implementation
Client Need: Safe, Effective Care Environment

16. **The correct answer is a.** Alprazolam (Xanax) is an antianxiety medication used for clients in panic levels of anxiety. Clomipramine (Anafranil) is a tricyclic antidepressant medication used primarily for obsessive-compulsive disorder. Doxepin (Sinequan) is a tricyclic antidepressant medication used in treatment for depression. Propanolol (Inderal) is a beta-blocker which may be used to prevent social phobia (Cook & Fontaine, 1991; pp. 132, 307).

Nursing Process: Analysis
Client Need: Psychosocial Integrity

17. **The correct answer is a.** Transmission in pain reception is compromised in older adults so they may take longer to recognize pain and act on it. Fear of dying in the hospital (option b) and organic brain changes causing misinterpretation of pain signals (option d) may be true but there is no assessment data offered to support either option. The client's son may have difficulty watching his mother's illness (option c) but this is not the point of the question (Lewis & Collier, 1992; p. 1502).

Nursing Process: Implementation
Client Need: Physiological Integrity

18. **The correct answer is d.** A barium contrast x-ray may show areas of lesion but will not show which area is bleeding. A urinary catheter (option a) will show kidney function which relates to fluid and electrolyte balance. Angiography (option b) will be useful in pinpointing the area of hemorrhage. Complete blood count (option c) shows the level of blood loss and dehydration (Lewis & Collier, 1992; pp. 1044-1045).

Nursing Process: Implementation
Client Need: Physiological Integrity

19. **The correct answer is a.** Lymph nodes generally are not able to be palpated unless an infections process has occurred. However, all lymph areas are palpated during a physical examination to rule out problems (option d). Areas where lymph nodes are found in the body should be softly palpated with the fingertips of the index and third fingers (options b and c) to check for tenderness and enlargement (Lewis & Collier, 1992; p. 655).

Nursing Process: Assessment
Client Need: Physiological Integrity

20. **The correct answer is c.** Rest periods should be programmed as part of the daily routine so fatigue is not overwhelming. A liquid (option a) or very chewy diet may cause problems with fatigue or possible aspiration because a concentrated effort is needed during meal times. Often medications are timed so they can reach peak action during stressful periods like mealtime but should not be increased without the physician's order (option d). Diversional activities and hobbies should

conserve energy. Basketball (option b) would expend a large amount of energy (Lewis & Collier, 1992; p. 1606).

Nursing Process: Evaluation
Client Need: Physiological Integrity

21. **The correct answer is a.** Clients with organic mental disorders are somewhat aware of what is happening. Undressing and bathing with assistance make the client aware of his inability to perform these basic tasks on his own. Options (b), (c) and (d) do not focus on the dynamics in organic disorders (Haber, Leach-McMahon, Price-Hoskins and Sideleau, 1992; p. 607).

Nursing Process: Analysis
Client Need: Psychosocial Integrity

22. **The correct answer is c.** Parents and children should have explanation of the reasons for restraints since it can be frightening to them. Option (c) explains why restraints are necessary and approximately when they will be removed. Option (a) is true but does not give reasons for the child's behavior which would assist the parents to understand the reason for the restraints. Option (b) is incorrect because falling asleep doesn't necessarily mean restraints can be removed since the child may still attempt to pull on the tubes. Option (d) is incorrect because it implies that the restraints would not be necessary if the nurse would be properly supervising the child (Marlow & Redding, 1988; p. 280).

Nursing Process: Implementation
Client Need: Safe, Effective Care Environment

23. **The correct answer is c.** The only reasons to cut the wires would be respiratory and cardiac arrest (options a and b). Other conditions such as choking or vomiting can be controlled through suction or nasogastric tubes. Cutting the wires poses problems and should only be done in an emergency situation because wire fragments can cause aspiration and respiratory problems. Mandibular fractures heal very quickly and wiring is usually released in four to five weeks (option d) (Lewis & Collier, 1992; p. 989).

Nursing Process: Planning
Client Need: Safe, Effective Care Environment

24. **The correct answer is c.** Clients are usually taught to return for post-procedure examination in two weeks. A post-abortion pregnancy test may still be positive up to two weeks after the procedure (option d). Douching (option b), sex, and tampon use should be avoided until after the post-procedure visit. Depression (option a) is normal after the procedure but should be monitored (Lewis & Collier, 1992; pp. 1424-1425).

Nursing Process: Implementation
Client Need: Physiological Integrity

25. **The correct answer is b.** Because this client is on immunosuppressant therapy, the additional immunosuppression caused by Cushing's syndrome makes the client vulnerable to microorganisms of all types. An elevated temperature is a clear indication of a possible life threatening infection in this client. Cushing's syndrome causes an increase

in the blood pressure; however, this reading is not severely elevated and the infectious process is the priority (option a). Mood swings are an expected symptom of Cushing's syndrome (option c). Stomach pain that is relieved by eating is an indication of a peptic ulcer, a symptom of Cushing's disorder; however, it is not the priority for this client (option d) (Black & Matassarin-Jacobs, 1993; pp. 1842-1847).

Nursing Process: Analysis
Client Need: Physiological Integrity

26. **The correct answer is a.** Electrolyte disturbances are usually evident in the QT interval when repolarization occurs. The PR interval (option b) often demonstrates a conduction problem with the AV node. The QRS complex (option c) demonstrates conduction problems in the bundle branch or ventricles. The PQRS interval (option d) is a mixed measurement not usually performed but would not indicate electrolyte problems (Lewis & Collier, 1992; p. 854).

Nursing Process: Analysis
Client Need: Physiological Integrity

27. **The correct answer is b.** Medications may affect the functioning during erections so this data may provide a clue towards the problem and would be one part of assessment. Since the client has secondary erectile dysfunction, this means he has been able to attain erection in the past and the dysfunction has limited the client's ability to attain erection now (option a). Testicular self-examination is important but knowledge of how to do the exam (option c) is not relevant. However, if the client has performed the exam, when it was done and if findings were normal or abnormal might be significant. Sex therapists (option d) may be needed but not until physical causes have been ruled out (Lewis & Collier, 1992; p. 1463).

Nursing Process: Assessment
Client Need: Physiological Integrity

28. **The correct answer is c.** Many Native American women believe that birth is "women's work" in which modesty must be preserved. They often feel more comfortable only if female attendants such as female nurses, aides and physicians are present during labor and birth. The husband assisting during delivery (option a) may be true for western culture. A long-sleeved gown or robe and a cap (option b) may be true for orthodox Jewish women who believe elbows, knees and hair are private parts of the body. Warm fluids during labor (option d) may be true for Vietnamese women (Olds, London & Ladewig, 1992; pp. 659).

Nursing Process: Planning
Client Need: Health Promotion & Maintenance

29. **The correct answer is c.** An antiseptic irrigation solution is ordered which means a medication is being given to irrigate the wound. The allergy sheet should be checked to ensure the client is not allergic to the antiseptic solution. Then the nurse should wash hands, don gloves, remove the dressing and discard it in a leakproof bag (option a). Soiled gloves should be discarded before

irrigation is continued (option d). The client should be medicated at least 30 minutes before the procedure (option b). Fifteen minutes is insufficient time for the medication to provide pain relief (Perry & Potter, 1986; pp. 1128-1129).

Nursing Process: Implementation
Client Need: Physiological Integrity

30. **The correct answer is a.** The mission states the purpose of an organization and the philosophy states the beliefs and values of that organization. A nurse may examine them to decide if that nurse's philosophy is compatible with the hospital's philosophy so that value clashes do not arise later. Statements that operationalize the function (option b) are goals. Statements that comprise a plan (option c) are policies. Statements that specify actions (option d) are rules (Marquis & Huston, 1992; pp. 45, 47, 52, 56).

Nursing Process: Analysis
Client Need: Safe, Effective Care Environment

PRACTICE SESSION: 20

Instructions:

Allow yourself 30 minutes to complete the following 30 practice questions. Use a timer to notify yourself when 30 minutes are over so that you are not constantly looking at your watch while completing the questions.

Situation:

A 25 year old man is brought by ambulance to the emergency room. He is strapped to the stretcher but is fighting against the restraints and shouting incoherently. He is accompanied by his live-in girlfriend. She reports that he seemed fine until he took some pills that he had purchased that afternoon. (The next two questions refer to this situation.)

1. The highest priority nursing action on this client's arrival in the emergency room is to:
   a. give syrup of ipecac.
   b. take his vital signs.
   c. start intravenous fluids.
   d. administer sedative medication.

2. The physician has ordered gastric lavage for the client. The best position for the client would be:
   a. supine with head turned toward the side.
   b. prone with head turned toward the side.
   c. reverse Trendelenburg.
   d. sidelying with head down.

3. A nurse has introduced several new changes to the staff over a short period of time: new scheduling procedures, new vacation policy, new retirement policy, new research project. Based on change theory the nurse would predict what effect on the staff?
   a. mild discomfort with eventual acceptance.
   b. acceptance of changes as inevitable.
   c. increased sick days and disorganization.
   d. grumbling but smooth transition.

4. The nurse is using an ophthalmoscope to visualize the optic disk but is having difficulty locating it. The best way to find it would be to:
   a. start with the macula and work toward the disk.
   b. make sure the ophthalmoscope lens is kept steady.
   c. follow a vessel until it gets to the disk.
   d. ask the client to look up toward the ceiling.

5. A client with an automatic implantable cardioverter/defibrillator (AICD) should be taught:
   a. not to take antiarrhythmic medication.
   b. to stay on a low sodium diet.
   c. to keep away from ovens.
   d. to avoid airport metal detectors.

6. The nurse takes a client's blood pressure but the pressure is difficult to hear. The initial action of the nurse should be to:
   a. take it again immediately.
   b. wait a few minutes then take it again.
   c. compare the reading to previous readings.
   d. take the blood pressure by palpation.

7. A student is assisting in the emergency room and blood is splashed onto her uniform. She looks panicked and asks the nurse what to do so she "doesn't catch anything". The best reply of the nurse would be:
   a. "Wash the uniform normally and nothing should happen."
   b. "Wash the uniform normally but add bleach to the wash."
   c. "Place the uniform in a plastic bag and dispose of it in the trash."
   d. "The uniform should be dry cleaned twice before wearing it again."

8. A client is undergoing arthroscopy for direct knee joint visualization. The client has reported for same day surgery and is being assessed by the nurse. The nurse would particularly assess for:
   a. amount of discomfort in the affected knee.
   b. degree of flexion in the affected knee.
   c. previous scars.
   d. present medications.

9. A client who has been taking tranylcypromine (Parnate) for depression calls the mental health clinic with complaints of headache, nausea, stiff neck and muscle twitching. The nurse understands that these symptoms are probably indicative of:
   a. tardive dyskinesia.
   b. hypertensive crisis.
   c. acute toxicity.
   d. akathisia.

10. Ruth Cubek, a nursing student, is caring for a 250 lb man who needs to be transferred from bed to a stretcher. Ruth is concerned she will not be able to lift him because she is only 5'0" and 110 lbs. herself. She therefore enlists the help of two other students to perform a three person carry. Ruth's instructor comes in the room and stops the procedure because:
    a. the students that are assisting Ruth are both men.
    b. one of the students is holding the head and shoulders, another is holding the thighs and legs.
    c. the students have pulled the client toward their chests.
    d. all of the students kept their feet together while lifting.

11. A young adult client, who has recently lost her mother, tearfully tells the nurse, "I am just so upset and sad, but I'm not sure I can talk about it." The most therapeutic response by the nurse would be:
    a. "When exactly did you lose your mother?"
    b. "I can see you are upset; I'll stay with you for awhile."
    c. "It's difficult to deal with loss but you're doing fine."
    d. "It sounds like you are not certain if you want to talk about this."

12. The nurse is preparing for a skin biopsy for culture. The nurse should:
    a. avoid cleaning the skin with antibacterial soap.
    b. instruct the client to keep bandage in place for two hours.
    c. prepare a sterile field for biopsy instruments.
    d. obtain a container with 10% formalin solution.

13. Sam is a 7 year old with attention deficit disorder with hyperactivity (ADHD). He is being treated with methylphenidate (Ritalin) 5 mg BID. Which of the following statements by Sam's parents would indicate a need for further teaching?
    a. "If Sam won't sit down for breakfast he should take his medication with a glass of juice and some toast."
    b. "Sam should take his second dose at lunch."
    c. "If Sam becomes extra talkative or alert we will call the doctor right away."
    d. "This drug will help Sam pay attention in class and be able to learn more."

14. A 28 year old female is receiving a combination of neostigmine (Prostigmin) and pyridostigmine (Mestinon) for maintenance therapy following a myasthenic crisis. In determining the effectiveness of these medications while she is receiving this course of therapy, the nurse should assess for:
    a. cholinergic crisis, which is treated with atropine sulfate (Atropine).
    b. cholinergic crisis, which is treated with anticholinesterase drugs.
    c. myasthenic crisis, which is treated with corticosteroids.
    d. myasthenic crisis, which is treated with thymectomy.

15. A client receiving electroconvulsive therapy (ECT) for depression is given atropine sulfate (Atropine) prior to the ECT procedure. The purpose of giving this drug is to:
    a. decrease oropharyngeal secretions.
    b. relax muscles.
    c. sedate the client.
    d. prevent apnea.

16. The role of the nurse in hospice care is:
    a. respite care.
    b. family support.
    c. pain relief as pain arises.
    d. inpatient nurse.

17. A post-operative client asks for pain medication. The physician has ordered one medication for mild pain and another medication for moderate pain. The nurse decides which medication to give the client based on:
   a. observations of the client's nonverbal behavior.
   b. the client's report of pain intensity.
   c. the number of days after surgery.
   d. the medication given the past few times.

18. A client calls the surgical clinic stating she has dizziness, sweating, nausea and diarrhea after eating. The client had a gastrectomy and is diagnosed with dumping syndrome. The nurse would teach the client to:
   a. force fluids to help dilute the food.
   b. eat a high carbohydrate diet.
   c. teach the client to eat several small meals a day.
   d. stay upright for at least one hour after meals.

19. A client in sickle cell crisis is admitted to the hospital. The nurse might call the physician with which of the following findings?
   a. Jaundice.
   b. Abdominal pain.
   c. Priapism.
   d. Aplastic anemia.

20. A client, hospitalized for chronic alcoholism, is being discharged on disulfiram (Antabuse). The nurse knows that her health teaching has been effective when the client states:
   a. "I must take my Antabuse every time I feel vulnerable to taking a drink."
   b. "If I drink I will become very sick."
   c. "Antabuse will curb my urge to drink."
   d. "I will have to avoid aged cheeses, raisins, yogurt and bananas."

21. A client is receiving pre-operative teaching for hiatal hernia repair using a thoracic incision. The client should be taught that:
   a. the surgery will prevent gas formation.
   b. he will lay in a flat supine position after surgery.
   c. smoking will be permitted only in designated areas.
   d. chest tubes may be inserted for drainage.

22. A 15 year old client is on the rehabilitation unit after a spinal cord injury affecting both legs. The nurse asks the client's family to buy high top athletic shoes for the client to wear. The shoes are necessary because:
   a. it increases the client's self-esteem.
   b. they will prevent foot drop.
   c. the client will wear the same shoes as his peer group.
   d. they will encourage the client to move his legs.

23. A client with pancreatitis is admitted to the medical unit. The nurse should also be alert for what complication?
    a. Hypoglycemia.
    b. Leg pain.
    c. Pancreatic tumor.
    d. Pleural effusion.

24. A nurse passes a room where she observes an aide performing mouth care on an unconscious client. The aide is not wearing gloves. The nurse should:
    a. ask the aide to talk with her in the hallway.
    b. go into the room and ask the aide to wear gloves.
    c. schedule an inservice on mouthcare.
    d. instruct the aide to read the procedure again.

25. A client's electrocardiograph monitor shows a normal QRS pattern and a pulse rate of 110. This describes which of the following heart patterns?
    a. Frequent premature atrial contractions (PAC).
    b. Wandering atrial pacemaker.
    c. Premature ventricular contractions (PVC).
    d. Sinus tachycardia.

26. A student nurse tells the charge nurse that her client's pulse is irregular. The initial response by the charge nurse should be to:
    a. ask the student to take the client's blood pressure.
    b. reassess the client's pulse.
    c. call the physician.
    d. ask the student to describe the irregularity.

27. A male client is brought to the emergency room with a head injury after a car accident. A subdural hematoma is confirmed by scan. After the scan, the client's blood pressure starts to drop and pulse becomes rapid. The nurse should:
    a. assess for other areas of bleeding.
    b. place the client in reverse Trendelburg position.
    c. wake the client every hour to check level of consciousness.
    d. perform a neurological assessment.

28. A 40 year old client with a history of polycystic kidney disease is admitted. The client is pregnant and wants to know if her child will contract the disease. The best answer of the nurse would be:
    a. "The child will have a 50% chance of getting the disease."
    b. "Children inherit the disease from their mothers."
    c. "Males usually contract the disease over women."
    d. "This disease is not genetically transmitted."

29. A client with bacterial meningitis is placed in isolation. Visitors have been restricted to immediate family members because:
    a. the disease will be transmitted to others.
    b. the environment must be kept quiet as possible.
    c. the client has probably requested the restriction.
    d. family members are probably immune.

30. A client is found to be deficient in beta-carotene. The nurse evaluates that teaching has been effective when the client states she will eat more:
   a. crackers and margarine.
   b. rice and noodles.
   c. eggs and chicken.
   d. yellow and orange vegetables.

STOP You have now completed Practice Session: 20. Now take a few minutes and correct your answers. Calculate your accuracy rate by dividing the number of questions you completed correctly by the total number of questions you completed (30).

Correct answers ÷ total number of questions completed = accuracy rate.

_____ ÷ _____ = _____

PRACTICE SESSION: 20

ANSWERS AND RATIONALES

1. **The correct answer is b.** The first action of the nurse would be assessment to determine the client's present condition. After a quick assessment, intravenous fluids (option c) may be started. Syrup of ipecac (option a) then may be given to rid the body of the toxic substances. Sedative medication (option d) may mask symptoms and cause further problems (Black & Matassarin-Jacobs, 1993; p. 2249).

   Nursing Process: Assessment
   Client Need: Physiological Integrity

2. **The correct answer is d.** The sidelying position prevents aspiration and head down promotes drainage. The other three positions (options a, b and c) may cause aspiration in the client (Black & Matassarin-Jacobs, 1993; p.2250).

   Nursing Process: Analysis
   Client Need: Safe, Effective Care Environment

3. **The correct answer is c.** Rapid changes in a relatively short period of time usually causes disorganization in staff and some demoralization which may result in taking time from work to sort through the changes. Options (a) and (d) may occur if one change is made and the staff is allowed to adjust before further change is made. Option (b) may be true of an apathetic staff (Gillies,

1989; p. 476).

   Nursing Process: Analysis
   Client Need: Safe, Effective Care Environment

4. **The correct answer is c.** If the optic disk is not readily visible, follow a vessel toward the disk. The macula (option a) should be the last to be examined since it requires direct light into the eye which is uncomfortable for the client. The ophthalmoscope lens should be adjusted (option b) for proper visualization. To observe the optic disk, the client should be asked to look straight ahead (option d) rather than upward so the light shines into the eye (Ignatavicius & Bayne, 1991; pp. 1004-1005).

   Nursing Process: Assessment
   Client Need: Physiological Integrity

5. **The correct answer is d.** Metal detectors, radio transmitters and similar objects may deactivate the automatic implantable cardioverter defibrillator (AICD). Conventional ovens (option c) should not pose a problem. A low sodium diet (option b) is not necessary because of the device unless edema is a problem. Clients are given the AICD due to a dysrhythmia and are often given antiarrhythmic medication (option a) (Ignatavicius & Bayne, 1991; pp. 2147-2149).

   Nursing Process: Implementation
   Client Need: Physiological Integrity

6. **The correct answer is b.** If the blood pressure is difficult to hear, wait 1 to 2 minutes and try to read the blood pressure again. Immediate reassessment of blood pressure (option a) may provide a falsely high reading and venous congestion. Since there is no present reading, a comparison to previous readings (option c) cannot be made. Blood pressure by palpation (option d) may be done if the second reading and readings on the other arm are also inaudible (Perry & Potter, 1986; p. 275).

Nursing Process: Implementation
Client Need: Physiological Integrity

7. **The correct answer is b.** First, the student should have used universal precautions so the incident didn't happen. However, if clothing is soiled with body fluids and the human immunodeficiency (HIV) status of the person is unknown, the clothes can be cleaned through usual washing procedures as long as bleach is used. Washing alone (option a) is insufficient. Dry cleaning (option d) and disposal (option c) are unnecessary (Black & Matassarin-Jacobs, 1993; p. 563).

Nursing Process: Implementation
Client Need: Safe, Effective Care Environment

8. **The correct answer is b.** A 40% degree of flexion is the minimum amount so the arthroscopy can be performed. Amount of discomfort (option a), previous scars (option c) and present medications (option d) may be relevant but degree of flexion may

prevent the procedure (Ignatavicius & Bayne, 1991; p. 730).

Nursing Process: Assessment
Client Need: Physiological Integrity

9. **The correct answer is b.** Hypertensive crisis is a major side effect of the monoamine oxidase inhibitors (MAOI's) (Parnate). Symptoms include high blood pressure, headache, nausea, vomiting, stiff neck, muscle twitching and chills. Symptoms of acute toxicity of the MAOI's include severe anxiety, convulsions, confusion, cool clammy skin, slowed reflexes and respiratory depression (option c). Tardive dyskinesia (option a), a serious side effect of the neuroleptic drugs, is characterized by irregular movements of the lower facial muscles, jaw, tongue, and extremities. Akathisia (option d) is also a side effect of antipsychotic or neuroleptic drugs and is described as restlessness, difficulty in sitting still, agitation and uncontrolled pacing (Rawlins, Williams & Beck, 1993; pp. 484-492).

Nursing Process: Analysis
Client Need: Physiological Integrity

10. **The correct answer is d.** To avoid back injury, the students should lift with their feet apart which distributes the weight more evenly. Options (a), (b) and (c) are all appropriate techniques in the use of a three person carry (Perry & Potter, 1986; pp. 1201, 1214-1215).

Nursing Process: Implementation
Client Need: Safe, Effective Care Environment

11. **The correct answer is b.** The nurse makes the observation that the client is upset and offers self by offering to stay with the client. Option (a) focuses on factual information rather than a feeling level. Option (c) is an example of false reassurance which is nontherapeutic communication. Option (d) is an interpretive response in that the client does not say she does not want to talk but is unsure if she is able (Varcarolis, 1990; pp. 117-122).

Nursing Process: Implementation
Client Need: Psychosocial Integrity

12. **The correct answer is c.** A skin biopsy for culture or histology requires a sterile field to prevent infection. The skin area for biopsy should be shaved and cleansed with an antibacterial soap (option a). The biopsy for culture is placed in sterile saline (option d). Formalin is used for histology specimens. The client should be instructed to keep the biopsy site bandage dry and in place for eight hours (option b) (Ignatavicius & Bayne, 1991; p. 1152).

Nursing Process: Implementation
Client Need: Safe, Effective Care Environment

13. **The correct answer is a.** Fruit juices acidify the urine, which enhances the methylphenidate (Ritalin) excretion thereby decreasing the effects of the medication. Methylphenidate (Ritalin) should be taken at mealtimes (option b) to minimize the side effect of anorexia. Hyperalertness and talkativeness (option c) are signs of amphetamine toxicity. Immediate attention is required

as amphetamine toxicity can be fatal. The desired effects of methylphenidate (Ritalin) therapy are increased attention span and ability to learn (option d) (Clunn, 1991; pp. 243-244).

Nursing Process: Evaluation
Client Need: Physiological Integrity

14. **The correct answer is a.** Myasthenic crisis in the client known to have myasthenia gravis is frequently associated with underdosage of the prescribed medication, stress or fatigue. Acute muscle weakness is seen in myasthenic crisis, which must be treated immediately with anticholinesterase medications. Cholinergic crisis (option b) is caused by overdosage of the anticholinesterase (cholinergic) medications. Atropine sulfate (Atropine), an anticholinergic drug, is the antidote for overdosage of anticholinesterase drugs and should be kept in close proximity to the client. During a myasthenic crisis, corticosteroids (option c) or thymectomy (option d) are not the treatment of choice (Baer & Williams, 1992; pp. 188-210).

Nursing Process: Evaluation
Client Need: Physiological Integrity

15. **The correct answer is a.** Atropine sulfate (Atropine) is given prior to electroconvulsive therapy (ECT) to decrease oropharyngeal secretions. Melhahexital sodium (Brevital) is given intravenously as a sedative (option c). Succinylcholine chloride (Anectine) is given as a muscle relaxant (option b). Oxygen is administered to the client because the muscle relaxant paralyzes the respiratory muscles and creates a

short period of apnea followed by snoring-like respirations (option d) (Rawlins, Williams & Beck, 1993; p. 268).

Nursing Process: Analysis
Client Need: Physiological Integrity

16. **The correct answer is b.** The role of the hospice nurse is to support the client and family in any way needed. Hospice care includes inpatient and home care (option d) including anticipatory guidance in bereavement as well as post-death bereavement counseling and support. The nurse can arrange for respite care through inpatient admission or through volunteers in the home (option a). Pain relief measures are usually aimed towards preventing or controlling pain (option c) rather than waiting for pain to arise (Ignatavicius & Bayne, 1991; pp. 213-215).

Nursing Process: Analysis
Client Need: Health Promotion & Maintenance

17. **The correct answer is b.** The client is the only true judge of pain intensity and how well the pain has responded to the medications. Therefore, the nurse should ask the client to describe pain intensity. Generally the same assessment tool should be used for measuring pain intensity. Observations by the nurse are not usually sufficient to classify a client's pain (option a). Number of days after surgery (option c) does not take the type of surgery or other factors into consideration. Medication given the past few times (option d) may not have been sufficient for pain relief. Also, the present pain

experience may be different, such as after ambulation rather than lying quietly in bed (Ignatavicius & Bayne, 1991; pp. 120-122).

Nursing Process: Analysis
Client Need: Physiological Integrity

18. **The correct answer is c.** The client should be taught to decrease the amount of food eaten at one time. Small meals decrease the incidence of dumping syndrome. Fluids are restricted (option a) during mealtime to delay gastric emptying. A low carbohydrate, high fat, high protein diet (option b) is recommended. The client is instructed to lay down after meals or even during meals (option d) to decrease the amount of food emptying out of the stomach (Ignatavicius & Bayne, 1991; p.1326).

Nursing Process: Implementation
Client Need: Physiological Integrity

19. **The correct answer is d.** Aplastic anemia occurs when there is abnormal development of red blood cells. It is a complication of sickle cell crisis requiring blood transfusion. Jaundice (option a) from destroyed blood cells, abdominal pain (option b) from infarcts and priapism (option c) from engorged blood vessels in the penis are severe but expected findings (Ignatavicius & Bayne, 1991; pp. 2252-2254).

Nursing Process: Analysis
Client Need: Physiological Integrity

20. **The correct answer is b.** Disulfiram (Antabuse) causes an unpleasant physical reaction when the client consumes any alcohol. It does not motivate the client

to stop drinking nor curb the urge to drink (option c). Disulfiram (Antabuse) must be taken every day (option a). Option (d) are the food instructions for a client who is taking a monoamine oxidase inhibitor antidepressant (Varacolis, 1990; p. 620).

Nursing Process: Evaluation
Client Need: Physiological Integrity

21. **The correct answer is d.** A thoracic incision would result in chest tube insertion. The head of the bed should be elevated after surgery (option b) to allow for lung expansion and the client should be ambulating as soon as possible. The client should be encouraged to stop smoking prior to surgery (option c). Gas formation is not prevented (option a) but gas bloat syndrome occurs where the client has problems ridding the body of the gas through belching (Ignatavicius & Bayne, 1991; p. 1284).

Nursing Process: Implementation
Client Need: Physiological Integrity

22. **The correct answer is b.** Foot drop may occur in clients who cannot exercise extremities and when muscles are not used. The high top athletic shoes will assist by supporting the feet and ankles in a functional position. Options (a) and (c) are possibilities but not the primary purpose of the shoes. The client cannot move his legs (option d) but the legs should be exercised with passive range of motion exercises (Black & Matassarin-Jacobs, 1993; p. 807).

Nursing Process: Analysis
0   **Client Need:** Physiological Integrity

23. **The correct answer is d.** Left pleural effusion can occur when pancreatic seepage flows through the lymph system into the pleural cavity. The client is then at risk for adult respiratory distress syndrome (ARDS). Hyperglycemia rather than low blood sugar (option a) may occur at times from damage to pancreatic islet cells. Abdominal pain, flank pain and back pain may occur from peritonitis. Leg pain (option b) generally doesn't occur. A pancreatic tumor (option c) may cause pancreatitis (Ignatavicius & Bayne, 1991; p. 1463).

Nursing Process: Analysis
Client Need: Physiological Integrity

24. **The correct answer is a.** If a staff member is doing something incorrectly, the nurse should interrupt the procedure if possible and ask to speak to the aide privately in the hallway (option b). The action should be corrected along with a rationale for why gloves should be worn which reinforces teaching. The action should be corrected immediately (options c and d) so that medical aesepis is maintained (Perry & Potter, 1986; p. 173).

Nursing Process: Implementation
Client Need: Safe, Effective Care Environment

25. **The correct answer is d.** In sinus tachycardia, the rate is usually 100-160. Both atrial and ventricular rhythms are regular. The QRS is normal. Conduction is normal. Premature atrial contractions (PAC) are irregular due to the earliness of the beat and a brief pause after the premature beat (option a). The identifying character-

istics of wandering atrial pacemaker (option b) include: a rate that is usually normal but may be slow, P waves are abnormal and change in size, shape and deflection. The P-R interval may vary or be constant. Premature ventricular contractions (PVC) occur due to an irritable focus in the ventricle that irritates a contraction before the normally expected beat. The rate is variable; rhythm is irregular. P waves are not present in the PVC, the P-R interval is immeasurable in the PVC complex. The QRS complex is wide and bizarre (option c) (Ignatavicius & Bayne, 1991; pp. 2117-2131).

Nursing Process: Analysis
Client Need: Physiological Integrity

26. **The correct answer is b.** When an irregular pulse is found, a second nurse should confirm the finding. Then characteristics of the pulse (option d) and vital signs are taken (option a). The physician (option c) should then be notified (Perry & Potter, 1986; p. 256).

Nursing Process: Analysis
Client Need: Physiological Integrity

27. **The correct answer is a.** Hypotension and rapid pulse are signs of hypovolemic shock. A subdural hematoma does not produce enough bleeding to cause hypovolemic shock so other areas of bleeding, such as the abdomen, must be explored. The subdural hematoma has already increased the intracranial pressure. Reverse Trendelenburg (option b) would increase it further. Checking for level of consciousness (option c) is part of a neurological assessment (option d). Both should be done but the shock is life threatening and should be assessed first (Ignatavicius & Bayne, 1991; p. 928).

Nursing Process: Implementation
Client Need: Physiological Integrity

28. **The correct answer is a.** Polycystic kidney disease is an inherited disorder (option d) which has an autosomal dominant trait. It also is not connected with the sex chromosomes so men and women have an equal chance of getting the disorder (options b and c). A child has a 50% chance of inheriting the gene that causes polycystic kidney disease (Ignatavicius & Bayne, 1991; p. 1828).

Nursing Process: Implementation
Client Need: Health Promotion & Maintainance

29. **The correct answer is b.** Because meningitis is an inflammation of the tissue surrounding the brain, seizures are a possibility. The environment should be kept quiet so as not to precipitate seizure activity. Family are not considered immune (option d) and may be asked to take medication as a preventive measure. The disease can be transmitted to others if proper precautions aren't taken (option a) including with family members. Isolation is usually ordered by the physician. The physician or the nurses (option c) may restrict visitors to keep the environment quiet (Ignatavicius & Bayne, 1991; pp. 900-901).

Nursing Process: Analysis
Client Need: Safe, Effective Care Environment

30. **The correct answer is d.** Beta-carotene is found in vegetables and fruits with yellow and orange coloring. The deeper the color, the more beta-carotene and Vitamin A are found. Options (a), (b) and (c) do not contain high levels of beta-carotene (Burtis, Davis & Martini, 1988; pp. 157, 159).

Nursing Process: Evaluation
Client Need: Physiological Integrity

REFERENCES

Baer, C. L. & Williams, B. R. (1992). Clinical pharmacology and nursing (2nd ed.). Springhouse, PA: Springhouse.

Bates, B. (1991). A guide to physical examination and history taking (5th ed.). Philadelphia: Lippincott.

Black, J. M. & Matassarin-Jacobs, E. (1993). Luckmannn and Sorensen's medical-surgical nursing: A psychophysiological approach (4th ed.). Philadelphia: Saunders.

Bobak, I. M., Jensen, M. D. & Zalar, M. K. (1989). Maternity and gynecologic care: The nurse and the family (4th ed.). St. Louis: Mosby.

Bomar, P. J. (ed.). (1989). Nurses and family health promotion: Concepts, assessment, and interventions. Philadelphia: Saunders

Bullock, B. L. & Rosendahl, P. P. (1992). Pathophysiology: Adaptations and alterations in function (3rd ed.). Philadelphia: Lippincott.

Burtis, G., Davis, J. & Martin, S. (1988). Applied nutrition and diet therapy. Philadelphia: Saunders.

Cardona, V. D., Hurn, P. D., Mason-Bastnagel, P. J., Schipp-Scanlon, A. M. & Berry-Veise, S. W. (1988). Trauma nursing from resuscitation through rehabilitation. Philadelphia: Saunders.

Carpenito, L. J. (1992). Nursing diagnosis: Application to clinical practice (4th ed.). Philadelphia: Lippincott.

Clunn, P. A. (ed.). (1991). Child psychiatric nursing. St. Louis: Mosby Year Book.

Cook, J. S. & Fontaine, K. L. (1991). Essentials of mental health nursing (2nd ed.). Redwood City, CA: Addison-Wesley.

Craven, R. F. & Hirnle, C. J. (1992). Fundamentals of nursing: Human health and function. Philadelphia: Lippincott.

D'Angelo, H. H. & Welsh, N. P. (Eds.). (1988). Medication administration and I.V. therapy manual: Process and procedures. Springhouse, PA: Springhouse.

Danielson, C. B., Hamel-Bissell, B. & Winstead-Fry, P. (1993). Families, health & illness: Perspectives on coping and intervention. St. Louis: Mosby.

Deglin, J. H., Vallerand, A. H. & Russin, M. M. (1991). <u>Davis's drug guide for nurses</u> (2nd ed.). Philadelphia: F. A. Davis.

Ellis, J. R. & Nowlis, E. A. (1989). <u>Nursing: A human needs approach</u> (4th ed.). Boston: Houghton Mifflin.

Fischbach, F. T. (1992). <u>A manual of laboratory and diagnostic tests</u> (4th ed.). Philadelphia: Lippincott.

Ford, R. D. (1987). <u>Diagnostic tests handbook</u>. Springhouse, PA: Springhouse.

Gillies, D. A. (1989). <u>Nursing management: A systems approach</u> (2nd ed.). Philadelphia: Saunders.

Haber, J., Leach-McMahon, A. Price-Hoskins, P. & Sideleau, B. F. (1992). <u>Comprehensive psychiatric nursing</u> (4th ed.). St. Louis: Mosby Year Book.

Hamilton, H. K. (ed.). (1982). <u>Diagnostics</u>. Springhouse, PA: Intermed Communications.

Hickey, J. R. (1986). <u>The clinical practice of neurological and neurosurgical nursing</u>. Philadelphia: Lippincott.

Ignatavicius, D. D. & Bayne, M. V. (1991). <u>Medical-surgical nursing: A nursing process approach</u>. Philadelphia: Saunders.

<u>Illustrated manual of nursing practice</u>. (1991). Springhouse, PA: Springhouse.

Jarvis, C. (1992). <u>Physical examination and health assessment</u>. Philadelphia: Saunders.

Johnson, B. S. (1993). <u>Psychiatric-mental health nursing: Adaptation and growth</u> (3rd ed.). Philadelphia: Lippincott.

Joiner, C. & Corkean, M. (1986). <u>Critical incidents in nursing management</u>. Norwalk, CT: Appleton-Century-Crofts.

Kee, J. L. & Marshall, S. M. (1992). <u>Clinical calculations: With applications to general and specialty areas</u> (2nd ed.). Philadelphia: Saunders.

Kenner, C. V., Guzzetta, C. E. & Dossey, B. M. (1985). <u>Critical care nursing: Body-mind-spirit</u> (2nd ed.). Boston: Little, Brown.

Ladewig, P. W., London, M. L. & Olds, S. B. (1990). <u>Essentials of maternal-newborn nursing</u>. Redwood City, CA: Addison-Wesley.

Lewis, S. M. & Collier, I. C. (1992). Medical-surgical nursing: Assessment and management of clinical problems (3rd ed.). St. Louis: Mosby Year Book.

Loeb, S. (Ed.) (1990). Nursing 90 drug handbook. Springhouse, PA: Springhouse.

Loeb, S. (Ed.) (1992). Nurse's book of advice. Springhouse, PA: Springhouse.

Long, B. C., Phipps, W. J. & Cassmeyer, V. L. (1993). Medical-surgical nursing: A nursing process approach (3rd ed.). St. Louis: Mosby.

Mandeville, L. K. & Troiano, N. H. (Eds.). (1992). High-risk intrapartum nursing. Philadelphia: Lippincott.

Marlow, D. R. & Redding, B. A. (1988). Textbook of pediatric nursing (6th ed.). Philadelphia: Saunders.

Marquis, B. L. & Huston, C. J. (1992). Leadership roles and management functions in nursing: Theory and application. Philadelphia: Lippincott.

Martin, L. L. & Reeder, S. J. (1991). Essentials of maternity nursing: Family-centered care. Philadelphia: Lippincott.

May, K. A. & Mahlmeister, L. R. (1994). Maternal and neonatal nursing (3rd ed.). Philadelphia: Lippincott.

McFarland, G. K. & Thomas, M. D. (Eds.) (1991). Psychiatric mental health nursing: Application of the nursing process. Philadelphia: Lippincott.

Olds, S. B., London, M. L. & Ladewig, P. W. (1992). Maternal-newborn nursing: A family-centered approach (4th ed.). Redwood City, CA: Addison-Wesley.

Pagana, K. D. & Pagana, T. J. (1994). Diagnostic testing and nursing implications: A case study approach (4th ed.). St. Louis: Mosby.

Pagana, K. D. & Pagana, T. J. (1992). Mosby's diagnostic and laboratory test reference. St. Louis: Mosby Year Book.

Perry, A. G. & Potter, P. A. (1986). Clinical nursing skills and techniques: Basic, intermediate, and advanced. St. Louis: Mosby.

Perry, A. G. & Potter, P. A. (1990). Clinical nursing skills and techniques (2nd ed.). St. Louis: Mosby.

Phipps, W. J., Long, B. C., Woods, N. F. & Cassmeyer, V. L. (1991). Medical-surgical nursing: Concepts and clinical practice (4th ed.). St. Louis: Mosby Year Book.

Poorman, S. G. (1988). Human sexuality and the nursing process. Norwalk, CT: Appleton & Lange.

Potter, P. A. & Perry, A. G. (1991). Basic nursing: Theory and Practice (2nd ed.). St. Louis: Mosby.

Potter, P. A. & Perry, A. G. (1989). Fundamentals of Nursing: Concepts, Process and Practice (2nd ed.). St. Louis: Mosby.

Rawlins, R. P., Williams, S. R. & Beck, C. K. (Eds.) (1993). Mental health - psychiatric nursing: A holistic life cycle approach (3rd ed.). St. Louis: Mosby Year Book.

Reiss, B. S. & Evans, M. E. (1990). Pharmacological aspects of nursing care (3rd ed.). Albany, NY: Delmar.

Smeltzer, S. C. & Bare, B. G. (1992). Brunner & Suddarth's textbook of medical-surgical nursing (7th ed.). Philadelphia: Lippincott.

Smith, S. & Duell, D. (1993). Clinical nursing skills: Nursing process model basic to advanced skills. Los Altos, CA: National Nursing Review.

Snyder, M. (1992). Independent nursing interventions (2nd ed.). Albany, NY: Delmar.

Spradley, B. W. (1990). Community health nursing: Concepts and practice (3rd ed.). Glenview, IL: Scott, Foresman/Little, Brown Higher Education.

Stuart, G. W. & Sundeen, S. J. (1991). Principles and practice of psychiatric nursing (4th ed.). St. Louis: Mosby Year Book.

Swanson, J. M. & Albrecht, M. (1993). Community health nursing: Promoting the health of aggregates. Philadelphia: Saunders.

Tappen, R. M. (1989). Nursing leadership and management: Concepts and practice (2nd ed.). Philadelphia: Davis.

Taylor, C., Lillis, C. & Lemone, P. (1989). Fundamentals of nursing: The art and science of nursing care. Philadelphia: Lippincott.

Timby, B. K. (1989). Clinical nursing procedures. Philadelphia: Lippincott.

Townsend, M. C. (1993). <u>Psychiatric mental health nursing: Concepts of care</u>. Philadelphia: Davis.

Vallerand, A. H. & Deglin, J. H. (1991). <u>Drug guide for critical care and emergency nursing</u>. Philadelphia: Lippincott.

Varcarolis, E. M. (1990). <u>Foundations of psychiatric-mental health nursing</u>. Philadelphia: Saunders.

Weaver, M. E. & Koehler, V. J. (1992). <u>Programmed mathematics of drugs and solutions</u> (5th ed.). Philadelphia: Lippincott.

Whaley, L. F. & Wong, D. L. (1989). <u>Essentials of pediatric nursing</u> (3rd ed.). St. Louis: Mosby.

Whaley, L. F. & Wong, D. L. (1991). <u>Nursing care of infants and children</u> (4th ed.). St. Louis: Mosby Year Book.

Williams, S. R. (1989). <u>Nutrition and diet therapy</u> (6th ed.). St. Louis: Mosby.

Wilson, H. S. & Kneisl, C. R. (1992). <u>Psychiatric nursing</u> (4th ed.). Redwood City, CA: Addision-Wesley.

Wong, D. L. (1993). <u>Whaley & Wong's essentials of pediatric nursing</u> (4th ed.). St. Louis: Mosby Year Book.

Wywialowski, E. F. (1993). <u>Managing client care</u>. St. Louis: Mosby.